To my wife Beth and our children Sarah and Emily
                    —ISN
To my wife Maria Angeles and our children Pablo and Silvia
                    —VF

  and

To all of the thousands of patients who participated in these
clinical trials
                    —ISN, VF

Foreword

The history of myocardial infarction is very old, and some of the greatest figures of medicine are associated with it. However, it was undoubtedly James B. Herrick who truly founded the concept of this disease as we know it today, during the twenty-seventh annual meeting of the Association of American Physicians in Atlantic City, May 14–16, 1912. Dr. Herrick presented his landmark, epoch-making contribution, "Certain Clinical Features of Sudden Obstruction of the Coronary Arteries." This may come as a surprise, but at the time no one paid much attention to his presentation. It is reported that, years later, Herrick commented:

> You know I never understood it. In 1912 when I rose to read my paper at the Association, I was elated, for I knew I had a substantial contribution to present. I read it and it fell flat as a pancake. No one discussed it except Emanuel Lippman, and he discussed every paper read that day. It was such a disappointment.

It is of further interest that Lippman responded, "I was the only one present who had enough knowledge of the subject to discuss the paper."

Fortunately, this did not discourage Herrick. In 1918 he again presented to the Association his work, then entitled "Concerning Thrombosis of the Coronary Arteries." The focus of this report was on the electrocardiogram alteration following coronary artery obstruction. He actually predicted: "May it perhaps be possible to localize a lesion in the coronary system with an accuracy comparable to that with which we locate obstructive lesions in the cerebral arteries."

Well! This is indeed history, but it took another 30 years for coronary artery disease to finally get the recognition and the attention it deserved. In 1948, under pressure from the medical/scientific community, as well as from an alarmed public, the U.S. government established the National Heart Institute to foster research on the diagnosis and treatment of heart disease—including, of course, myocardial infarction, which, with its ever-increasing death rate, was the main cause of the alarm.

Eventually, the death rate plateaued and then started to decrease. Today, although we must remain vigilant and cognizant that myocardial infarction is still a critical public health problem, we can also marvel at what has been accomplished and at the many hundreds of thousands of lives that have been saved as a result.

Primary prevention has contributed to our progress, but, unfortunately, only modestly. There is no question that most of the credit for this decline in the death rate is due to the development and the application of interventional and pharmacological therapies. Cardiologists—and, when necessary, general physicians—now have an arsenal of weapons to combat myocardial infarction. This volume is a visit to that arsenal. To my knowledge, there is no other volume in which one can so readily find in such accessible form all the information concerning the many interventions that are available today. Clinical trials are described, explained, and evaluated, thus giving the physician the ability to apply effectively the remarkable knowledge that is available.

Since Herrick's day, times have changed. The presentations of any new study on myocardial infarction elicits much discussion, which never falls "flat as a pancake." These discussions are frequently like a battleground, and often lead to confusion rather than clarification. Much credit must be given to the editors, Ira S. Nash and Valentin Fuster, and the many contributors for providing the medical community with such a lucid and helpful review.

Claude Lenfant, M.D.
Bethesda, Maryland

Preface

All physicians want to do what is best for their patients. Whenever possible, the clinical decisions we make should be informed by credible research that has established the utility and safety of our treatments. This is the fundamental principle of evidence-based medicine. Although we would like to have evidence supporting all our treatments, for all our patients, for all their conditions, such will obviously never be the case. Clinical research can never address the infinite variety of circumstances that may confront the practicing physician. Many conditions will never be rigorously studied, because of limits on time and resources. Many patients we treat may not be exactly like the patients who participated in the clinical trials, for reasons of age, gender, ethnicity, or comorbid conditions. The number of potential treatments is always likely to exceed the number of well-studied ones, especially for those conditions where understanding of the underlying pathophysiology is expanding rapidly and treatment modalities develop at a pace that clinical trials cannot match. The net result is that successful navigation in the sea of uncertainty will forever require clinical judgment and skill in the ''art'' of medicine.

We are fortunate, however, to have in hand a wealth of information about what is ''best'' for many of our options, concerning many of our patients, for some of their most serious conditions. There is, perhaps, no arena where this is more true than in the care of patients with acute myocardial infarction. The clinical trials that are discussed in this book provide the knowledge base of rigorously obtained, reliable, and relevant data upon which informed treatment ought to be based. They have also served as a model for how such information should be obtained.

Our goal in presenting this volume is to improve the quality of care of patients with myocardial infarction by detailing the strength of evidence in favor of using some therapies and against using others. We also present the lack of definitive evidence pertaining to yet other therapeutic options.

We have divided the book into three major parts. Part I is devoted to an examination of the clinical trials that have established the efficacy of particular therapies: acute coronary reperfusion by either pharmacological or mechanical means, the use of aspirin, the early and late use of beta-blockers, the early and late use of ACE inhibitors, and the reduction of blood cholesterol. Part II is devoted to reviewing the trials that have cast doubt on the efficacy of other therapies, which must therefore be considered of questionable value as part of the standard treatment strategy for infarct patients: early and late use of calcium channel blockers and the routine use of heparin, nitroglycerin, and magnesium. Finally, Part III deals with alternative overall strategies for myocardial infarction care rather than particular therapies: invasive versus conservative management and the interplay of thrombolysis and PTCA.

A word about the title. Efficacy refers to how well a particular treatment works under idealized circumstances, as are typically achieved in randomized clinical trials. Efficacious therapies are those which can, under the right conditions, lead to measurable benefits. So, for instance, studies of primary angioplasty for acute myocardial infarction that are performed at premier, high-volume centers with experienced operators tell us what the greatest potential benefit from primary PTCA may be. Efficacy should be distinguished from effectiveness, which refers to how well a treatment works when generally applied under ''real world'' conditions. To the extent that large clinical trials are able to mimic clinical choices encountered in everyday practice, are performed in a community setting, and include a broad cross-section of the population, their results speak to both efficacy and effectiveness. Studies of acute PTCA done in community hospitals on a relatively unselected population of patients by operators who represent a more typical profile of interventional cardiologists would define its effectiveness.

Completing this volume could never have succeeded without the support and encouragement of the professionals at Marcel Dekker, to whom we owe our gratitude. We are also indebted to all of our talented contributors, not only for their participation in this project, but for their lasting contribution to the care of patients with myocardial infarction. Many people around the world literally owe their lives to the pioneering work of these investigators. It is no exaggeration to say that many more lives will be saved if we consistently apply the knowledge generated by these clinical trials.

Ira S. Nash, M.D.
Valentin Fuster, M.D., Ph.D.
New York, New York

Contents

Contents

Contributors

Ettore Ambrosioni, M.D. Professor of Medicine and Director, Third Department of Internal Medicine, University of Bologna, Bologna, Italy

Stephen G. Ball, Ph.D., F.R.C.P. Professor of Cardiology, Institute for Cardiovascular Research, University of Leeds, Leeds, England

Solomon Behar, M.D. Professor of Cardiology, Heart Institute, Sheba Medical Center, Tel-Hashomer, Israel

Claudio Borghi, M.D. Medical Director, Department of Internal Medicine, University of Bologna, Bologna, Italy

Eugene Braunwald, M.D. Distinguished Hersey Professor of Medicine, Department of Medicine, Brigham and Women's Hospital, Boston, Massachusetts

Robert P. Byington, Ph.D. Associate Professor of Epidemiology, Department of Public Health Science, Wake Forest University School of Medicine, Winston-Salem, North Carolina

Robert M. Califf, M.D. Professor of Medicine, Duke Clinical Research Center, Duke University Medical Center, Durham, North Carolina

Christopher P. Cannon, M.D. Assistant Professor of Medicine, Harvard Medical School, and Associate Physician, Cardiovascular Division, Brigham and Women's Hospital, Boston, Massachusetts

David P. de Bono, M.D., F.R.C.P. Professor of Cardiology and Head, Department of Medicine, Glenfield General Hospital and University of Leicester Medical School, Leicester, England

Rafael Díaz, M.D. Co-Director, Cardiovascular Medicine, Instituto Cardiovascular de Rosario, Rosario, Argentina

Stephen G. Ellis, M.D. Director, Sones Cardiac Catheterization Laboratory, Department of Cardiology, The Cleveland Clinic Foundation, Cleveland, Ohio

Raymond J. Gibbons, M.D.   Arthur M. and Gladys D. Gray Professor of Medicine, Mayo Medical School, and Co-Director, Nuclear Cardiology Laboratory, Mayo Clinic, Rochester, Minnesota

Robert P. Giugliano, M.D., S.M.   Cardiovascular Division, Brigham and Women's Hospital, Boston, Massachusetts

Robert E. Goldstein, M.D.   Professor of Medicine and Physiology and Chair, Department of Medicine, Uniformed Services University of the Health Sciences, Bethesda, Maryland

Alistair S. Hall, Ph.D., M.R.C.P.   Senior Lecturer in Cardiology, Institute for Cardiovascular Research, University of Leeds, Leeds, England

John R. Hampton, D.M., D. Phil., F.R.C.P.   Professor, Department of Cardiovascular Medicine, Queens Medical Centre, Nottingham, England

Jørgen Fischer Hansen, M.D., Ph.D.   Head, Department of Cardiovascular Medicine, Bispebjerg University Hospital, Copenhagen, Denmark

Åke Hjalmarson, M.D., Ph.D.   Professor, Department of Medicine, Institute of Heart and Lung Diseases, Sahlgrenska Hospital and Göteborg University, Göteborg, Sweden

David R. Holmes, Jr., M.D.   Professor of Medicine, Mayo Clinic, Rochester, Minnesota

Neeraj Jolly, M.D.   Interventional Cardiology Fellow, The Cleveland Clinic Foundation, Cleveland, Ohio

John Kjekshus, M.D., Ph.D.   Professor, Section of Cardiology, Department of Medicine, Rikshospitalet, University of Oslo, Oslo, Norway

Lars Køber, M.D.   TRACE Study Office, Copenhagen, Denmark

Aldo P. Maggioni, M.D.   Director, Research Center, Italian Association of Hospital Cardiologists, Florence, Italy

David T. Nash, M.D.   Clinical Professor of Medicine, State University of New York Health Science Center, Syracuse, New York

William W. O'Neill, M.D.   Director, Division of Cardiology, Department of Internal Medicine, William Beaumont Hospital, Royal Oak, Michigan

Ernesto Paolasso, M.D.   Director, Cardiovascular Medicine, Instituto Cardiovascular de Rosario, and Co-Director ECLA, Rosario, Argentina

Terje R. Pedersen, M.D.   Professor of Clinical Cardiology, University of Oslo, and Cardiology Department, Aker Hospital, Oslo, Norway

1

GISSI-1

GIANNI TOGNONI and ALDO P. MAGGIONI

Gruppo Italiano per lo Studio della Streptochinasi nell'Infarto Miocardico (GISSI). Effectiveness of intravenous thrombolytic treatment in acute myocardial infarction. Lancet 1986; ii: 397–402.

PROTOCOL

The best way of summarizing the characteristics, results, and implications of the GISSI study would, perhaps, be to reproduce the original reports (1,2). The conciseness of the text and the discussion accurately reflected the philosophy that led to its formulation and implementation, as well as the atmosphere that surrounded the communication of its results. The questions present in the international arena were straightforward (Table 1). The overall design of the study protocol was a close reproduction of the population-oriented pragmatic approach of very large-scale clinical trials proposed some years before (3) to provide reliable answers to clinically and epidemiologically relevant questions (Fig. 1).

The main results, presented in Table 2, can be presented as answers to the questions formulated in the protocol:

The administration of streptokinase (SK) produced a statistically highly significant 18% decrease in the overall mortality of the treated population.

The beneficial effect was even more impressive in the predefined subpopulation treated soon after onset of pain (Fig. 2).

The incidence of feared cerebrovascular events (defined as the sum of ischemic and hemorragic episodes) in the SK and control groups was very low (<1%) and comparable between the two groups.

The impact of the doubling of the in-hospital reinfarction rate was clearly out- weighed by and is included in the overall benefit of decreased mortality.

The hemorrhagic complications were not specifically worrisome.

Other SK-related adverse events (e.g., hypotension and allergic reactions) did occur, but they did not lead to an important proportion of clinically relevant compli- cations.

The time-dependent size of the beneficial effect on in-hospital mortality, represented by the survival curves in Figure 2, appears today to be even more suggestive than in the original report, as it anticipates what years later the overall meta-analysis of thrombolytic trials proposed as an established fact (4).

Table 1   Questions Addressed in the GISSI Protocol

Does intravenous streptokinase infusion produce a clinically relevant benefit in terms of reduction of in-hospital and one-year mortality?

Is the effect, if any, dependent on the interval from onset of pain to streptokinase administration?

Are the risks associated with the treatment acceptable?

Several other points set out in GISSI need to be emphasized:

1. The absence of benefit shown in non-Q AMI led to the exclusion of this class of patients from subsequent thrombolytic trials.
2. What later became the "early hazard" issue (4) specifically in the elderly population, had appeared already in the interim analysis (data nonpublished).
3. The higher mortality of women was suggested as a question requiring specific in-depth analysis.

COMMENTS

GISSI has often been referred to as a landmark trial and is regarded as the beginning of the thrombolytic era, because systemic thrombolysis was shown to be not only effective, but remarkably safe. The closeness of the GISSI protocol to the conditions of usual care gave the findings additional strength and perspective: thrombolysis had been shown to be practicable in every type of coronary care unit (CCU), provided essential diagnostic procedures (pain and electrocardiogram) were applied, with the only caveat being explicit well-known contraindications. The epidemiological approach adopted to recruit patients,

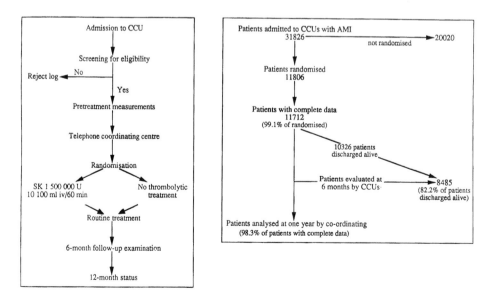

Figure 1   GISSI protocol and flow diagram.

Table 2 Efficacy and Safety Results of GISSI

A. Efficacy: Mortality by Hours from Onset of Symptoms

Hours	SK % (deaths/n)	C % (deaths/n)	p	RR (95% CI)	Total % (deaths/n)
Hour ≤ 3	9.2 (278/3016)	12.0 (369/3078)	0.0005	0.74 (0.63–0.87)	10.6 (647/6094)
Hour > 3–6	11.7 (217/1849)	14.1 (254/1800)	0.03	0.80 (0.66–0.98)	12.9 (474/3649)
Hour > 6–9	12.6 (87/693)	14.1 (93/659)	NS	0.87 (0.64–1.19)	13.3 (180/1352)
Hour > 9–12	15.8 (46/292)	13.6 (41/302)	NS	1.19 (0.75–1.87)	14.6 (87/594)
Hour < 1	8.2 (52/635)	15.4 (99/642)	0.0001	0.49 (0.34–0.69)	11.8 (151/1277)
All patients	10.7 (628/5860)	13.0 (758/5852)	0.0002	0.81 (0.72–0.90)	11.8 (1386/11,712)

B. Safety

Symptom	AR leading to withdrawal of SK infusion		AR attributed to SK after completion of infusion	
	No	%	No	%
Major bleeds	0	—	19	0.3
Allergic reactions	99	1.6	42	0.7
Anaphylactic shock	7	0.1	0	—
Hypotension	96	1.6	82	1.4

SK = streptokinase; C = control; RR = relative risk; n = number of patients; NS = not significant; AR = adverse reaction.

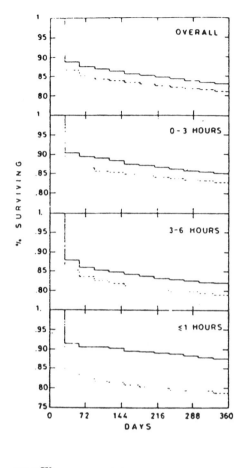

Figure 2 One-year cumulative percentage survival of overall population and survival by hours from onset of symptoms.

with no restrictive inclusion criteria (no limit of age, a fair representation of women, and an extended time spectrum), proved to be a very effective strategy with respect to (1) the efficiency of recruitment; (2) the possibility of exploring the information that could be derived from the analysis of subgroups; and (3) the timely transferability of the experimental results to the routine practice.

Another benefit of the GISSI trial was that the majority of the Italian patients were exposed to the advantage of thrombolysis at least 2–3 years before patients in other countries.

Well before the ISIS-2 results could be interpreted as indicating a more generalized use of thrombolysis (with the fundamental addition of aspirin), the GISSI findings were the basis for the approval of the thrombolytic indication by the U.S. Federal Drug Administration.

REFERENCES

1. Gruppo Italiano per lo Studio della Streptochinasi nell' Infarto Miocardico (GISSI). Effectiveness of intravenous thrombolytic treatment in acute myocardial infarction. Lancet 1986; ii:397–402.
2. Gruppo Italiano per lo Studio della Streptochinasi nell' Infarto Miocardico (GISSI). Long-term effects of intravenous thrombolysis in acute myocardial infarction: final report of the GISSI study. Lancet 1987; ii:871–874.
3. Yusuf S, Collins R, Peto R. Why do we need some large simple randomized trials? Stat Med 1984; 3:409–420.
4. Fibrinolytic Therapy Trialists' (FTT) Collaborative Group. Indications for fibrinolytic therapy in suspected acute myocardial infarction: collaborative overview of early mortality and major morbidity results from all randomised trials of more than 1000 patients. Lancet 1994; 343:311–322.

2

ISIS-2

PETER SLEIGHT

Second International Study of Infarct Survival Collaborative Group. Randomized trial of intravenous streptokinase, oral aspirin, both or neither, among 17,187 cases of suspected acute myocardial infarction. ISIS–2. Lancet 1988; ii: 349–360.

INTRODUCTION

At the time when ISIS-2 was designed, streptokinase (SK) had been available for many years as a fibrinolytic agent. Although it had been shown to dissolve clots by Sherry and colleagues, fear of hemorrhage and the mixed clinical benefit seen in a series of small trials limited its use.

However, a systematic overview by Yusuf et al. (1) suggested that its use might reduce mortality in acute myocardial infarction (AMI) by about 25%. This, coupled with angiographic demonstration of thrombolysis by intracoronary thrombosis or by intravenous streptokinase by Rentrop, Schroder, and colleagues (2,3), set the stage for several large trials of intravenous SK in AMI.

ISIS-2

The second international study of infarct survival (ISIS-2) built on the worldwide collaborative group developed in ISIS-1. This group was expanded to 417 hospitals in 16 countries; 17,187 patients with suspected AMI were randomized to SK, aspirin, both, or neither within 24 hours of the onset of symptoms (4). (The aspirin arm of this trial will be described separately in Chapter 12.) A similar study was carried out (5) coordinated by the Mario Negri Institute in Milan; the GISSI group in Italy had originated as part of the ISIS-1 collaboration. These studies used the intravenous regimen developed by Schroeder et al. (3) of 1.5 million units of streptokinase (Behringwerke–Streptase®) given over one hour. As in ISIS-1 (6), telephone randomization reduced bias and, together with minimal data collection at entry, ensured rapid recruitment over about 2½ years. A single-sided discharge form, together with a prerandomization ECG, were returned on discharge.

Patients were eligible if thought on clinical grounds (by their own physicians) to be within 24 hours of the onset of AMI and to have no clear indication for, or contraindication against, SK (or aspirin). Computer "minimization" algorithms were used to favor balance between the groups on treatment. Subsequent posthospital mortality was gathered from government records.

RESULTS

As in ISIS-1, results were analyzed by use of observed-expected methods and log rank time to death analyses. There were 791 vascular deaths by 5 weeks in the group allocated SK and 1029 on SK placebo (9.2 vs. 12.0%, reduction 25%, $p = < 0.00001$) (Fig. 1). Nonvascular mortality was balanced (32 deaths in each group) so the reduction in total mortality was also highly significant. Compliance with allocated SK was 92% or more.

At the then median follow-up of 15 months, the early 25% difference from placebo continued. A 10-year follow-up has, remarkably, shown, no convergence or divergence from the result at 5 weeks (ISIS-2 group, unpublished).

ISIS-2 showed the expected reduction in benefit with delayed treatment. However, contrary to opinion at that time there was still an effect in patients treated 6–12 hours from onset and a nonsignificant benefit in those randomized 12–24 hours from onset. There was no particularly large benefit in those randomized within 1 hour of onset.

Mortality at 5 weeks was more than halved in the large group randomized to SK

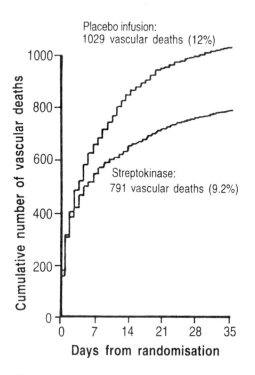

Figure 1 Cumulative vascular mortality in days 0–35. All patients allocated active streptokinase versus all allocated a placebo infusion. (From Ref. 4.)

and aspirin less than 4 hours from onset. Patients with ST depression did not appear to benefit, whereas benefit was clear in those with ST elevation or bundle branch block.

The downside of SK treatment was a small but significant 0.1% excess of cerebral hemorrhage and 0.3% excess in major bleeds with SK, which occurred largely in those in whom heparin treatment was planned. Despite the excess of cerebral hemorrhage, total stroke was reduced in those receiving SK due to a shortfall in ischemic stroke. SK significantly increased the risk of reinfarction in hospital (2.8% vs. 2.0%); this excess was not seen in those also receiving aspirin.

Hypotension was also much more common on SK (10% vs. 2%) and was unrelated to initial blood pressure. No cases of anaphylactic shock were reported. ISIS-2 imposed no age limit on the patients eligible and so (unusually for a clinical trial in those days) included over 3000 patients over age 70. Significant benefit was seen in elderly subjects. The proportional reduction in mortality was slightly less than in middle-aged subjects, but since their absolute risk was much higher than in younger patients, the numbers of lives saved per 1000 treatments was considerably higher. Of course the subjects randomized were selected at the discretion of the randomizing physician, and no doubt some patients with other complicating diseases were excluded. Nevertheless, since the incidence of MI increases very steeply with age and since many elderly patients were well and active before their MI, it is important not to deny them the benefit of thrombolysis because of fear of increased risk of hemorrhagic stroke.

In fact, in the Fibrinolytic Therapy Trialists' overview, there was surprisingly no increase in stroke with age in the SK group, although there was a fivefold increase with age using tPA. This difference may be a result of the protective effect of the hypotension associated with SK.

There was a small increase in risk of stroke with increasing entry blood pressure in SK-treated patients, but again this was less than with tPA.

Overall in ISIS-2 and in the FTT overview, thrombolytic therapy was consistently beneficial over a large number of subgroups, characterized by sex, age, diabetes, entry blood pressure, entry heart rate, and planned treatment with beta blockers, aspirin, or anticoagulants. The only subgroups not to benefit were those with ST depression on the ECG and those with normal ECG or only T-wave changes. The placebo group mortality in those with near-normal ECGs was very low and so benefit might not be expected. But the mortality in those with ST depression was high, around 18–19% at 5 weeks; they were undoubtedly undergoing infarction and so the lack of benefit was unexpected. This may reflect the differing pathology in patients with ST depression (more prior infarction, more multivessel disease) or may be (as Peto believes) the play of chance from many subgroup analyses. Perhaps one of the most important findings in ISIS-2 has, in retrospect, been treated too much as a joke. This was the analysis by patient star sign; those born under Gemini or Libra derived no benefit from aspirin. It is easy to laugh at this, but clinicians and trialists regularly carry out subgroup analyses and then believe them when they produce odd results (e.g., men versus women, or anterior versus inferior MI).

DISCUSSION

ISIS-2 and GISSI-1 were planned together; GISSI-1 reported first (8). GISSI-1 was a simple comparison of SK versus open control and gave strong evidence overall for the benefit of thrombolysis by SK. However, it was a smaller trial, and so it was inevitable

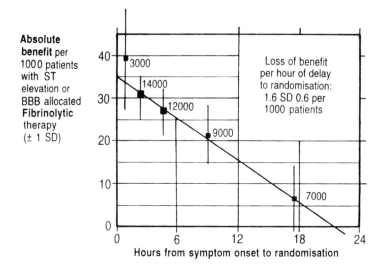

Figure 2 Absolute reduction in 35-day mortality versus delay from symptom onset to randomization among 45,000 patients with ST elevation or bundle branch block (BBB). (All patients in ASSET and LATE are included.) For patients whose delays were recorded as 0–1, 2–3, 4–6, 7–12, and 13–24 hours, absolute benefit (±1 SD) is plotted against mean recorded delay time (0.98, 2.50, 4.79, 9.11, and 17.48 hours, respectively). Area of black square and extent to which it influences line drawn through five points is approximately proportional to the number of patients it is based on. (Formally, the area is inversely proportional to the variance of absolute benefit it describes, and the slope is inverse-variance-weighted least squares regression line.) (From Ref. 4.)

that some subgroups would not show benefit, e.g., those over age 65, those randomized over 6 hours, and those with a history of prior MI. These findings were shown to be false by ISIS-2 and more convincingly by the FTT overview—a good illustration of the dangers of overinterpretation of subgroup results. As the ISIS-2 publication stated, "lack of evidence of benefit" just in one subgroup is not "evidence of lack of benefit," but physicians do often make this error in transferring trial results to clinical practice.

The striking 45% reduction in mortality seen in GISSI-1 in patients randomized within one hour of onset of MI gave birth to the "golden hour" hypothesis. However, this was a retrospective analysis that was not borne out by ISIS-2 (which examined this prospectively) or by the FTT overview of all large trials of thrombolysis (Fig. 2).

A later analysis by Simoons (9) revived the golden hour by suggesting that the inverse relation between time to treatment and benefit was not linear (as in Fig 2) but was strongly curvilinear. However, this later analysis may be criticized for publication bias in that not all the small trials quoted by Simoons gave results for the first hour: it is likely that those trials that did not report their data for this period saw no such strikingly different results. The largest direct study of this problem—the European Myocardial Infarction Project (EMIP) study of treatment in the ambulance versus one hour delayed thrombolysis in hospital—showed the greatest benefit for earlier treatment in those randomized 3 hours after onset, with no benefit of earlier treatment in those randomized in less than 3 hours from onset (10). The Myocardial Infarction Triage and Intervention (MITI) study (11), which did support the "golden hour," was only one-tenth the size of EMIP and is therefore much less reliable. Nevertheless, despite this controversy it is clear that early treatment is extremely important and that relatively simple and cheap organizational changes to produce a "fast track" for MI patients are very beneficial (12).

REFERENCES

1. Yusuf S, Peto R, Lewis J, Collins R, Sleight P. Beta blockade during and after myocardial infarction: an overview of the randomised trials. Prog Cardiovasc Dis 1985; 27:335–371.
2. Rentrop P, Blanke H, Kostering H, Karsch KR. Intrakoronare Streptokinase-Applikation bei akutem Infarkt und instabiler Angina pectoris. Dtsch Med Wschr 1990; 105:221–228.
3. Schroeder R. Systemic versus intracoronary streptokinase infusion in the treatment of acute myocardial infarction. J Am Coll Cardiol 1983; 1:1254–1261.
4. ISIS-2 (Second International Study of Infarct Survival) Collaborative Group. Randomised trial of intravenous streptokinase, oral aspirin, both or neither among 17,187 cases of suspected acute myocardial infarction: ISIS-2. Lancet 1988; ii:349–360.
5. GISSI (Gruppo Italiano per lo Studio della Streptochinasi nell'Infarcto Miocardico). Effectiveness of intravenous thrombolytic treatment in acute myocardial infarction. Lancet 1986; I: 397–401.
6. ISIS-1 (International Studies of Infarct Survival) Collaborative Group. Randomised trial of intravenous atenolol among 16,027 cases of suspected acute myocardial infarction: ISIS-1. Lancet 1986; ii:57–66.
7. Fibrinolytic Therapy Trialists' (FTT) Collaborative Group. Indications for fibrinolytic therapy in suspected acute myocardial infarction: collaborative overview of early mortality and major morbidity results from all randomised trials of more than 1000 patients. Lancet 1994; 343: 311–322.
8. Gruppo Italiano per lo Studio della Streptochinasi nell'Infarto Miocardico (GISSI). Long term effects of intravenous thrombolysis in acute myocardial infarction: final report of the GISSI study. Lancet 1987; ii:872–874.
9. Boersma E, Maas AC, Deckers JW, Simoons ML. Early thrombolytic treatment in acute myocadial infarction: reappraisal of the golden hour. Lancet 1996; 348:771–775.
10. The European Myocardial Infarction Project Group. Prehospital thrombolytic therapy in patients with suspected acute myocardial infarction. N Engl J Med 1993; 329:383–389.
11. Weaver WD, Cerqueira M, Hallstrom AP, Litwin PE, Martin JS, Kudenchuk PJ, Eisenberg M. Prehospital-initiated vs hospital-initiated thrombolytic therapy. The Myocardial Infarction Triage and Intervention trial. JAMA 1993; 270:1211–1216.
12. Pell AC, Miller HC, Robertson CE, Fox KA. Effect of "fast track" admission for acute myocardial infarction on delay to thrombolysis. Br Med J 1992; 304:83–87.

3

ASSET

ROBERT G. WILCOX

Wilcox RG, Olsson CG, Skene AM, Von Der Lippe G, Jensen G, Hampton JR for the ASSET Study Group. Trial of tissue plasminogen activator for mortality reduction in acute myocardial infarction. Anglo-Scandinavian study of early thrombolysis (ASSET). Lancet 1988; ii: 525–530.

INTRODUCTION

Until the early 1960s, the care of patients with acute myocardial infarction comprised pain relief, oxygen, prolonged bed rest, and reaction to complications as they emerged, particularly arrhythmias and heart failure. The gradual acceptance of the coronary care unit (CCU) concept, the description of closed chest cardiopulmonary resuscitation, and the increasing availability of electrical defibrillation initiated a fundamental change in philosophy. As researchers using animal models showed that the amount of irreversibly damaged myocardium could be substantially reduced by a wide variety of agents (usually given before experimental coronary artery occlusion) or by early restoration of coronary flow, clinicians were eager to test some of these interventions in patients (1).

For pragmatic purposes, the initial clinical investigations were concerned more with "metabolic support" of the jeopardized myocardium. With the eventual acceptance that in the majority of cases acute myocardial infarction was caused by complete or subtotal occlusion of a coronary artery by a fresh thrombus, usually in the vicinity of an existing atherosclerotic plaque, attention returned to reperfusion (2–4). There had been earlier attempts to effect clot dissolution using the bacterial extract streptokinase, but only with the publication of large well-designed controlled clinical trials was chemical reperfusion with thrombolytic agents accepted into everyday clinical use (5,8). Streptokinase, the thrombolytic drug used in all these trials, is not clot specific and thus causes a generalized hypocoagulable defect, is antigenic, and thus occasionally is associated with acute allergic phenomena and the formation of antibodies that could render subsequent exposures ineffective, dangerous, or both.

Tissue plasminogen activator (tPA) is a naturally occurring substance having greater selectivity for plasminogen-plasmin conversion at the clot site. There is therefore less likelihood of precipitating allergic phenomena or as much disturbance of systemic coagulation, with the theoretical ability to produce more complete clot lysis (9). Originally extracted from melanoma cell culture, most clinical experience has been with the recombinant preparation (tPA). In randomized trials, tPA was shown to produce better early patency than either placebo or streptokinase, especially with an initial higher infusion rate, and there was an effect against reocclusion with a prolonged low-dose infusion (10–12).

However, the optimum treatment schedule had not been agreed upon, and caution was expressed about expecting too much from these theoretical or largely inconclusive pilot studies (13). Despite these uncertainties and reservations, we designed and conducted a clinical study comparing tPA against placebo in patients with suspected acute myocardial infarction with death as the primary endpoint (14,15).

PATIENTS AND METHODS

Recruitment began in November 1988, eventually involving 52 centers in Denmark, Norway, Sweden, and the United Kingdom. Patients aged 18–75 years, of either sex, and with the clinical suspicion of an acute myocardial infarction, (AMI) within the previous 5 h were considered for inclusion. No electrocardiographic criteria were mandatory. An attempt was made to register all patients admitted to the participating CCUs with a working diagnosis of AMI and to record their eventual diagnosis and outcome for one month wherever possible. Patients were excluded if they had a medical or surgical history that might predispose them to a bleeding risk if allocated tPA, if local follow-up was difficult, or if consent was refused.

TRIAL MEDICATION AND PERMITTED COTREATMENTS

Patients were randomized double-blind to receive either tPA or matching placebo. tPA was given as a 10-mg bolus followed by an infusion of 50 mg in the next hour, then 20 mg in each of the next 2 h. All patients received an initial bolus dose of intravenous heparin 5000 units, then an infusion of 1000 U/h for the next 21 h commencing immediately after the 3-h study infusion. No target aPTT levels were stipulated.

During the course of the study all centers agreed to follow a common therapeutic policy for uncomplicated included patients. Thus, intravenous beta-blockers, antiarrhythmics, anticoagulants, and antiplatelet agents were prescribed only for agreed clinical events. Prophylactic oral beta-blockers, however, were encouraged according to local practice.

Clinic follow-up was scheduled for 1 and 6 months. Survival status at 12 months was by postal or telephone enquiry in order to assess symptomatic status, readmission diagnosis, drug usage, and interventions.

TRIAL COORDINATION AND DATA HANDLING

The trial was coordinated from the Department of Medicine, University Hospital, Nottingham, with each participating country also having a national clinical coordinator. The data base was handled by the Statistical Data Centre in the Department of Mathematics, University of Nottingham. Only the independent ethical committee (now called a Data and Safety Monitoring Board) periodically received unblinded progress reports.

STATISTICAL CONSIDERATIONS

The only endpoint was death. It was assumed that the 1-month overall fatality rate in the placebo group would be 12% and that the 6-month overall fatality rate in the placebo group would be 15%. A trial in 5000 patients would thus have greater than 90% power to detect a relative difference of 20% between the tPA and placebo groups at 6 months and would be large enough to examine mortality both at 6 months and at 1 month.

DIAGNOSTIC DEFINITIONS

The following definitions were used:

Definite myocardial infarction (MI)—Convincing history plus pathological Q waves in the ECG and peak enzyme levels exceeding twice the upper limit of normal.

Probable myocardial infarction—Convincing history plus either pathological Q waves or raised cardiac enzymes to twice the upper limit of normal.

Possible myocardial infarction—Convincing history plus ECG abnormalities not diagnostic of myocardial infarction and an increase of cardiac enzymes but to less than twice the upper limit of normal.

Ischemic heart disease (IHD)—Previous myocardial infarction or angina without new ECG or enzyme changes.

Chest pain of unknown cause (CP?C)—No history of previous myocardial infarction or angina and no ECG or enzyme evidence to suggest an event at this admission. No other cause for chest pain found.

Bleeding complications were divided into major or minor categories, irrespective of the need for blood transfusion. Major bleeds comprised any hematemesis, melena, severe hemoptysis, or hematuria. Minor bleeds comprised slight hemoptysis or trace hematuria and skin or gum bleeding.

RESULTS

Recruitment

Recruitment began in November 1986 and ended in February 1988, by which time 13,282 consecutive patients with suspected AMI were assessed for study entry. Of these 8269 (62%) were excluded—74% because of symptoms > 5 hours previously; 8% > 75 years of age; 6% recent hemorrhage, known ulcer, or bleeding diathesis; and 4% refused consent.

Included Patients: Mortality

Of the 5013 randomized patients, 2499 received placebo plus heparin and 2514 alteplase (tPA) plus heparin. The two treatment groups were well matched for baseline demographic variables (Table 1). There were no differences in diagnostic categorization for the index admission, but fatality was significantly lower in those given alteplase both at 1 and at 6 months (Table 2). Overall, by 1 month there was a 26% relative reduction in mortality (95% CI 11–39%, $p = 0.0011$) and 21% at 6 months (95% CI 8–32%, $p = 0.0026$).

Outcome at 12 months was available for 2103 (84%) patients given alteplase and for 2127 (85%) controls. Estimates for overall 12-month mortality are 13.2% and 15.1%, respectively, a relative reduction of 12.6% ($p = 0.05$). The corresponding figures for patients with a confirmed initial diagnosis of myocardial infarction are 15.7% and 18.9%, a relative reduction of 16.9% ($p = 0.01$).

The survival curves show that the difference between the groups was established early in the hospital phase with little difference thereafter (Fig. 1). Subset analysis showed a consistent trend in favor of thrombolytic treatment (Table 3). Paradoxically, smokers had a better outcome than those who had never smoked. Despite not requiring ECG entry criteria, there was no evidence of harm to those who had a normal ECG at entry (alteplase

Table 1   Preadmission Characteristics and Clinical Status on Admission (%)

	tPA (2514)	Placebo (2499)
Sex (Male/Female)	77/23	77/23
Age		
≤45	9	9
46–65	58	57
>65	33	34
History		
MI	27	27
Angina	49	46
Hypertension	26	24
Diabetes	7	6
Smoking		
Never	33	33
Ex-(>6 months)	20	20
Current	47	46
Drugs		
Beta blockers	23	23
Calcium blockers	15	13
Diuretics (hypertension)	11	10
Diuretics (heart failure)	9	8
Glycosides	6	5
ECG		
Normal	18	17
Abnormal (any reason)	82	83
Treatment for heart failure on admission		
Nil	77	76
Nitrate	4	5
Frusemide 40 mg	12	13
Frusemide 80 mg	4	4
Frusemide + vasodilator	1.6	1.4
Missing data	1.4	1.4

Table 2 Outcome at 1 and 6 Months by Diagnosis and Treatment

	Alteplase		Placebo	
Outcome	1 month	6 month	1 month	6 month
Overall death	7.2	10.4	9.8	13.1
M.I. 72%	9.4	12.6	13.1	17.1
I.H.D. 17%	1.1	5.3	1.6	4.0
CP?C/other 11%	2.6	4.2	1.1	1.7

MI = myocardial infarction; IHD = ischemic heart disease; CP?C = chest pain of un-known cause; other = other proven diagnosis.

patients ECG abnormal vs. normal 82% vs. 18%, 1-month mortality 8.5% vs. 1.6%; control patients ECG abnormal vs. normal 83% vs. 17%, 1-month mortality 11.2% vs. 3.0%).

Included Patients: Morbidity

Strokes

Where possible strokes were classified as embolic or hemorrhagic according to clinical, imaging, or necropsy data (but most remained unclassified). By 1 month the incidence of total stroke was 1.1% in the alteplase group and 1.0% in the placebo group. The corresponding figures at 6 months were 2% and 1.3%. Most strokes occurred in patients with an in-hospital diagnosis of acute myocardial infarction.

Bleeds

Bleeding from a noninfusion site occurred in 100 patients given alteplase but only 10 given placebo: blood transfusion was necessary in only 5 and 3 patients, respectively.

Other Clinical Events

There were no major differences for in-hospital complications other than for the incidence of cardiogenic shock (Table 4).

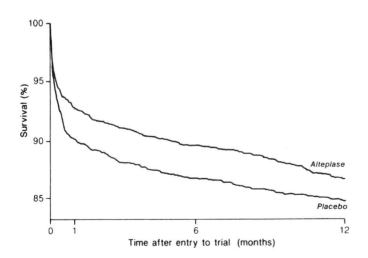

Figure 1 Life-table survival curves by intention-to-treat analysis.

Table 3   Six-Month Mortality (%) by Subgroup

	Alteplase	Placebo
Sex		
Male	10.2	12.9
Female	11.1	14.2
Time to treatment (hr)		
0–3	11.1	14.0
>3	9.9	12.2
Age (yr)		
≤55	5.1	5.9
56–65	10.2	11.8
66–75	15.4	20.9
Electrocardiograph		
Normal	3.2	3.7
Abnormal	12.0	15.1
Cigarette smoker		
Nonsmoker	11.8	14.9
Smoker	9.1	11.2
Ex-smoker	10.6	13.8
Country		
United Kingdom	10.3	12.0
Sweden	10.8	13.3
Norway	10.2	14.3
Denmark	9.8	15.1
Previous history		
MI		
No	9.1	12.1
Yes	14.0	16.0
Angina		
No	8.4	10.9
Yes	12.5	15.8
Hypertension		
No	10.1	11.8
Yes	11.2	17.3
Diabetes mellitus		
No	9.9	12.7
Yes	17.1	19.5
Previous treatment		
Beta blocker		
No	9.9	11.9
Yes	12.2	17.3
Calcium antagonist		
No	9.3	12.6
Yes	16.4	16.7
Antifailure		
No	8.7	10.5
Yes	16.4	21.6

Table 4 In-Hospital Complications Other Than Strokes

Complication	tPA	Placebo
Recurrent MI	99 (3.9%)	114 (4.5%)
Ventricular arrhythmias (day 1)	146 (5.8%)	108 (4.3%)
Ventricular fibrillation	94 (3.7%)	116 (4.6%)
Asystole	100 (3.9%)	122 (4.8%)
Pulmonary embolism	11 (0.4%)	14 (0.5%)
Other embolism	12 (0.4%)	19 (0.7%)
Cardiogenic shock	96 (3.8%)	129 (5.1%)*
Heart failure	446 (17.7%)	461 (18.4%)

* $p < 0.05$.

At 6 months approximately 30% of patients in both groups were considered to have angina pectoris and 22–23% were treated with diuretics for heart failure. There were no significant differences in cardiovascular treatment regimens between groups at 6 months despite the significant survival difference.

Of the 2361 discharged patients in the alteplase group, 730 (30.9%) were readmitted at least once in the first 6 months, compared with 623 of 2300 (27.0%) controls; 174 (7.3%) and 131 (5.7%), respectively, had evidence of at least one reinfarction.

One hundred and seven discharged patients (4.5%) in the alteplase group and 101 (4.4%) in the placebo group underwent coronary angiography; 49 and 59 patients, respectively, had coronary artery bypass surgery; and 9 patients in each group underwent percutaneous coronary angioplasty.

Excluded Patients

Of the 8148 fully documented excluded patients, the index diagnosis was AMI 61%, IHD 23%, CP?C 10%, and other diagnoses 6%. In most centers, excluded patients were followed to 1 month; in a few this was confined to in-hospital data. Overall mortality was 13.1%; in those with AMI the mortality was 17.5%, IHD 2.4%, CP?C <1%, other diagnoses 6.5%. Excluded patients with an index diagnosis of AMI therefore had a much higher early mortality than both included AMI patients randomized to placebo (13.1%) and included patients randomized to alteplase (9.4%).

DISCUSSION

The ASSET study remains the only placebo-controlled assessment of the early use of alteplase in patients with acute myocardial infarction. The observed reduction in both early and medium-term mortality is similar to that reported for streptokinase (7,8).

The 95% CIs for the reduction in overall early fatality were 11–39% for alteplase compared with 10–28% for streptokinase in GISSI-1 and 12–20% for streptokinase alone in ISIS-2, suggesting that when given in the schedules used in these controlled studies, the two drugs are unlikely to produce strikingly different outcomes. This expectation was eventually realized in two large comparative studies (GISSI 2/International and ISIS-3) (16,17).

The study also provided important safety as well as outcome data for alteplase, especially bleeding risk and the increased but not delayed risk of hemorrhagic stroke, which has been a constant feature of all subsequent trials of a tissue plasminogen activator.

ASSET did not separately assess either the contribution of the intravenous heparin cotreatment or the role of aspirin when coadministered with a tissue plasminogen activator. The strength of the aspirin effect observed in ISIS-2 has been accepted as proof that this is mandatory in all nonsensitive patients with AMI, irrespective of whether or which thrombolytic schedule is employed. Only now in the mid-1990s is the position of aspirin being challenged by other antiplatelet agents (clopidogrel, platelet glycoprotein IIb/IIIa receptor antagonists).

The ASSET study highlighted a number of other issues that have subsequently undergone further scrutiny. Current smokers had a better outcome than either never or ex-smokers, itself not an original observation, but a difference we attributed to younger age and less previous cardiovascular morbidity, which was confirmed in a subsequent study (18,19). As in GISSI-1, we found a similar pattern of cardiovascular drug usage and of new clinical events (angina, heart failure, reinfarction) in the two randomized groups during the medium-term follow-up period. One could argue for differences either way (better left ventricular function should require less treatment; increased survival of some higher risk patients), and much longer follow-up may be needed for further clarification (20).

The participating CCUs in the ASSET study kept a register of patients admitted with suspected acute MI, the reasons for not randomizing into the study (time delay being responsible for 74% of exclusions), and the short-term outcome of such patients. Excluded patients comprised 62% of the total registered patients: those with an index diagnosis of AMI had a 1-month fatality of about 17% as compared with 13% for the included control group. The register thus demonstrated the selection of lower-risk patients for treatment and suggested the need to keep the overall expectations from thrombolysis in perspective.

The ASSET trial organization and execution also confirmed the willingness of colleagues from many countries to enthusiastically contribute to important questions in cardiovascular therapy. This tremendous cooperation was of course also seen in ISIS-2 and no doubt encouraged the spirit of international mega-trials over the next decade, in which trials of tens of thousands of patients could be recruited in 12–18 months of endeavor. Such collaboration has advanced the evaluation of both newer schedules for old drugs (GUSTO-I) and new drugs in comparison with established comparators (INJECT) (21,22).

We are now in the era of new antiplatelets, antithrombins, and ''coagulation cascade inhibitors'': there are newer thrombolytic drugs entering phase III trials, and the issue of primary angioplasty as the preferred reperfusion strategy is hotly debated. We have come a long way indeed from prolonged bed rest, oxygen, and pain relief.

ACKNOWLEDGMENTS

In this invited historical appreciation of the ASSET study, the author wishes to thank his co-investigators, all of whom are included in the original papers, and *The Lancet* for permission to reproduce and quote liberally from the trial publications. The study was supported by a grant from Boehringer Ingelheim.

REFERENCES

1. Reimer KA, Lowe JE, Rasmussen MM, Jennings RB. Myocardial infarct size vs. duration of coronary occlusion in dogs. Circulation 1977; 56:786–794.
2. Davies MJ, Woolf N, Robertson WB. Pathology of acute myocardial infarction with particular reference to occlusive coronary thrombi. Br Heart J 1976; 38:659–664.
3. DeWood MA, Spores, J, Notske R, Mouser LT, Burroughs R, Golden MS, Lang HT. Prevalence of total coronary occlusion during the early hours of transmural myocardial infarction. N Engl J Med 1980; 303:897–902.
4. Falk E. Coronary thrombosis: pathogenesis and clinical manifestations. Am J Cardiol 1991; 68:28–35B.
5. Fletcher AP, Alkjaersig N, Smymiotis FE, Sherry S. Treatment of patients suffering from early myocardial infarction with massive and prolonged streptokinase therapy. Trans Assoc Am Phys 1958; 71:287–296.
6. The ISAM Study Group. A prospective trial of intravenous streptokinase in acute myocardial infarction (ISAM): mortality, morbidity, and infarct size at 21 days. N Engl J Med 1986; 314: 1465–1471.
7. GISSI. Effectiveness of intravenous thrombolytic treatment in acute myocardial infarction. Lancet 1986; i:397–402.
8. ISIS-2 (Second International Study of Infarct Survival) Collaborative Group. Randomised trial of intravenous streptokinase, oral aspirin, both, or neither among 17187 cases of suspected acute myocardial infarction: ISIS 2. Lancet 1988; ii:349–360.
9. van de Werf F, Collen D. Coronary thrombolysis with tissue-type plasminogen activator: an overview. Eur Heart J 1985; 6:902–904.
10. Verstraete M, Bernard R, Bony M, Collen D, Erbel R, Lennane RJ, Mathey D, Michels HR, Schartl M, Vebis R, Braver RW, de Bono DP, Huhmann W, Lubsen J, Meyer J, Rutsch W, Schmidt W, Von Essen R. Randomised trial of intravenous recombinant tissue-type plasminogen activator versus intravenous streptokinase in acute myocardial infarction. Lancet 1985; i:842–847.
11. Verstraete M, Bleifeld N, Brower RW, Collen D, Dunning AJ, Lubsen J, Michel PL, Schafer J, Vanhaecke J, Van de Werf F, Charbonnier B, de Bono DP, Lennane RJ, Mathey DG, Raynaud P, Vahanian A, van de Kley G, Von Essen R. Double blind randomised trial of intravenous tissue-type plasminogen activator versus placebo in acute myocardial infarction. Lancet 1985; ii:965–969.
12. Gold HK, Leinbach RC, Johns JA, Yasuda T, Garabedian HD, Collen D. Prevention of coronary reocclusion and reduction in late coronary stenosis by maintenance recombinant tissue-type plasminogen activator (rt-PA) infusion. Circulation 1986; 74:II-368.
13. Sherry S. Recombinant tissue plasminogen activator (rtPA): Is it the thrombolytic agent of choice for an evolving acute myocardial infarction? Am J Cardiol 1987; 59:986–989.
14. Wilcox RG, Olsson CG, Skene AM, Von Der Lippe G, Jensen G, Hampton JR, for the ASSET Study Group. Trial of tissue plasminogen activator for mortality reduction in acute myocardial infarction. Anglo-Scandinavian Study of Early Thrombolysis (ASSET). Lancet 1988; 2:525–530.
15. Wilcox RG, Von Der Lippe G, Olsson CG, Jensen G, Skene AM, Hampton JR. Effects of alteplase in acute myocardial infarction: 6-month results from the ASSET study. For the Anglo-Scandinavian Study of Early Thrombolysis. Lancet 1990; 335:1175–1178.

16. GISSI-2 and International Study Group. Six-month survival in 20891 patients with acute myocardial infarction randomised between alteplase and streptokinase with or without heparin. Eur Heart J 1992; 13:1692–1697.

17. ISIS-3. A randomised comparison of streptokinase vs. tissue plasminogen activator vs. anistreplase and of aspirin plus heparin vs. aspirin alone among 41229 cases of suspected acute myocardial infarction. Lancet 1992; 339:753–770.

18. Sparrow D, Dawber TR, Cotton T. The influence of cigarette smoking on prognosis after a first myocardial infarction. A report from the Framingham Study. J Chron Dis 1978; 31:425–428.

19. Barbash GI, White HD, Modam M, Diaz R, Hampton JR, Heikkila J, Kristinsson A, Moulopoulos S, Paolasso EAC, Van der Werf T, Pehrsson K, Sandoe E, Simes J, Wilcox RG, Verstraete M, von der Lippe G, van de Werf F, for the investigators of the International Tissue Plasminogen Activator/Streptokinase Mortality Trial. Acute myocardial infarction in the young—the role of smoking. Eur Heart J 1995; 16:313–316.

20. Van de Werf F. Thrombolysis for acute myocardial infarction. Why is there no extra benefit after hospital discharge? Circulation 1995; 91(12):2862–2864.

21. The GUSTO Investigators. An international randomised trial comparing four thrombolytic strategies for acute myocardial infarction. N Engl J Med 1993; 329:673–682.

22. The INJECT Trial Study Group. Randomised, double-blind comparison of reteplase double-bolus administration with streptokinse in acute myocardial infarction (INJECT): trial to investigate equivalence. Lancet 1995; 346:329–336.

4

ISIS-3

PETER SLEIGHT

Third International Study of Infarct Survival Collaborative Group. ISIS-3:
A randomized comparison of streptokinase vs. tissue plasminogen
activator vs. anistreplase and of aspirin plus heparin vs. aspirin alone
among 41,299 cases of suspected acute myocardial infarction. Lancet
1992; 339: 753–770.

ISIS-3 compared streptokinase, tissue plasminogen activator duteplase (tPA), and anis-treplase in a randomized trial in 41,229 patients with suspected myocardial infarction (MI) up to 24 hours from the onset of symptoms (1). All the patients received aspirin (162 mg/day) in an enteric-coated formulation, with the first tablet chewed for rapid effect.

At the time ISIS-3 was planned, there was wide experience with streptokinase but a slightly more convenient formulation of streptokinase had been developed—anysolated plasminogen streptokinase activated complex (APSAC or anistreplase)—which could be given as a slow bolus. There was also some evidence that anistreplase might lyse intracoronary thrombi more rapidly (2). At the same time, two equally effective genetically engineered forms of recombinant human tPA—alteplase and duteplase—were shown to lyse thrombi more rapidly, as judged by angiograms at 90 minutes after onset, but it was not known how safe they would prove to be in widespread use, especially since a higher dose of alteplase had had to be abandoned because of high cerebral hemorrhage rates (3). ISIS-3 was therefore designed to assess the risks or benefits of the three regimens and also the risks or benefits of adding high-dose subcutaneous heparin to 162 mg of aspirin daily. (The latter is discussed separately in Chap. 33.)

Indirect comparisons of the previous large trials of the three lytic agents [ISIS-2 (4), GISSI-1 (5), ISAM (6), ASSET (7), and AIMS (8)] suggested that it was unlikely that large differences between them would emerge.

As in the previous ISIS trials, entry procedures, drug delivery, and reporting were streamlined in order to facilitate recruitment of large numbers of patients. Telephone randomization (with no forms) ensured the collection of full baseline data and identification for follow-up through government records.

In those instances where the physician was certain he or she wished to use lytic therapy, the randomization was between the three thrombolytic agents, but where the physician was uncertain of the benefit of lysis (perhaps because of a relatively normal ECG or only ST depression on the initial ECG), randomization was between one of the three lytic agents and open control. As a result 45,856 patients were randomized from

914 hospitals in 20 countries over the 18 months or so between September 1989 and January 1991. In 36,381 patients the physicians were "certain" of the indications for thrombolysis. In the remaining 9475 patients, half received thrombolysis. A total of 41,299 patients therefore received thrombolysis, and this report concerns only this group. The remaining patients were reported as part of the Fibrinolytic Therapy Trialists (FTT) overview (9).

Compliance to allocated treatment was high, with around 97% starting the fibrinolytic and 93% (streptokinase), 94.3% (tPA), and 97.4% (APSAC) completing the infusion; the higher APSAC figure probably reflects the shorter infusion period for this formulation.

There were no significant differences in mortality at 35 days or at 3 and 6 months between the different fibrinolytic regimens for either vascular or nonvascular death (Fig. 1).

There was a significant ($p < 0.01$) excess of stroke with tPA compared with streptokinase (1.39% vs. 1.04%); much of this was early and due to cerebral hemorrhage. The difference in cerebral hemorrhage was highly significant in patients both with and without heparin added to aspirin ($p < 0.001$ and 0.002, respectively) (Fig. 2).

Allergic reactions were more frequent in both streptokinase (3.6%) and anistreplase (5.1%, $p < 0.00001$) than with duteplase (0.8%, $p < 0.00001$). Very few were troublesome, but as expected hypotension was reported more commonly with streptokinase than with tPA (11.8% vs. 7.1%, $p < 0.00001$). Compared with control (in the uncertain arm), tPA was still associated with hypotension (4.14% vs. 1.5%, $p < 0.00001$). Reinfarction in hospital was significantly less with tPA 2.93% than with streptokinase (3.47%) ($p < 0.02$).

The overall results of the fibrinolytic comparison of streptokinase and duteplase in ISIS-3 were similar to those of GISSI-2 (10) and its international arm (11), which compared streptokinase with alteplase. In this trial there were nonsignificantly more deaths with alteplase than streptokinase (9.6% vs. 9.2%, respectively). There was no difference

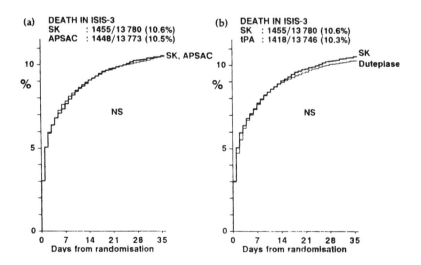

Figure 1 Cumulative percentage dead in days 0-35 in ISIS-3: fibrinolytic comparison (a) of streptokinase and APSAC; (b) of streptokinase and tPA. (From Ref. 1.)

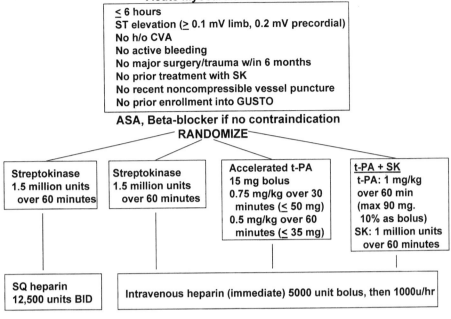

Acute Myocardial Infarction

≤ 6 hours
ST elevation (≥ 0.1 mV limb, 0.2 mV precordial)
No h/o CVA
No active bleeding
No major surgery/trauma w/in 6 months
No prior treatment with SK
No recent noncompressible vessel puncture
No prior enrollment into GUSTO

ASA, Beta-blocker if no contraindication
RANDOMIZE

Streptokinase
1.5 million units
over 60 minutes

Streptokinase
1.5 million units
over 60 minutes

Accelerated t-PA
15 mg bolus
0.75 mg/kg over 30
  minutes (≤ 50 mg)
0.5 mg/kg over 60
  minutes (≤ 35 mg)

t-PA + SK
t-PA: 1 mg/kg
over 60 min
(max 90 mg.
10% as bolus)
SK: 1 million units
over 60 minutes

SQ heparin
12,500 units BID

Intravenous heparin (immediate) 5000 unit bolus, then 1000u/hr

Primary endpoint: 30 day mortality

Figure 1   The GUSTO trial design. (From Ref. 24.)

3. Combination tPA (1.0 mg/kg over a 60-minute period, not to exceed 90 mg,
    with 10% of the dose being given as a bolus) and streptokinase (1.0 million
    units over 60 minutes) given via separate infusion catheters along with the same
    intravenous heparin regimen.

After the first 1160 patients were enrolled in the study, preliminary results from
the ISIS-3 trial suggested that the best results with streptokinase came with concomitant
administration of subcutaneous (SQ) heparin. To test this streptokinase regimen, a fourth
limb was added to the GUSTO trial, with infusion of 1.5 million units of intravenous
streptokinase over 60 minutes followed by 12,500 units of SQ heparin beginning 4 hours
after initiation of thrombolytic therapy (26). This would allow for an adequate reference
population to the ISIS-3 and GISSI-2 trials, incorporating the best treatment results
achieved with streptokinase.

Eligible patients included those who presented within 6 hours of an acute myocardial
infarction with ST elevation (≥0.1 mV in two or more limb leads or ≥0.2 mV in two or
more contiguous precordial leads). Patients were excluded for a prior history of stroke,
active bleeding, recent trauma or major surgery, prior enrollment in trial, prior treatment
with streptokinase, or having had noncompressible vascular punctures. Patients with severe uncontrolled hypertension (systolic blood pressure ≥ 180 mmHg) were felt to have
a relative contraindication to enrollment. Following informed consent, eligible patients
were randomized to one of the four treatment strategies. All received chewable aspirin,
and those without contraindication received beta-blocker therapy. All other medications

and revascularization strategies were at the discretion of the attending physician. Of note, patients were not excluded on the basis of advanced age on the presence of cardiogenic shock (26).

A vital component of the GUSTO trial was the prospectively designed angiographic substudy (27), the purpose of which was to test whether early and complete vessel patency is the mechanism underlying thrombolytic efficacy. A subset of patients was randomized to four different timing patterns of angiography at the same time they were enrolled into the four thrombolytic treatment strategies. The angiography intervals were 90 minutes, 180 minutes, 24 hours, and 5–7 days. Patients assigned to the 90-minute time frame also underwent a follow-up study at 5–7 days. Such a substudy allowed for the assessment of patency at different time points and its association with ventricular function and survival. GUSTO was the first megatrial to incorporate such a mechanistic approach to establish a link between survival and the underlying angiographic findings (23,27).

RESULTS

A total of 41,021 patients were enrolled into the GUSTO study, 2431 of whom were also entered into the angiographic substudy. Enrollment took place between December 27, 1990, and February 22, 1993, with 1081 hospitals in 15 countries and 4 continents participating in the study. The angiographic substudy involved 75 of these centers.

Primary Endpoints

The primary endpoint of the trial was 30-day all-cause mortality (Table 1; Fig. 2). Patients treated with tPA had an absolute reduction in mortality of 1.0% (from 7.3 to 6.3%) as compared with those given streptokinase (combined IV and SQ heparin arms, $p = 0.001$) The relative risk reduction was 14.6%. This translates into an additional 10 lives saved per 1000 patients treated, or the prevention of 1 out of 7 deaths that would be expected

Table 1   Major Clinical Endpoints

	Patients (%)				
Endpoint	Streptokinase + SQ heparin ($n = 9796$)	Streptokinase + IV heparin ($n = 10,377$)	Accelerated tPA + IV heparin ($n = 10,344$)	Combination SK/tPA + IV heparin ($n = 10,328$)	p value: tPA vs. both SK groups
30-day mortality	7.2	7.4	6.3	7.0	0.001
Nonfatal stroke	7.9	8.2	7.2	7.9	0.006
Nonfatal hemmorrhagic stroke	7.4	7.6	6.6	7.4	0.004
Nonfatal disabling stroke	7.7	7.9	6.9	7.6	0.006

Source: Ref. 26.

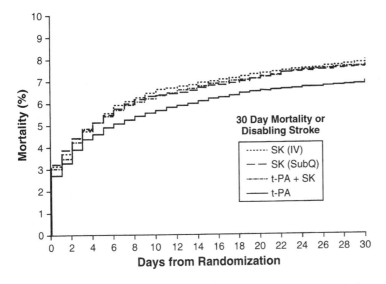

Figure 2 Kaplan-Meier curves of 30-day mortality or disabling stroke by treatment group. (From Ref. 26.)

with streptokinase therapy. The tPA arm was also superior to the combination thrombolytic regimen, which had a 7.0% mortality at 30 days (26).

Similarly, significant differences were also found for the combined endpoints of death and nonfatal stroke. The magnitude and significance of these differences were similar whether the streptokinase arms were compared individually or in combination (26).

Angiographic Substudy

The angiographic substudy helped to delineate the mechanism of this benefit (Fig. 3). Patients receiving tPA had significantly improved 90-minute complete vessel reperfusion (thrombolysis and myocardial infarction or TIMI grade 3 flow) than those treated with streptokinase ($p < 0.001$). TIMI 3 flow was established in 54% of patients at 90 minutes

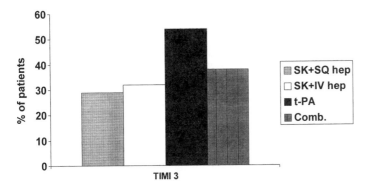

Figure 3 Ninety-minute complete vessel patency (TIMI 3 flow) by treatment group. (From Ref. 27.)

with tPA, in 29 and 32% in the streptokinase groups, and in 38% of patients with combination thrombolytic treatment (27).

No residual differences in patency existed at 180 minutes, 24 hours, or 5–7 days. There were no significant differences among the four treatment groups in the incidence of reocclusion (5.9% for tPA, 5.5% for SK/IV heparin, 6.4% for SK/SQ heparin, and 4.9% for combination tPA/SK) (27).

Ventriculography at 90 minutes (Table 2) demonstrated significantly less widespread and less severe wall motion abnormalities in those receiving tPA alone. The tPA group also had a lower end systolic volume index ($p = 0.037$) and a higher percentage of patients with preserved regional wall motion. A similar trend (not statistically significant) for improved global ejection fraction existed in the tPA group (27).

The most revealing result of the angiographic substudy was the association between 90-minute patency (irrespective of treatment assignment) and mortality (Fig. 4). TIMI grade 0 or 1 flow was associated with an 8.9% mortality rate at 30 days, TIMI 2 flow with a 7.4% mortality. Complete reperfusion (TIMI 3 flow) was associated with a 30-day mortality of 4.4% ($p = 0.08$ for TIMI 3 vs. TIMI 2, $p = 0.009$ for TIMI 3 vs. TIMI 0-1) (27).

In addition, all indices of left ventricular function were better in patients that achieved TIMI 3 flow (higher ejection fraction, lower end systolic volume index, fewer abnormal chords, less wall motion abnormality in the ischemic zone and higher percentage of those with preserved regional wall motion, with $p < 0.001$ for all parameters, as compared with TIMI grades 0,1, or 2) (Table 3) (27).

Ventricular function at 90 minutes (independent of treatment assignment) was also related to survival (Fig. 4). Among those with an ejection fraction of greater than 45%, 30-day mortality was 3.9%. But in those with an ejection fraction of less than 45%, mortality rate increased to 14.7% ($p < 0.001$) (27).

The GUSTO trial demonstrated a reduced 30-day mortality rate with accelerated

Table 2 Left Ventricular Function According to Treatment Group

Ventriculography at 90 minutes	SK + SQ heparin	SK + IV heparin	Accelerated tPA	tPA + SK	p value: tPA vs. both SK groups
Ejection fraction (%)	58 ± 15	57 ± 15	59 ± 15	58 ± 15	NS
ESVI (ml/m²)	28 ± 15	30 ± 17	27 ± 16	29 ± 16	0.037*
Wall motion (SD/chord)	−2.5 ± 1.5	−2.7 ± 1.4	−2.4 ± 1.4	−2.4 ± 1.5	0.018
Abnormal chords (no.)	23 ± 17	25 ± 18	21 ± 19	24 ± 19	0.027
Preserved RWM (percent of group)	18	19	29	21	<0.001

Values are expressed as means ± standard deviation (SD). ESVI denotes end-systolic volume index, and RWM denotes regional wall motion. Wall motion is expressed as the mean magnitude of depressed infarct-zone chords; wall motion was considered preserved if all infarct zone chords were normal. Chords in the infarct zone were considered abnormal if they were more than 2 SD below the norm.
*p value given for tPA vs. SK/intravenous heparin group.
Source: Ref. 24.

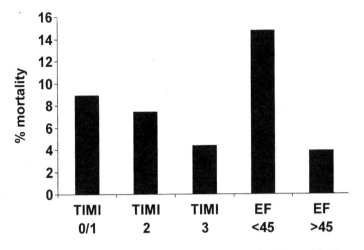

Figure 4   Relationship between TIMI grade, LV function at 90 minutes, and mortality. (From Ref. 27.)

tPA compared with streptokinase (with either SQ or IV heparin) or the combination thrombolytic regimen (24). The angiographic substudy revealed that tPA resulted in improved 90-minute patency and left ventricular function. Furthermore, TIMI 3 flow and left ventricular function at 90 minutes were independent predictors of 30-day mortality (27). This supports the concept that the superiority of tPA over streptokinase results from earlier and more complete restoration of flow, with improved myocardial salvage.

In accord with this, Simes et al. developed a model to predict the mortality differences in the main GUSTO trial based on the findings of the angiographic substudy (28).

Table 3   Left Ventricular Function According to TIMI Grade

Ventriculography at 90 minutes	TIMI 0	TIMI 1	TIMI 2	TIMI 3	p value: TIMI 3 vs TIMI 0 & 1 or TIMI 2
Ejection Fraction (%)	55 ± 15	55 ± 15	56 ± 15	62 ± 14	<0.001
ESVI (ml/m²)	31 ± 17	33 ± 21	29 ± 14	26 ± 14	<0.001
Wall motion (SD/chord)	-2.8 ± 1.3	-2.7 ± 1.4	-2.6 ± 1.4	-2.2 ± 1.5	<0.001
Abnormal chords (no.)	26 ± 17	26 ± 19	27 ± 19	18 ± 17	<0.001
Preserved RWM (percent of group)	11	17	19	31	<0.001

Values are expressed as means ± standard deviation (SD). ESVI denotes end-systolic volume index, and RWM denotes regional wall motion. Wall motion is expressed as the mean magnitude of depressed infarct-zone chords; wall motion was considered preserved if all infarct zone chords were normal. Chords in the infarct zone were considered abnormal if they were more than 2 SD below the norm.
Source: Ref. 27.

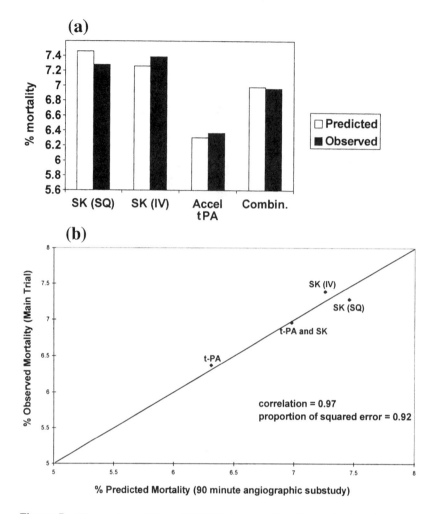

Figure 5 Observed mortality in GUSTO trial vs. predicted mortality based on angiographic substudy: (a) histogram by treatment group; (b) plot of predicted vs. observed mortality. (From Ref. 28.)

The model assumed that the differences in mortality could be accounted for entirely by differences in the 90-minute patency rate. The correlation between predicted and observed mortality was striking (Fig. 5), with a correlation coefficient of 0.97 and a proportion of squared error of 0.92 (28)

The lack of superiority of the combination thrombolytic arm can be explained by the angiographic substudy, which documented lower 90-minute patency rates as compared with tPA alone (27). This may have been secondary to a plasminogen steal (29), which was also demonstrated when tPA and anistreplase were combined (TIMI-IV) (30); plasminogen levels may have been too low for these enzymes to exert their therapeutic effect.

Mortality Within 24 Hours

The GUSTO trial prespecified mortality within 24 hours as a secondary endpoint of the study to gain insight into the association between reperfusion and early death (31). There were a total of 2851 deaths in the GUSTO trial during the 30-day follow-up period. Of these, 1125 (39%) occurred within the first 24 hours and 641 (22%) occurred within the first 6 hours after initiating thrombolytic therapy. As with 30-day mortality, significant differences existed between the four treatment groups with regard to early deaths. The 24-hour or early mortality rate was significantly lower in the tPA group (2.3%) as compared with the streptokinase arms (2.8–2.9%, $p = 0.005$). This 0.5% absolute reduction in mortality for the first 24 hours represents half of the benefit demonstrated in the main 30-day GUSTO results. This substantive early benefit again suggests the important role of early reperfusion (31).

A breakdown of the timing of early mortality helps to further delineate the effects of early reperfusion (Fig. 6). For the first 6 hours after the initiation of thrombolytic therapy, there are no differences in mortality across the four treatment groups. Beginning at hour 6, however, there is a sustained reduction in the mortality rate with tPA. Parallel to these findings are those of the angiographic substudy, which demonstrates that around this sixth hour, a distinct survival benefit becomes apparent for those patients who had TIMI-3 flow at 90 minutes (regardless of treatment arm) (31). These results again point to the beneficial effects of early and complete restoration of antegrade flow, which begins to produce a mortality benefit within a few hours. The equivalence for the first 6 hours post therapy is unclear, but it may represent the time required for stunned myocardium to recover.

The patients who died within the first 6 hours clinically demonstrated pretreatment signs of significant LV dysfunction, with greater incidence of hypotension and tachycardia (31). This group may not have had sufficient LV reserve to await recovery of LV function and may represent those who could benefit from more aggressive hemodynamic support.

Enzyme Substudy

A European substudy of GUSTO involving 553 patients looked at the patterns of enzyme release in the four treatment groups (32). The plasma activity of α-hydroxybutyrate dehydrogenase (HBDH) was analyzed at the initiation of thrombolytic therapy and at prespecified intervals up to 96 hours following lytic therapy. Infarct size was then determined as the cumulative HBDH release over 72 hours.

Patients receiving tPA had accelerated release of the myocardial enzyme ($p < 0.0001$) and smaller infarct size ($p = 0.04$) than patients receiving streptokinase. A subgroup of these patients were also enrolled in the GUSTO angiographic substudy. In these patients, a marked association was found between TIMI grade at 90 minutes and infarct size, with the smaller infarcts in patients with TIMI 3 flow ($p = 0.024$). Multivariate linear regression analysis revealed that the effect of treatment on the pattern of enzyme release (with superiority of tPA) could be explained by the differential effects on 90-minute patency (32).

Though it involves only a relatively small number of patients, the results of the enzyme substudy are consistent with the findings of the main GUSTO trial. Treatment with tPA results in limitation of infarct size, via improved early and complete infarct artery patency.

Cardiac Complications

Although not primary endpoints, other clinical parameters analyzed in the GUSTO trial further emphasize the benefit of tPA in improving myocardial salvage (Table 4). Patients

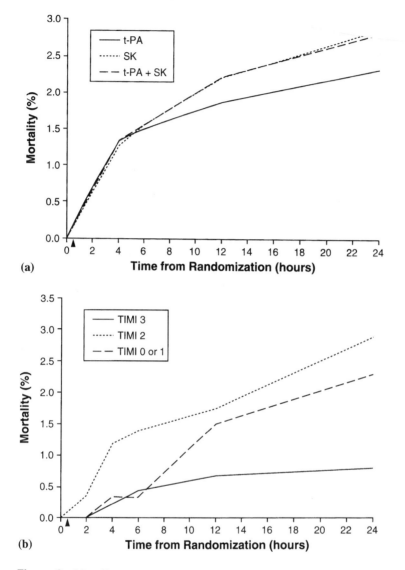

Figure 6 Mortality according to time from randomization: (a) by treatment group; (b) by TIMI grade. (From Ref. 31.)

receiving tPA were less likely to develop cardiogenic shock, congestive heart failure, or sustained hypotension. There were fewer arrhythmic complications in the tPA group, with less atrioventricular block or asystole, and less sustained ventricular tachycardia or ventricular fibrillation (24).

The GUSTO trial provides an important insight into the role of reperfusion therapy for cardiogenic shock. Unlike many prior thrombolytic trials, GUSTO did not exclude patients with shock. In addition, a prospective plan was designed to identify and analyze these patients (33).

Cardiogenic shock was identified in 2972 (7.2%) of the 41,021 patients enrolled

Table 4 Cardiac Complications by Treatment Group

Complications	Patients (%)				
	Streptokinase + SQ Heparin	Streptokinase + IV Heparin	Accelerated tPA + IV Heparin	Combination SK/tPA + IV Heparin	*p*-value: tPA vs. both SK groups
Congestive heart failure	17.5	16.8	15.2	16.8	<0.001
Cardiogenic shock	6.9	6.3	5.1	6.1	<0.001
Sustained hypotension	13.3	12.5	10.1	12.4	<0.001
Atrioventricular block	9.5	8.7	7.3	8.4	<0.001
Asystole	6.0	6.4	5.3	6.4	0.003
Sustained ventricular tachycardia	6.8	6.5	5.6	6.1	0.001
Ventricular fibrillation	7.1	6.9	6.3	6.9	0.02

Source: Ref. 26.

into GUSTO (33). Only a minority of these, 315 (11%), presented in shock; the remainder developed shock during the hospitalization (the majority within 48 hours of randomization).

Among patients who presented in cardiogenic shock, or in those who developed it during the hospitalization, there was a tendency for a lower mortality rate with streptokinase. Among those who developed shock after admission, 30-day mortality was 51% in the streptokinase and subcutaneous heparin group compared to 57% in the tPA group ($p = 0.061$). Thirty-day mortality for those presenting with shock was 54% in those receiving streptokinase and intravenous heparin, compared with to 61% for tPA. This may have been related to the greater dependence on tissue perfusion for clot lysis with tPA (33).

The GUSTO trial confirmed the high morality rates associated with cardiogenic shock, and its contribution to overall mortality following myocardial infarction. Among all deaths in the GUSTO trial, 58% (1647 of 2851) occurred in the context of cardiogenic shock. A critical finding of the study was that mortality in those who developed shock during hospitalization was as high as in those who presented in shock (55% vs. 57%) (33). This emphasizes the need to identify signs of incipient shock and suggests that more aggressive use of adjunctive reperfusion strategies (such as angioplasty and intraaortic balloon pumping) should be considered. Indeed, patients with cardiogenic shock who underwent percutaneous transluminal coronary angioplasty (PTCA) did have a substantially lower mortality than those who did not (31% vs. 61%, $p < 0.001$), although this substudy was not a controlled trial of PTCA.

Subgroup Analyses

Numerous secondary analyses have been performed within the GUSTO study to analyze thrombolytic therapy in various population subgroups. It must be emphasized that the trial was powered only for the primary endpoints among the whole population studied. There fore, all the ~~~~~~~

~~~~~~~~ suggested by these analyses, rather than focus solely on the statistical significance of these differences (23).

The GUSTO trial prespecified three major subgroups for analyses, according to age (>75 vs. ≤75 years), infarct location (anterior vs. inferior), and time to treatment.

Age

The majority of patients (88%) in the GUSTO trial were under the age of 75. In this group, there was a 21% relative reduction in mortality with tPA over streptokinase (4.4% vs. 5.5%, odds ratio of 0.79 with 95% CI 0.70–0.89%). In patients over the age of 75, there was still a reduction in mortality with tPA (19.3% vs. 20.6%), although the confidence intervals crossed unity (odds ratio of 0.92 with 95% CI 0.78–1.10%). There was a higher incidence of hemorrhagic stroke in the older patients with tPA than with streptokinase (2.08% vs. 1.23%, odds ratio 1.71 with 95% CI 1.01–2.88%). Despite this, the composite endpoint of death or nonfatal disabling stroke still favored tPA (20.2% vs. 21.5%, odds ratio 0.93 with 95% CI 0.78–1.10%) (26).

A more detailed analysis of the effect of age on outcome with thrombolytic therapy has been performed by White et al. (35). Clinical outcomes were examined for patients under the age of 65, for those aged 65–74, for those aged 75–85, and for patients older than 85 years. Thirty-day mortality increased with age (3.0% in those under age 65, 9.5% in those 65–74 years, 19.6% in those 75–85 years, and 30.3% in those over the age of 85). Similarly, the incidence of stroke, cardiogenic shock and heart failure also increased with age.

Except in patients older than age 85, there was a consistent survival advantage for the tPA-treated group (Table 5). Despite the increased stroke risk with tPA, the composite endpoint of death or nonfatal disabling stroke still favored tPA. Only in the few patients older than age 85 ($n = 412$) did streptokinase appear to have an advantage, but the numbers were quite small.

These findings suggest that the elderly are at much higher risk for death and other complications of myocardial infarction. Even after adjustment for comorbid conditions, patients in the upper quartile of age in the GUSTO population had a fourfold increase in mortality compared with those in the lowest quartile (36), with age being the strongest independent clinical predictor of 30-day mortality ($\chi^2 = 717$, $p < 0.00001$) (35,36). It is precisely because of this that early and complete infarct vessel patency is so important in this group. Due to the higher frequency of adverse events in the elderly, the net incremental clinical benefit of tPA over streptokinase is actually highest in the 75- to 85-year-old age group (with 17 fewer deaths or disabling strokes per 1000 patients treated, as compared to 5 fewer events per 1000 treated in the <65 years age group) (35).

Infarct Location

Patients with both anterior and inferior infarctions benefited from tPA, although those with anterior infarcts derived a proportionately greater benefit. For anterior infarcts (39% of patients), 30 day mortality was 8.6% in the tPA group compared to 10.5% in the streptokinase groups (odds ratio 0.81, 95% CI 0.71–0.92%). Mortality rate for inferior infarcts was 4.7% with tPA and 5.3% with streptokinase (odds ratio 0.89, 95% CI 0.78–1.03%) (26).

Table 5 Major Clinical Endpoints by Age and Treatment Group

Age (yr)	tPA (%)	SK-SQ heparin (%)	Odds ratio (95% CI) tPA vs. SK/SQ heparin	SK-IV heparin (%)	Odds ratio (95% CI) tPA vs. SK/IV heparin
<65					
Death	2.7	3.2	0.83 (0.67, 1.03)	3.4	0.78 (0.64, 0.96)
Any stroke	0.75	0.67	1.12 (0.73, 1.71)	0.73	1.03 (0.68, 1.55)
Death or disabling stroke	3.0	3.5	0.86 (0.7, 1.05)	3.6	0.82 (0.68, 1.00)
65–74					
Death	8.3	10.4	0.77 (0.64, 0.93)	10.3	0.79 (0.66, 0.94)
Any stroke	2.18	1.46	1.5 (1.00, 2.24)	2.22	0.99 (0.69, 1.41)
Death or disabling stroke	9.1	10.8	0.83 (0.69, 0.98)	11.0	0.8 (0.68, 0.96)
75–85					
Death	18.2	20.2	0.88 (0.71, 1.08)	19.2	0.93 (0.76, 1.15)
Any stroke	4.19	3.24	1.31 (0.84, 2.03)	2.5	1.71 (1.07, 2.71)
Death or disabling stroke	19.2	21.1	0.89 (0.72, 1.09)	19.8	0.96 (0.79, 1.18)
>85					
Death	30.0	26.4	1.19 (0.64, 2.23)	32.0	0.91 (0.51, 1.64)
Any stroke	1.82	2.3	0.79 (0.11, 5.7)	6.0	0.29 (0.06, 1.47)
Death or disabling stroke	30.0	27.6	1.13 (0.6, 2.1)	34.0	0.83 (0.47, 1.49)

Source: Ref. 35.

Time to Treatment

0–2 hours and 2–4 hours, this benefit was greater (4.3% vs. 5.4% and 5.5% vs. 6.7%, respectively) than the benefit seen 4–6 hours after the onset of symptoms (8.9% vs. 9.3%). Only in the 4% of patients in GUSTO who were enrolled more than 6 hours after the onset of symptoms did streptokinase appear to have a survival advantage. This may represent a point in time when myocardium is irreversibly injured, so that the benefit of more aggressive regimens for achieving earlier and more complete vessel patency is lost.

Coronary Artery Bypass Graft Surgery

There were small variations in the incidence of surgical revascularization (done at the discretion of the attending physician) among the four treatment groups in GUSTO. To ensure that this did not contribute to the observed mortality differences seen in the trial, further analysis was performed on this subgroup of patients (37).

A total of 3526 patients in the GUSTO trial underwent coronary artery bypass graft (CABG) surgery during their initial hospital admission. Nine percent of the tPA group and 8.3% of the combined streptokinase groups underwent surgical revascularization ($p = 0.05$). However, further analysis reveals that a 15% reduction in mortality was already apparent with tPA within the first week of enrollment, at a time when the incidence of CABG did not differ among the four treatment groups. It was only after one week that patients in the tPA group began to undergo CABG at a significantly higher rate. Thus the mortality benefit with tPA cannot be attributed to bypass surgery. The increased use of CABG after the first week in the tPA group may reflect the enhanced survival with tPA and hence a larger number of patients that could be referred for bypass (37).

Gender

Prior trials of thrombolytic therapy have demonstrated that women have a higher mortality rate after myocardial infarction than men (2,38). A variety of clinical variables have been suggested to explain this; women presenting with infarcts tend to be older and have a greater frequency of hypertension and diabetes than their male counterparts (39). The GUSTO trial included one of the largest number of women (10,315) in a trial of myocardial infarction, and hence allows for a more detailed analysis of the effect of gender on outcome with thrombolytic therapy.

Women did have a significantly higher 30-day mortality rate than did men (11.3% vs. 5.5%, $p < 0.001$) (40). There was also a greater incidence of nonfatal complications, such as congestive heart failure (22% vs. 14%, $p < 0.001$), shock (9% vs. 5%, $p < 0.001$), and reinfarction (5.1% vs. 3.6%, $p < 0.001$) (40). These differences could be partially accounted for by differences in baseline characteristics (age, time to present to the hospital, time to treatment upon arrival, incidence of hypertension and diabetes). However, even after adjustment for these clinical differences, female sex remained a marginal independent risk factor for death (relative risk of 1.15 with 95% CI of 1.0–1.31%) (36,40).

The relative benefit of tPA over streptokinase was of similar magnitude in women

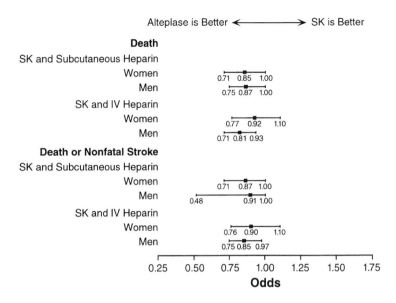

Figure 7 Point estimates and 95% confidence intervals for major endpoints: men vs. women. (From Ref. 40.)

as it was in men, both for 30-day mortality and the composite endpoint of death or nonfatal disabling stroke (Fig. 7). After correction for baseline clinical variables, gender was not an independent risk factor for stroke (40).

The angiographic substudy further examined the effects of gender (41). Five hundred and forty-three (22.3%) of the patients in the substudy were women. There were no differences between women and men in regard to the achievement of complete infarct artery patency (TIMI-3 flow) at 90 minutes (38.5% vs. 37.8%). Women did have a higher incidence of reocclusion of an initially patent artery (8.7% vs. 5.1%, $p = 0.14$); however, there was insufficient power to verify the significance of this difference. There were no differences in global or regional left ventricular function, either at 90 minutes or at 5–7 days, between women and men. The fact that, despite this, female sex remains an independent risk factor for death is intriguing. The suggestion of increased reocclusion in women may deserve further attention and, if confirmed, may relate to the smaller caliber coronary vessels and increased tortuosity.

Twelve women in the GUSTO trial were actively menstruating at the time of enrollment (42). Despite the small number in this cohort, the lack of deaths, stroke, or hemodynamically significant bleeding in this group (three patients had moderate bleeding requiring transfusion) suggests that the use of thrombolytic therapy should not be automatically dismissed in this population.

Diabetes

The results of the GUSTO angiographic substudy demonstrated that diabetes was an independent risk factor for mortality, even after correction for angiographic and other clinical variables ($p = 0.02$) (43). The substudy, however, did not establish a clear pattern of

Global ejection fraction and ventricular function in the region of the infarct vessel were similar in diabetics and nondiabetics. This subgroup analysis, however, may not have been powered to detect true differences in vessel patency or left ventricular function between diabetics and nondiabetics.

Diabetics did have blunting of the compensatory hyperkinetic response in the noninfarct zone. Diabetic patients also had a tendency towards more frequent reocclusion of an initially patent vessel (9.2% vs. 5.3%, $p = 0.17$). However, this was based on a small number of clinical events, so the significance of this finding is unclear. Further studies need to be done to clarify the reasons behind the poorer outcome with thrombolytic therapy in the diabetic population.

Prior Cardiac History

Sixteen percent of the patients enrolled in the GUSTO trial had a history of prior myocardial infarction (44). These patients were older, with a higher incidence of multivessel disease and lower ejection fractions. As such, this group had a higher 30-day mortality rate than those without prior history (11.7% vs. 5.9%, $p = 0.001$). Consistent with the main GUSTO results, this cohort of patients fared better with tPA than they did with streptokinase (30-day mortality 10.4% vs. 12.2%, $p = 0.049$). Thrombolytic therapy was as efficacious in this group as it was in those without MI, with similar incidence of TIMI 3 flow at 90 minutes (38% vs. 37.7) (44).

The GUSTO angiographic trial included 48 patients with saphenous vein graft (SVG) thromboses (45). Although this is a very small sample size, it nonetheless represents one of the largest series available for analysis. The 90-minute patency rate (TIMI 2 or 3) in vein graft thrombosis was significantly lower than for native vessels (48% vs. 69%, $p = 0.01$). Though obviously underpowered, these results suggest that thrombolytic therapy is less efficacious in this subgroup of patients.

Stroke After Thrombolysis

Intracranial hemorrhage remains the most feared adverse outcome of thrombolytic therapy. In the GUSTO trial, all suspected strokes were reviewed by an independent committee, and vigorous attempts were made in every instance to categorize the stroke with brain imaging. Detailed information about the functional status of survivors of stroke was also obtained. The GUSTO trial thus provides one of the largest and most complete databases characterizing stroke following thrombolytic therapy.

There was a total of 592 strokes among the 41,021 patients enrolled (incidence of 1.4%). In 549 of these (93%), either a CT scan, MRI, or cerebral angiogram was performed. There were differences in the incidence of stroke among the four treatment arms ($p = 0.007$) (Fig. 8). In the streptokinase groups, the incidence was 1.19% with adjunctive SQ heparin and 1.39% with IV heparin. The incidence was 1.55% in the tPA group and 1.64% in the combination thrombolytic arm. Much of the difference was accounted for by the difference in the incidence of primary intracranial hemorrhage. The incidence of such bleeds was 0.46% in the streptokinase/SQ heparin arm, 0.57% in the streptokinase/

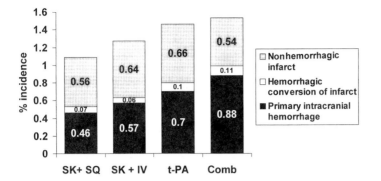

Figure 8 Stroke type and incidence by treatment group. (From Ref. 46.)

IV heparin arm, 0.70% in the tPA arm, and 0.88% in the combination arm ($p < 0.001$) (46).

The majority of primary intracranial hemorrhages (77.1%) occurred within the first 24 hours after the initiation of therapy. The median time for development of hemorrhage was significantly lower with tPA than it was for the streptokinase groups (10 hours vs. 17 and 18 hours, for the streptokinase groups with IV heparin and SQ heparin, respectively, $p = 0.0113$). Age, diastolic blood pressure, weight, and prior cerebrovascular disease were the strongest independent predictors of subsequent intracranial hemorrhage (46).

Forty-one percent of all strokes resulted in death, with 59.7% of primary intracranial hemorrhages and 17% of nonhemorrhagic infarcts being fatal. There were no significant differences in the functional outcomes after stroke by treatment assignment, though there was a trend for better recovery (with only minor or no residual deficit) in the streptokinase groups (46).

The incidence of stroke with thrombolytic therapy partly offsets the benefit gained by early restoration of infarct vessel patency. Treatment with streptokinase resulted in five deaths due to stroke per 1000 patients treated, compared to seven deaths per 1000 treated with tPA. Nevertheless, there is substantial benefit in terms of overall net clinical benefit with thrombolytic therapy as a whole, with tPA yielding a greater proportionate benefit than streptokinase (46).

One-Year Follow-Up

One-year follow-up data is available for 96% of the patients enrolled into GUSTO (47). The overall 1-year mortality rate in the streptokinase groups was 10.1%: 9.1% in those who received tPA and 9.9% in the combination group ($p = 0.011$ for tPA vs. SK/SQ heparin, $p = 0.009$ for tPA vs. SK/IV heparin, and $p = 0.05$ for tPA vs. combination). Thus the 1.0% absolute reduction in mortality with tPA was sustained at one year (Fig. 9). The mortality rate after 30 days was essentially the same across all four treatment groups. Among 30-day survivors, those treated with tPA had significantly fewer in-hospital complications, such as shock, heart failure, sustained hypotension, atrioventricular block, and atrial fibrillation (47).

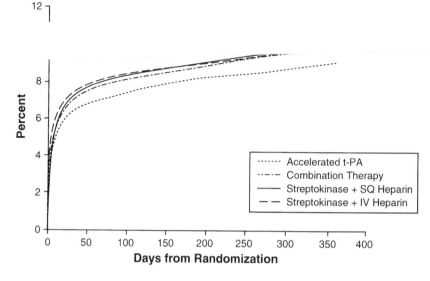

Figure 9   One-year mortality by treatment group. (Adapted from Ref. 47.)

CONCLUSION

Trials such as GISSI-1 and ISIS-2 firmly established the efficacy of thrombolytic therapy in the treatment of acute myocardial infarction. Based on pathophysiology, this benefit appeared to be mediated by early restoration of flow through the infarct vessel. Although intuitively logical, no large-scale trial had been able to verify this. The GUSTO trial was undertaken to validate the hypothesis that early, complete and sustained vessel patency results in improved survival in myocardial infarction.

The results of the GUSTO trial established that treatment with accelerated tPA results in lower mortality as compared with streptokinase (with either adjunctive SQ or IV heparin). Tissue plasminogen activator conferred an absolute 1.0% reduction in mortality, which translates into preventing one of seven deaths that would have otherwise occurred with standard therapy. These results were consistent across almost all subgroups tested (including age, gender, infarct location, and time to treatment within 6 hours), with the greatest clinical benefit seen in those with anterior infarcts who presented early in the course of their infarction. There was a slightly higher incidence of stroke with tPA (0.2% absolute increase), but the composite endpoint of death or nonfatal disabling stroke still favored tPA. Treatment with tPA also resulted in fewer complications of infarction, including cardiogenic shock, hypotension, atrioventricular block, and ventricular tachyarrhythmias.

More importantly, the GUSTO trial established the mechanism of this benefit. The angiographic study proved that TIMI 3 flow at 90 minutes was associated with improved survival and with improved LV function. Accelerated tPA yielded better results because it was more likely than streptokinase to establish early TIMI 3 flow. The enzyme substudy was entirely consistent with this, with treatment with tPA resulting in smaller infarct size. This benefit was sustained since the incidence of reocclusion with accelerated tPA and intravenous heparin was comparable to streptokinase with either subcutaneous or intravenous heparin.

While confirming the benefits of thrombolytic therapy, the results of GUSTO also highlight the shortcomings of such therapy. Treatment with accelerated tPA and intravenous heparin resulted in 90-minute TIMI 3 flow in only 54% of patients. Though this was better than that achieved by other thrombolytic regimens, it nonetheless means that nearly half of patients did not achieve timely and complete reperfusion. Thrombolytic therapy appeared to be less effective in certain subgroups of patients, particularly in cardiogenic shock or in patients with vein graft occlusions. Women and diabetics appeared to benefit less from thrombolytic therapy, although TIMI 3 flow was achieved at similar rates as in the population as a whole. The possibility of reocclusion accounting for this diminished benefit in these subgroups may warrant further investigation.

The GUSTO trial demonstrated the benefit of establishing early, complete, and sustained infarct vessel patency. It also highlighted the need to develop further strategies for the attainment of this goal. This represents the greatest contribution of this trial to the evolving knowledge about thrombolytic therapy and treatment for myocardial infarction.

REFERENCES

1. Koren GK, Weiss AT, Hasin Y, Applebaum D, Welber S, Rozenman Y, Lotan C, Mosseri M, Sapoznikov D, Luria MH, Gotsman MS. Prevention of myocardial damage in acute myocardial ischemia by early treatment with intravenous streptokinase. N Engl J Med 1985; 313:1384–1389.

2. Gruppo Italiano per lo Studio della Streptochinasi nell'Infarto Miocardico (GISSI): effectiveness of intravenous thrombolytic treatment in acute myocardial infarction. Lancet 1986; I: 397–401.

3. Bates ER. Is survival in acute myocardial infarction related to thrombolytic efficacy or the open-artery hypothesis? A controversy to be investigated with GUSTO. Chest 1992; 101(4 Suppl):140S–150S.

4. Gruppo Italiano per lo Studio della Sopravvivenza nell'Infarto Miocardico. GISSI-2: a factorial randomised trial of alteplase versus streptokinase and heparin versus no heparin among 12,490 patients with acute myocardial infarction. Lancet 1990; 336:65–71.

5. ISIS-3 (Third International Study of Infarct Survival) Collaborative Group. ISIS-3: a randomised comparison of streptokinase vs. tissue plasminogen activator vs. anistreplase and of aspirin plus heparin vs. aspirin alone among 41,299 cases of suspected acute myocardial infarction. Lancet 1992; 339:753–770.

6. Granger CB, Califf RM, Topol EJ. Thrombolytic therapy for acute myocardial infarction: A review. Drugs 1992; 44:293–325.

7. Topol EJ. Validation of the early open infarct vessel hypothesis. Am J Cardiol 1993; 72:40G–45G.

8. Van de Werf F, Califf RM, Armstrong PW, Bates ER, Ross AM, Kleinman NS, Topol EJ. Progress culminating from ten years of clinical trials on thrombolysis for acute myocardial infarction. GUSTO-I Steering Committee. Global Utilization of Streptokinase and Tissue Plasminogen Activator for Occluded Coronary Arteries. Eur Heart J 1995; 16:1024–1026.

9. The International Study Group. In-hospital mortality and clinical course of 20,891 patients with suspected acute myocardial infarction randomised between alteplase and streptokinase with or without heparin. Lancet 1990; 336:71–75.

10. Neuhaus KL, Feuerer W, Jeep-Tebbe S, Niederer W, Vogt A, Tebbe U. Improved thrombolysis with a modified dose regimen of recombinant tissue-type plasminogen activator. J Am Coll Cardiol 1989; 14:1566–1569.

11. Neuhaus KL, Van Essen R, Tebbe U, Vogt A, Roth M, Riess M, Niederer W, Forycki F,

13. Topol EJ. Which thrombolytic agent should one choose. Prog Cardiovasc Dis 1991; 34(3): 165–178.

14. Rao AK, Pratt C, Berke A, Jaffe A, Ockene I, Schreiber TL, Bell WR, Knatterud G, Robertson TL, Terrin ML. Thrombolysis in Myocardial Infarction (TIMI) Trial-Phase I: hemorrhagic manifestations and changes in plasma fibrinogen and the fibrinolytic system in patients treated with recombinant tissue plasminogen activator and streptokinase. J Am Coll Cardiol 1988; 11:1–11.

15. Rapold HJ, de Bono D, Arnold AER, Arnout J, De Cock F, Collen D, Verstraete M, for the European Cooperative Study Group. Plasma fibrinopeptide A levels in patients with acute myocardial infarction treated with alteplase. Correlation with concomitant heparin, coronary artery patency, and recurrent ischemia. Circulation 1992; 85:928–934.

16. Garabedian HD, Gold HK. Coronary thrombolysis, conjunctive heparin infusion, and the effect on systemic thrombin activity. Circulation 1992; 85:1205–1207.

17. Eisenberg PR. Role of heparin in coronary thrombolysis. Chest 1992; 101(4 suppl):131S–139S.

18. Becker RC, Gore JM. The challenge of maintaining coronary arterial patency with intravenous heparin following tissue plasminogen activator administration. Cardiology 1993; 83:100–106.

19. Hsia J, Hamilton WP, Kleiman N, Roberts R, Chaitman BR, Ross AM, for the Heparin-Aspirin Reperfusion Trial (HART) investigators. A comparison between heparin and low-dose aspirin as adjunctive therapy with tissue plasminogen activator for acute myocardial infarction. N Engl J Med 1990; 323:1433–1437.

20. De Bono DP, Simoons ML, Tijssen J, Arnold AER, Betriu A, Burgersdijk C, Lopez Bescos L, Mueller E, Pfisterer M, Van de Werf F, Zijlstra F, Verstraete M. Effect of early intravenous heparin on coronary patency, infarct size, and bleeding complications after alteplase thrombolysis: results of a randomised double blind European Cooperative Study Group trial. Br Heart J 1992; 67:122–128.

21. Bleich SD, Nichols TC. Schumacher RR, Cooke DH, Tate DA, Teichman SL. Effect of heparin on coronary arterial patency after thrombolysis with tissue plasminogen activator in acute myocardial infarction. Am J Cardiol 1990; 66:1412–1417.

22. Ohman EM, Califf RM, Topol EJ, Candela R, Abbottsmith C, Ellis SG, Sigmon KN, Kereiakes D, George B, Stack R, and the TAMI study group. Consequences of reocclusion after successful reperfusion therapy in acute myocardial infarction. Circulation 1990; 82:781–791.

23. Holmes DR Jr, Califf RM, Topol EJ. Lessons we have learned from the GUSTO trial. Global utilization of streptokinase and tissue plasminogen activator for occluded arteries. J Am Coll Cardiol 1995; 25(7 suppl):10S–17S.

24. Aylward P. The GUSTO trial: background and baseline characteristics. Aust NZ J Med 1993; 23:728–730.

25. Califf RM, Topol EJ, Stack RS, Ellis SG, George BS, Kereiakes DJ, Samaha JK, Worley SJ, Anderson JL, Harrleson-Woodlief L, Wall TC, Phillips HR III, Abbottsmith CW, Candela RJ, Flanagan WH, Sasahara AA, Mantell SJ, Lee KL for the TAMI study group. Evaluation of combination thrombolytic therapy and timing of cardiac catheterization in acute myocardial infarction. Results of thrombolysis and angioplasty in myocardial infarction—phase 5 randomized trial. Circulation 1991; 83:1543–1556.

26. The GUSTO Investigators. An international randomized trial comparing four thrombolytic strategies for acute myocardial infarction. N Engl J Med 1993; 329:673–682.

27. The GUSTO Angiographic Investigators. The effects of tissue plasminogen activator, strepto-kinase, or both on coronary-artery patency, ventricular function, and survival after acute myo-cardial infarction. N Engl J Med 1993; 329:1615–1622.

28. Simes RJ, Topol EJ, Holmes DR Jr, White HD, Rutsch WR, Vahanian A, Simoons ML, Morris D, Betriu A, Califf RM, Ross AM, for the GUSTO-I Investigators. Link between the angio-graphic substudy and mortality outcomes in a large randomized trial of myocardial reperfusion. Importance of early and complete infarct artery reperfusion. Circulation 1995; 91:1923–1928.

29. Torr SR, Nachowiak DA, Fujii S, Sobel BE. ''Plasminogen steal'' and clot lysis. J Am Coll Cardiol 1992; 19:1085–1090.

30. Cannon CP, McCabe CH, Diver DJ, Herson S, Greene RM, Shah PK, Sequeira RF, Leya F, Kirshenbaum JM, Magorien RD, Palmeri ST, Davis V, Gibson CM, Poole WK, Braunwald E, and the TIMI-4 investigators. Comparison of front-loaded recombinant tissue-type plasmin-ogen activator, anistreplase and combination thrombolytic therapy for acute myocardial in-farction: results of the Thrombolysis in Myocardial Infarction (TIMI-4) trial. J Am Coll Cardiol 1994; 24:1602–1610.

31. Kleiman NS, White HD, Ohman EM, Ross AM, Woodlief LH, Califf RM, Holmes DR Jr, Bates E, Pfisterer M, Vahanian A, Topol EJ, for the GUSTO Investigators. Global utilization of streptokinase and tissue plasminogen activator for occluded coronary arteries. Mortality within 24 hours of thrombolysis for myocardial infarction. The importance of early reperfu-sion. Circulation 1994; 90:2658–2665.

32. Baardman T, Hermens WT, Lenderink T, Molhoek GP, Grollier G, Pfisterer M, Simoons ML. Differential effects of tissue plasminogen activator and streptokinase on infarct size and on rate of enzyme release: influence of early infarct related artery patency. The GUSTO Enzyme Substudy. Eur Heart J 1996; 17:237–246.

33. Holmes DR Jr, Bates ER, Kleiman NS, Sadowski Z, Horgan JH, Morris DC, Califf RM, Berger PB, Topol EJ, for the GUSTO-I Investigators. Global utilization of streptokinase and tissue plasminogen activator for occluded coronary arteries. J Am Coll Cardiol 1995; 26:668–674.

34. Yusuf S, Wittes J, Probstfield J, Tyroler HA. Analysis and interpretation of treatment effects in subgroups of patients in randomized clinical trials. J Am Med Assoc 1991; 266:93–98.

35. White HD, Barbash GI, Califf RM, Simes RJ, Granger CB, Weaver D, Kleiman NS, Aylward PE, Gore JM, Vahanian A, Lee KL, Ross AM, Topol EJ, for the GUSTO-I investigators. Age and outcome with contemporary thrombolytic therapy-results from the GUSTO-I Trial. Circulation 1996; 94:1826–1833.

36. Lee KL, Woodlief LH, Topol EJ, Weaver WD, Betriu A, Col J, Simoons M, Aylward P, Van de Werf F, Califf RM, for the GUSTO-I Investigators. Predictors of 30-day mortality in the era of reperfusion for acute myocardial infarction. Results from an international trial of 41,021 patients. Circulation 1995; 91:1659–1668.

37. Tardiff BE, Califf RM, Morris D, Bates E, Woodlief LH, Lee KL, Green C, Rutsch W, Betriu A, Aylward P, Topol EJ, for the GUSTO-I investigators. Coronary revascularization surgery after myocardial infarction: impact of bypass surgery on survival after thrombolysis. J Am Coll Cardiol 1997; 29:240–249.

38. ISIS-2 (Second International Study of Infarct Survival) Collaborative Group. Randomized trial of intravenous streptokinase, oral aspirin, both or neither among 17,187 cases of suspected acute myocardial infarction: ISIS-2. Lancet 1988; ii:349–360.

39. White HD, Barbash GI, Modam M, Simes J, Diaz R, Hampton JR, Heikkila J, Kristinsson A, Moulopoulus S, Paolasso EAC, Van der Werf T, Pehrsson K, Sandoe E, Wilcox RG, Vers-traete M, von der Lippe G, Van der Werf F, for the Investigators of the International Tissue Plasminogen Activator/Streptokinase Mortality Study. After correcting for worse baseline characteristics, women treated with thrombolytic therapy for acute myocardial infarction have the same mortality and morbidity as men except for a higher incidence of hemorrhagic stroke. Circulation 1993; 88:2097–2103.

40. Weaver WD, White HD, Wilcox RG, Aylward PE, Morris D, Guerci A, Ohman EM, Barbash

GI, Betriu A, Sadowski Z, Topo EJ, Califf RM, for the GUSTO-I investigators. Comparisons of characteristics and outcomes among women and men with acute myocardial infarction treated with thrombolytic therapy. J Am Med Assoc 1996; 275:777–782.

41. Woodfield SL, Lundergran CF, Reiner JS, Thompson MA, Rohrbeck SC, Deychak Y, Smith JO, Burton JR, McCarthy WF, Califf RM, White HD, Weaver WD, Topol EJ, Ross AM. Gender and acute myocardial infarction: is there a different response to thrombolysis? J Am Coll Cardiol 1997; 29:35–42.

42. Karnash SL, Granger CB, White HD, Woodlief LH, Topol EJ, Califf RM, for the GUSTO-I investigators. Treating menstruating women with thrombolytic therapy: insights from the global utilization of streptokinase and tissue plasminogen activator for occluded coronary arteries (GUSTO-I) trial. J Am Coll Cardiol 1995; 26:1651–1656.

43. Woodfield SL, Lundergran CF, Reiner JS, Greenhouse SW, Thompson MA, Rohrbeck SC, Deychak Y, Simoons ML, Califf RM, Topol EJ, Ross AM, for the GUSTO-I Angiographic Investigators. Angiographic findings and outcome in diabetic patients treated with thrombolytic therapy for acute myocardial infarction: the GUSTO-I experience. J Am Coll Cardiol 1996; 28:1661–1669.

44. Brieger DB, Mak KH, Miller DP, for the GUSTO-I investigators. Second MI patients derive particular benefit from aggressive establishment of infarct artery patency. Insights from GUSTO-I (abstr). Circulation 1996; 94 (suppl):I–441.

45. Reiner JS, Lundergrar CF, Kopecky SL, Topp H, Boyle D, Ross AM. Ineffectiveness of thrombolysis for acute MI following vein graft occlusion (abstr). Circulation 1996; 94(suppl):I–570.

46. Gore JM, Granger CB, Simoons ML, Sloan MA, Weaver WD, White HD, Barbash GI, Van de Werf F, Aylward PE, Topol EJ, Califf RM, for the GUSTO-I investigators. Stroke after thrombolysis. Mortality and functional outcomes in the GUSTO-I trial. Circulation 1995; 92: 2811–2818.

47. Califf RM, White HD, Van de Werf F, Sadowski Z, Armstrong PW, Vahanian A, Simoons ML, Simes PJ, Lee KL, Topol EJ, for the GUSTO-I investigators. One year results from the Global Utilization of Streptokinase and tPA for Occluded Coronary Arteries (GUSTO-I) Trial. Circulation 1996; 94:1233–1238.

alteplase regimen, the results of late thrombolysis would actually be better than was suggested by the LATE study.

That, of course, is pure speculation, and it may well be that neither the EMERAS nor the LATE results represent a true picture of thrombolytic efficacy in patients seen late in their illness. The truth can only be derived from a specific comparative trial of the two agents.

UNRESOLVED QUESTIONS IN THE LATE STUDY

In any clinical trial the results of subgroup analyses must be regarded with extreme caution. This is true when the subgroups are prespecified in the protocol, but any conclusions drawn from subgroups selected after the trial has been completed and the basic results are known may well be highly misleading and should be regarded only as hypothesis-generating. Nevertheless, post hoc analysis of some subgroups of the LATE patients did provide some puzzling, and possibly important, results.

During the course of the trial an apparently minor protocol change was approved by the Steering Committee, the members of which were of course ignorant of the trial results at that time. The original protocol required that included patients had to be admitted to the hospital more than 6 hours after the onset of symptoms, because in many centers LATE was running in parallel with the GISSI-2 International Study (18), for which all myocardial infarction patients admitted within 6 hours were being considered. After this early study had been completed, patients were included in LATE who had been admitted to the hospital within 6 hours of the onset of symptoms, but whose treatment had for some reason been delayed so that thrombolysis was initiated in the 6 to 24-hour time window. Because of this protocol change it was decided that a separate analysis should be made of patients included according to the original protocol and those admitted under the terms of the changed protocol; it was not anticipated that these groups would behave differently. To the surprise of the Steering Committee, it was found that patients admitted within 6 hours but treated between 6 and 24 hours after the onset of symptoms received no benefit from thrombolysis (35-day fatality 7.0% alteplase, 6.25% placebo). However, among the patients who were admitted more than 6 hours after the onset of symptoms, the benefit of alteplase treatment was clear (fatality 9.7% alteplase, 12.0% placebo, relative risk reduction 19.2%, $p = 0.03$). This finding suggested that the protocol change had somehow defined two different populations of patients, and this led to further analyses specifically designed to develop a hypothesis that might explain the difference.

It seemed likely that patients who were admitted within 6 hours but were not treated did not have the criteria that would indicate immediate thrombolysis, or treatment would have been given. Among these patients the delay from hospital admission to randomization was 11.7 hours, representing the time needed for the ECG to change or cardiac enzymes to rise, so that the trial's inclusion criteria were fulfilled. The patients admitted more than 6 hours after the onset of pain were, however, treated a mean of 1.25 hours after admission, and presumably these patients had criteria for thrombolysis on admission. When the patients were arbitrarily divided into groups given thrombolysis within 3 hours of admission to hospital or more than 3 hours after admission (whether they had been admitted in less than 6 hours or more than 6 hours after onset of symptoms), it was found that in the first group thrombolysis caused marked reduction in fatality at 35 days (alteplase 8.6%, placebo

12.0%, $p = 0.005$), whereas in the second group alteplase had no effect (alteplase 8.6%, placebo 7.9%).

Combining the delay from onset of symptoms and the delay in treatment after admission, it was found that of the patients who were treated within 12 hours of the onset of symptoms, and after a hospital delay of less than 3 hours, alteplase reduced fatality by 29%. Among patients treated within 12 hours, but including a delay of more than 3 hours, the risk reduction was only 9%.

Among the patients treated between 12 and 24 hours after the onset of pain, the risk reduction with alteplase was 22% if treatment was begun within 3 hours of admission, but where the delay was more than 3 hours (a group of 1968 patients) alteplase treatment was associated with an *increased* risk of death of 15%. Further analyses failed to identify clear differences between the patients whose treatment was or was not delayed after hospitalization, but this may simply reflect the way data were collected.

All these subgroup analyses may be providing totally spurious results, but it does seem that some patients benefit from alteplase treatment as late as 12–24 hours after the onset of symptoms. It seems likely that these are patients who, on admission to hospital, had the standard clinical and electrocardiographic indications for immediate thrombolysis. If these indications are present neither on admission nor 3 hours later, then there seems no point in giving alteplase. Clearly this hypothesis could be tested in a clinical trial, but this would be difficult and expensive, and it is therefore extremely unlikely that such a study will ever be done.

CONCLUSIONS

The FTT meta-analysis, suggesting that there is little point in giving a thrombolytic agent more than 12 hours after the onset of symptoms, is probably an oversimplification, as is often the case with meta-analysis. Late treatment with streptokinase may well be ineffective, but the LATE trial suggests that it is worth giving alteplase up to 24 hours after the onset of symptoms, particularly patients who have clinical and electrocardiographic indications for thrombolysis on admission to hospital.

REFERENCES

1. Weaver WD. Time to thrombolytic treatment: factors affecting delay and their influence on outcome. J Am Coll Cardiol 1995; 25:3S–9S.
2. Birkheard JS, on behalf of the joint audit committee of the British Cardiac Society and a cardiology committee of Royal College of Physicians of London. Time delays in provision of thrombolytic treatment in six district hospitals. Br Med J 1992; 305:445–448.
3. Maggioni AP, Franzosi MG, Santoro E, White H, Van de Werf F, Tognoni G, the Gruppo Italiano Per Lo Studio De la Sopravvivenza Nell'Infarto Miocardico II (GISSI-2), and the International Study Group. The risk of stroke in patients with acute myocardial infarction after thrombolytic and antithrombotic treatment. N Engl J Med 1992; 327:1–6.
4. LATE Study Group. Late Assessment of Thrombolytic Efficacy (LATE) study with alteplase 6-24 hours after onset of acute myocardial infarction. Lancet 1993; 342:759–766.
5. EMERAS (Estudio Multicéntrico Estreptoquinasa Repúblicas de América del Sur) Collaborative Group. Randomised trial of late thrombolysis in patients with suspected acute myocardial infarction. Lancet 1993; 342:767–772.

6. Davies MJ. Successful and unsuccessful coronary thrombolysis. Br Heart J 1989; 61:381–384.

7. The GUSTO Angiographic Investigators. The effects of tissue plasminogen activator, streptokinase, or both on coronary-artery patency, ventricular function, and survival after acute myocardial infarction. N Engl J Med 1993; 329:1615–1622.

8. The GUSTO Investigators. An international randomised trial comparing four thrombolytic strategies for acute myocardial infarction. N Engl J Med 1993; 329:673–682.

9. The GUSTO-III Investigators. A comparison of reteplase with alteplase for acute myocardial infarction. N Engl J Med 1997; 337:118–123.

10. Bode C, Smalling RW, Sen S. Recombinant plasminogen activator angiographic phase II international dose finding study (RAPID): patency analysis and mortality endpoints. Circulation 1993; 88:1–292 (abstr 1562).

11. European Working Party. Streptokinase in recent myocardial infarction: a controlled Multicentre Trial. Br Med J 1971; 3:325–331.

12. Gruppo Italiano per lo Studio Della Streptochinasi Nell'Infarto Miocardico (GISSI). Effectiveness of intravenous thrombolytic treatment in acute myocardial infarction. Lancet 1986; i: 397–401.

13. ISIS-2 (Second International Study of Infarct Survival) Collaborative Group. Randomised trial of intravenous streptokinase, oral aspirin, both, or neither among 17,187 cases of suspected acute myocardial infarction: ISIS-2. Lancet 1988; ii:349–360.

14. AIMS Trial Study Group. Effect of intravenous APSAC on mortality after acute myocardial infarction: preliminary report of a placebo-controlled clinical trial. Lancet 1988; i:545–549.

15. Wilcox RG, Von der Lippe G, Olsson CG, Jensen G, Skene AM, Hampton JR, for the ASSET Study Group. Trial of tissue plasminogen activator for mortality reduction in acute myocardial infarction. Anglo-Scandinavian Study of Early Thrombolysis (ASSET). Lancet 1988; ii:525–530.

16. Fibrinolytic Therapy Trialists' (FTT) Collaborative Group. Indications for fibrinolytic therapy in suspected acute myocardial infarction: collaborative overview of early mortality and major morbidity results from all randomised trials of more than 1000 patients. Lancet 1994; 343: 311–322.

17. Boersma E, Maas ACP, Deckers JW, Simoons ML. Early thrombolytic treatment in acute myocardial infarction: reappraisal of the golden hour. Lancet 1996; 348:771–775.

18. GISSI-2 and International Study Group. Six-month survival in 20,891 patients with acute myocardial infarction randomized between alteplase and streptokinase with or without heparin. Eur Heart J 1992; 13:1692–1697.

19. ISIS-3 (Third International Study of Infarct Survival). Collaborative Group. ISIS-3: a randomised comparison of streptokinase vs tissue plasminogen activator vs anistreplase and of aspirin plus heparin vs aspirin alone among 41,299 cases of suspected acute myocardial infarction. Lancet 1992; 339:753–770.

7

EMERAS

ERNESTO PAOLASSO and RAFAEL DÍAZ

Estudio Multicentrico Estreptoquinasa Republicas de America del Sur (EMERAS) Collaborative Group. Randomized trial of late thrombolysis in patients with suspected acute myocardial infarction. Lancet 1993; 342: 767–772.

During the late 1980s it became clear that fibrinolytic therapy reduces mortality among patients treated within a few hours of the onset of symptoms of acute myocardial infarction (AMI) (1–5). However, many patients with suspected AMI do not reach the hospital until several hours after symptoms begin.

Several controlled trials of fibrinolytic therapy—mainly using intravenous streptokinase (SK)—were conducted during the 1960s and 1970s. These studies were so small—none involving more than 750 patients—that they yielded apparently conflicting results, but an overview of their findings with appropriate methodology (6) suggested that mortality could be reduced not only among patients treated early (0–6 hours after the onset of pain) but also among those presenting later (between 6 and 12 hours, or even after a delay of more than 12 hours). To test this hypothesis, two large-scale high-dose SK trials—GISSI-1 (1) and ISIS-2 (2)—included patients from 0 to 12 and from 0 to 24 hours after the onset of symptoms, respectively, during the late 1980s. An overview of these studies left little doubt that mortality is reduced considerably among patients treated within 0–3 hours (31%) and 3–6 hours (22%), but the benefit was less evident among patients treated more than 6 hours after symptom onset (10.8% death among SK patients vs. 12.3% among controls) (2). The apparent avoidance of 15 deaths per 1000 patients treated after 6 hours might seem medically worthwhile, but the 95% confidence interval (CI) around this 14% reduction was 1–24%, consistent with there being little or even no effect on mortality.

A reliable determination of the value of late thrombolysis is of utmost importance, because an extension of the time window for treatment would make such therapy available to more patients; there is laboratory and clinical evidence that late reperfusion of the occluded artery is possible (7,8). Although myocardial salvage is doubtful after a few hours of coronary occlusion, the late patency of occluded coronary vessels may have salutary effects by improving healing of infarcted myocardium, reducing left ventricular dilatation and remodeling, and reducing arrhythmic substrate (9,10).

THE STUDY

To help determine more reliably the time window for worthwhile benefit from fibrinolytic therapy, EMERAS (Estudio Multicéntrico Estreptoquinasa Repúblicas de América del Sur) (11) randomized to SK versus placebo patients presenting up to 24 hours from the onset of pain in whom there was not thought to be a clear indication for fibrinolytic therapy. It was also planned that the results would contribute to a collaborative overview of trials addressing the late thrombolysis issue (12).

Between 1988 and 1991, 4534 patients were enrolled in a network of 236 hospitals in 6 South American countries under the coordination of the EMERAS Coordinating Centre in Argentina. Initially, patients were eligible if they were thought to be within 24 hours of the onset of suspected AMI [with or without electrocardiographic (ECG) changes] and to have—in light of previous trials—no clear indication for, or clear contraindication to, SK. Soon after the study began it became clear that thrombolytic therapy was of benefit for patients presenting within 6 hours (1,2), so the entry criteria were altered to include only those patients presenting between 6 and 24 hours from onset. The only absolute contraindications to SK treatment specified by the protocol were a history of stroke, gastrointestinal hemorrhage, or peptic ulcer within the previous 6 months. Relative contraindications suggested by the protocol were the usual ones in fibrinolytic trials: major surgery, head injury or biopsy within the previous 2 weeks, more than 10 minutes of cardiopulmonary resuscitation during the previous 24 hours, valvulopathy or cardiomyopathy with atrial fibrillation, active pericarditis, known allergy to SK, SK treatment within the previous 6 months, pregnancy, severe renal or hepatic impairment, or some other life-threatening disease.

After informed consent was obtained, eligible patients were randomized to receive an intravenous infusion of SK 1.5 MU or matching placebo over about 1 hour in 100 ml of saline. The trial infusion was to be interrupted only if it was thought by the responsible physician to be clearly indicated. At the beginning of the study, because of the lack of evidence of benefit conferred by aspirin, patients were randomly allocated to oral aspirin or placebo in a 2 × 2 factorial design (Fig. 1). The emergence of clear evidence of benefit

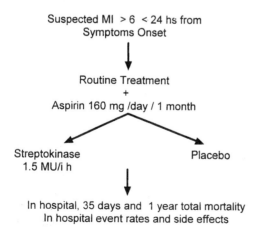

Figure 1 EMERAS design.

from aspirin use in AMI and the confirmation of clear benefit conferred by fibrinolytic therapy to patients treated within 6 hours of symptoms onset in ISIS-2 (2) led to the discontinuation of the aspirin comparison in May 1988. Daily low-dose aspirin (160 mg) was strongly recommended for all patients unless there was a clear contraindication, and patients presenting within 6 hours of pain onset were not to be randomized between active and placebo infusions, but treated actively with SK. In all other respects physicians were free to use whatever additional therapy (including anticoagulants) they considered indicated. Whether or not the correct trial treatment was given, patients remained in the group to which they have been allocated for an intention-to-treat analysis (13). ECGs were read blind to treatment allocation by three observers. ECG abnormalities were classified as (1) bundle branch block, (2) ST elevation, (3) anterior, inferior, other, (4) ST depression, (5) other abnormality, or (6) normal ECG.

Confirmation or refutation of any stroke and its etiology was based on blind central review of records by a committee comprising a neurologist, a cardiologist, and a general physician. Strokes were classified as probably hemorrhagic or probably ischemic. For any stroke, the day on which it occurred was recorded, allowing separate examination of strokes on day 0–1 (when an excess was observed with SK in ISIS-2) or later (when a shortfall with SK had previously been reported) (2). Disability following a stroke was classified as significant or not significant.

In-hospital follow-up was based on discharge forms, and 35-day and 1-year follow-up (vital status) were obtained by national coordinators. Discharge alive was at a median of 11 days, and the completeness of mortality follow-up was 99% at discharge, 97% at 5 weeks, and 90% at 1 year.

The main endpoints were to be mortality in hospital and at the end of the first year. In the light of results from the previous overview (6) and from more recent trials (1,2), it seemed reasonable that fibrinolytic therapy might reduce early mortality by at least 15–20 deaths per 1000 patients treated. For reasonable power to detect such an effect, it was planned to randomize 4000 patients by EMERAS. The principal subsidiary analyses were to be of the effects of SK on in-hospital mortality subdivided by hours from pain onset (7–12,13–24) and a similar analysis for 5 week mortality to allow for comparisons with other major fibrinolytic trials.

Comparisons of survival to 1 year involve time-to-death analysis with log-rank methods (13), but for events in hospital and deaths during the first 5 weeks, comparisons were by simple analysis of total numbers affected. Probability values are two-sided throughout, and $2p > 0.05$ is not significant (NS).

During recruitment, interim results for events in hospital were reviewed three times by an independent data-monitoring committee, which, in the light of these analyses or any other evidence or advice, would tell the coordinators if, in their view, there was at any time proof beyond a reasonable doubt (i.e., at least 35D) that for all or for some types of patients either treatment was clearly indicated or clearly contraindicated in terms of a net difference in mortality. Otherwise, the collaborators, organizing committee, and sponsors were to remain ignorant of the interim results. The demonstration in another trial (2) of a survival benefit with aspirin for AMI patients and with SK for those treated within 6 hours of symptom onset led to the discontinuation of these comparisons. For fibrinolytic comparison in patients treated at 6–24 hours, however, randomization continued until January 31, 1991, by which time almost all the SK and matching placebos provided for the trial had been used.

RESULTS

Of 8124 consecutive patients admitted to the participating hospitals with a diagnosis of suspected AMI, 4543 were randomized, with 663 (15%) presenting within 6 hours of symptom onset—before ISIS-2 (2) results became available—2080 (46%) between 7 and 12 hours, and 1791 (40%) between 13 and 24 hours. The main reasons for exclusion are shown in Table 1. Two thousand two hundred and fifty-seven patients were allocated to receive SK and 2277 placebo, and baseline characteristics were well balanced. The median time to entry was 11 hours, which is, as intended, longer than in previous trials, and half of the patients were still symptomatic at the time of randomization. A high proportion of older patients was included in the trial.

Adherence to study medication was high; among those patients discharged alive (at a median of 11 days) the infusion was completed in 98% of patients allocated placebo and 96% of those allocated SK. After the use of daily aspirin was recommended by the protocol amendment, 82% of patients received aspirin or some other antiplatelet regimen. Anticoagulation use was optional with 23% receiving intravenous heparin and an additional 14% receiving subcutaneous heparin alone. Antiplatelet and anticoagulant use was similar in both treatment groups.

Table 1   Baseline Characteristics (% of number randomized)

Characteristic	SK	Placebo	Characteristic	SK	Placebo
Hours from pain onset			Diastolic BP		
0–3	2.2	3.4	<70	13.8	13.7
4–6	12.7	10.9	70–108	80.9	81.3
7–12	46.3	45.4	≥110	5.3	4.9
13–24	38.8	40.2	Heart rate (/min)		
Pain at entry	57.7	57.5	<60	5.9	7.0
Female	23.4	23.5	60–91	74.9	73.9
History			≥100	19.2	19.0
Diabetic	16.4	17.0	Prerandomization		
Previous MI	12.7	12.2	ECG		
Previous angina	57.0	55.9	BBB	6.8	7.5
Previous	42.9	44.3	Anterior ST elevation	36.7	37.3
hypertension			Inferior ST elevation	31.3	29.4
Age (yr)			Other ST elevation	6.3	5.3
<55	31.5	32.3	ST depression	4.1	4.5
55–64	32.5	31.2	Other abnormality	13.3	14.0
65–74	25.8	25.8	Normal ECG	1.5	1.9
>75	10.2	10.7	Reasons for exclusion		
Systolic BP			<6 or >24 hours presentation	66	
<100	6.6	5.9	Doubtful AMI	8	
100–174	89.6	90.0	Contraindications to SK	13	
≥175	3.9	4.1	Administrative reasons	10	
			NA	3	

BP = blood pressure; NA = not available.

function, and improved survival (20). However, there is increasing evidence that relatively late myocardial reperfusion may also exert a favorable influence on clinical outcome that is time independant and not related to myocardial salvage (20–22). If myocardial salvage resulting from thrombolytic treatment were the only mechanism responsible for the benefit conferred by fibrinolytics, it would be anticipated that left ventricular function would be substantially better in actively treated patients than in those receiving placebo, with this improvement in function resulting in improved survival. However, in several of the early placebo-controlled trials of fibrinolytic therapy in which patients were entered relatively late in their course (4–6 hours after symptoms onset), left ventricular ejection fraction (LVEF) was not improved by active treatment, yet mortality was reduced (23,24). In contrast, the patency of the infarct-related artery (IRA) evaluated angiographically correlated strongly with survival (25,26). These observations and those from other trials, taken together, suggested that even when thrombolytic therapy does not salvage sufficient myocardium to improve LVEF, it may improve survival.

Several studies in the thrombolytic era showed that the patent IRA achieved even too late to limit infarct size (6–24 hours after symptom onset) is associated with smaller increases in end-diastolic and end-systolic left ventricular volumes, better LVEFs, and reduced wall motion abnormalities (26–29). This observation strongly suggests that reperfusion, even late (>6 hours), of myocardium at risk after the IRA occlusion reduces ventricular dilatation and, to a lesser extent, improves left ventricular function as compared with no reperfusion. This concept is consistent with the open artery hypothesis (25).

Infarct expansion and ventricular remodeling contribute to the late deleterious effects of AMI on left ventricular function either in animals (30) or in patients (31,32). Systolic expansion of the infarcted region, caused by slippage of necrotic fibers and wall thinning, is counteracted by hyperfunction of the nonischemic, noninfarcted myocardium, and stroke volume and LVEF are maintained. Progressively, the hemodynamic burden on the residual viable myocardium resulting from the combination of loss of contractile tissue and infarct causes remodeling of the ventricle, which dilates, hypertrophies, and becomes more spherical (33–36).

Late reperfusion may exert a number of protective actions on the infarcted ventricle. Intramyocardial hemorrhage and edema and acceleration of scar formation result in stiffening of the infarcted tissue and reduced infarct expansion, ventricular dilatation, and remodeling (37). In addition to accelerating myocardial scar formation, late reperfusion provides a blood-filled coronary vascular bed that might serve as a scaffold, reducing systolic expansion and aneurysm of the necrotic area, thereby reducing ventricular dilatation. Experiments in different species have shown that late reperfusion is associated with immediate reduction of diastolic ventricular volumes (36,38) and a thick scar (34). Similar observations have been made in patients. Reperfusion has been demonstrated to exert a restraining effect on infarct expansion (39), while persistent occlusion of the IRA is associated with greater infarct expansion, aneurysm, and more severe impairment of left ventricular function (40,41).

There are other mechanisms not related, or indirectly related, to improved myocardial healing and left ventricular remodeling by which late thrombolysis may be of benefit. It has been observed that the patency of the IRA is associated with greater electrical stability, and this may account in part for fewer tachyarrhythmias, such as spontaneous late ventricular tachycardia and ventricular fibrillation (42–44), late potentials detected by signal-averaged electrocardiography (45–47), and less frequently induced sustained ventricular tachycardia by electrophysiologic studies in patients with AMI who have received fibrinolytic therapy (48,49).

CONCLUSION

It can be concluded, based on the large body of evidence emerging from the results of EMERAS (11), LATE (14), and the Fibrinolytic Therapy Trialists Overview (15), that the time window for routine fibrinolytic therapy must be extended to 12 hours after the onset of symptoms of acute myocardial infarction. Some patients (e.g., those still in pain or with persistence of ST elevation) might benefit from even more delayed fibrinolytic therapy, but more evidence is needed in this category of patients (15).

The absolute reduction in mortality in patients treated 7–12 hours after the onset of symptoms, although moderate, is worthwhile, as 20 premature deaths can be avoided per 1000 patients treated. As myocardial infarction is a common disease with high prevalence and still high mortality rates, the extension of the time window for fibrinolytic therapy beyond the first few hours after onset may save thousands of lives annually worldwide.

REFERENCES

1. GISSI (Gruppo Italiano per lo Studio della Streptochinasi nell' Infarto Miocardico). Effectiveness of intravenous thrombolytic treatment in acute myocardial infarction. Lancet 1986; i: 397–401.
2. ISIS-2 (Second International Study of Infarct Survival). Collaborative Group. Randomised trial of intravenous streptokinase, oral aspirin, both, or neither among 17,197 cases of suspected acute myocardial infarction: ISIS-2. Lancet 1988; ii:349–360.
3. ISAM (Intravenous Streptokinase in Acute Myocardial Infarction) Study Group. A prospective trial of intravenous streptokinase in acute myocardidal infarction (ISAM): mortality, morbidity, and infarct size at 21 days. N Engl J Med 1986; 314:1465–1471.
4. AIMS (APSAC Intervention Mortality Study) Trial Study Group. Effects of intravenous APSAC on mortality after acute myocardial infarction: preliminary report of a placebo-controlled clinical trial. Lancet 1988; i:545–549.
5. Wilcox RG, Von der Lippe G, Olsson CG, Jensen G, Skene AM, Hampton JR for the ASSET (Anglo-Scandinavian Study of Early Thromboysis) Study Group. Trial of tissue plasminogen activator for mortality reduction in acute myocardial infarction (ASSET). Lancet 1988; ii: 525–530.
6. Yusuf S, Collins R, Peto R, et al. Intravenous and intracoronary fibrinolytic therapy in acute myocardial infarction: overview of results on mortality, reinfarction and side-effects from 33 randomized controlled trials. Eur Heart J 1985; 6:556–585.
7. Collen D, Stassen JM, Verstraete M. Thrombolysis with human extrinsic (tissue-type) plasminogen activator in rabbits with experimental jugular vein thrombosis. J Clin Invest 1983; 71: 368–376.
8. van't Hof AW, Zijltra F, de Boer MJ, Liem AL, Hoorntje JC, Suryapranata H. Patncy and reinfarction in late-entry myocardial infarct patients treated with reperfusion therapy. Angiology 1997; 48(3):215–222.
9. Golia G, Marino P, Rametta F. Reperfusion reduces left ventricular dilatation by preventing infarct expansion in the acute and chronic phases of myocardial infarction. Am Heart J 1994; 127:499–509.
10. Gang E, Hong M, Wang F, Velazquez I, Nalos P, Myers M, Lew AS. Does reperfusion influence the incidence of ventricular late potentials in acute myocardial infarction (abstr)? Circulation 1987; 76 (suppl IV):342.
11. EMERAS (Estudio Multicéntrico Estreptoquinasa Repúblicas de América del Sur) Collabora-

tive Group. Randomised trial of late thrombolysis in patients with suspected acute myocardial infarction. Lancet 1993; 342:767–772.

12. Comité Organizador de EMERA. Estudio Multicéntrico Estreptoquinasa—República Argentina (EMERA). Rev Fed Arg Cardiol 1987; 16:238–240.

13. Peto R, Pike MC, Armitage P, et al. Design and analysis of randomized clinical trials requiring prolonged observation of each patient II: analysis and examples. Br J Cancer 1977; 35:1–39.

14. LATE Study Group. Late Assessment of Thrombolytic Efficacy (LATE) study with alteplase 6–24 hours after onset of acute myocardial infarction. Lancet 1993; 342:759–766.

15. Fibrinolytic Therapy Trialists' (FTT) Collaborative Group. Indications for fibrinolytic therapy in suspected acute myocardial infarction: collaborative overview of early mortality and major morbidity results from all randomised trials of more than 1000 patients. Lancet 1994; 343: 311–322.

16. ISIS Pilot Study Investigators. Randomised factorial trial of high-dose intravenous streptokinase, of oral aspirin and of intravenous heparin in acute myocardial infarction. Eur Heart J 1987; 8:634–642.

17. Schaper W. Natural defense mechanism during ischaemia. Eur Heart J 1983; 4(suppl D):73–78.

18. Banka VS, Chadda KD, Helfant RH. Limitation of myocardial revascularization in restoration of regional contraction anomalies by coronary occlusion. Am J Cardiol 1974; 34:164–170.

19. Reimer KA, Lowe JE, Resmussen MM, Jennings RB. The wave front phenomenon in ischemia cell death I: myocardial infarct size versus duration of coronary occlusion. Circulation 1977; 56:786–794.

20. Braunwald E. Myocardial reperfusion, limitation of infarct size, reduction of left ventricular dysfunction and improved survival: should the paradigm be expanded? Circulation 1989; 79: 441–444.

21. Van de Werf F. Discrepancies between the effects of coronary reperfusion on survival and left ventricular function. Lancet 1989; i:1367–1369.

22. Califf RM, Topol EJ, Gersh BJ. From myocardial salvage to patient salvage in acute myocardial infarction. The role or reperfusion therapy. J Am Coll Cardiol 1989; 14:1382–1388.

23. White HD, Norris RM, Brown MA, et al. Effect of intravenous streptokinase on left ventricular function and early survival after acute myocardial infarction. N Engl J Med 1987; 317:850–855.

24. Kennedy JW, Ritchie JL, Davies KB, et al. The Western Washington randomized trial of intracoronary streptokinase in acute myocardial infarction; a 12-month follow up report. N Engl J Med 1985; 312:1073–1078.

25. Dalen JE, Gore JM Braunwald E, et al., and the TIMI Investigators. Six- and twelve-month follow of the phase I Thrombolysis in Myocardial Infarction (TIMI) Trial. Am J Cardiol 1988; 62:179–185.

26. Harrison JK, Califf RM, Woodlief LH, et al., and the TAMI Study Group. Systolic left ventricular function after reperfusion therapy for acute myocardial infarction: an analysis of determinants of improvement. Circulation 1993; 87:1531–1541.

27. Topol EJ, Califf RM, Vandormael M, et al., and the Thrombolysis and Angioplasty in Myocardial Infarction-6 Study Group. A randomized trial of late reperfusion for acute myocardial infarction. Circulation 1992; 85:2090–2099.

28. Leung W-H, Lau C-P. Effects of severity of the residual stenosis of the infarct-related artery coronary artery on left ventricular dilatation and function after acute myocardial infarction. J Am Coll Cardiol 1992; 20:307–313.

29. Hirayama A, Nashidi K, Kodama K. Prevention of left ventricular dilation without infarct size limitation by late reperfusion in patients with acute myocardial infarction. Jpn Circ J 1992; 56(suppl 5):1438–1441.

30. Pfeffer JM, Pfeffer MA, Fletcher PJ, Braunwald E. Progressive ventricular remodeling in rat with myocardial infarction. Am J Physiol 1991; 260:H1406–HJ1414.

31. McKay RG, Pfeffer MA, Pasternak RL, et al. Left ventricular remodeling following myocardial infarction. Circulation 1986; 74:693–702.

32. Mitchell GF, Lamas Ga, Vaughen DE, Pfeffer MA. Left ventricular remodeling in the year after first anterior myocardial infarction: a quantitative analyses of contractile segment lengths and ventricular shape. J Am Coll Cardiol 1992; 19:113–144.

33. Lamas GA, Pfeffer MA, Braunwald E. Patency of the infarct-related coronary artery and ventricular geometry. Am J Cardiol 1991; 68:41D–51D.

34. Hochman JS, Choo H. Limitation of myocardial infarct expansion by reperfusion independent of myocardial salvage. Circulation 1987; 75:299–306.

35. Bonaduce D, Petretta M, Villari B, et al. Effects of late administration of tissue-type plasminogen activator on left ventricular remodeling and function after myocardial infarction. Am J Coll Cardiol 1990; 16:1561–1568.

36. Hale SL, Kloner RA. Left ventricular topographic alterations in the completely healed rat infarct caused by early and late coronary artery reperfusion. Am Heart J 1988; 116:1508–1513.

37. Pirzada FA, Weiner JM, Hood WB Jr. Experimental myocardial infarction: accelerated myocardial stiffening related to coronary reperfusion following ischemia. Chest 1987; 74:190–195.

38. Brown W, Swinford RD, Gadde P, Lillis O. Acute effects of delayed reperfusion on infarct shape and left ventricular volume: a potential mechanism of additional benefits from thrombolytic therapy. J Am Coll Cardiol 1991; 17:1641–1650.

39. Marino P, Destro G, Barbieri E, Bicego D. Reperfusion of the infarct-related coronary artery limits left ventricular expansion beyond myocardial salvage Am Heart J 1992; 123:1157–1165.

40. Meizlish JL., Berger HJ, Plankey M, et al. Functional left ventricular aneurysm formation after acute anterior transmural myocardial infarction: incidence, natural history and prognostic implication. N Engl J Med 1984; 311:1001–1006.

41. Froman MB, Collins HW, Kopelman HA, et al. Determinants of left ventricular aneurysm formation after acute myocardial infarction: A clinical and angiographic study. J Am Coll Cardiol 1986; 8:1256–1262.

42. Schroeder R. Ventricular fibrillation complicating myocardial infarction (letter). N Engl J Med 1988; 318:381–382.

43. Arnold JMO, Antman EM, Przyklenk K, et al. Differential effects of reperfusion on incidence of ventricular arrhythmias and recovery of ventricular function at 4 days following coronary occlusion. Am Heart J 1987; 113:1055–1065.

44. Horvitz LL, Pietrolungo JF, Suri RS, et al. An open infarct-related artery is associated with a lower risk of lethal ventricular arrhythmias in pateints with a left ventricular aneurysm. Circulation 1992; 86 (suppl. I):1–315.

45. Aguirre FV, Kern MJ, Hsia J, et al. Importance of myocardial infarct artery patency on the prevalence of ventricular arrhythmias and late potentials after thrombolysis in acute myocardial infarction. Am J Cardiol 1991; 68:1410–1416.

46. McClements BM, Adgey AAJ. Value of signal-averaged electrocardiography, radionuclide ventriculogrphy, Holter monitoring and clinical variables for prediction of arrhythmic events in survivors of acute myocardial infarction in the thromboytic era. J Am Coll Cardiol 1993; 21:1419–1427.

47. Gomes JA, Mehra R, Barreaca P, et al. Quantitative analysis of the high-frequency components of the signal-averaged QRS complex in patients with acute myocardial infarction: a prospective study. Circulation 1985; 72:105–111.

48. Kersschot LE, Brugada P, Ramentol M, et al. Effects of early reperfusion in acute myocardial infarction on arrhythmias induced by programmed stimulation: a prospective, randomized study. J Am Coll Cardiol 1986; 7:1234–1242.

49. Sager PT, Perlmutter RA, Rosenfeld LE, et al. Electrophysiologic effects of thrombolytic therapy in patients with a transmural anterior myocardial infarction complicated by left ventricular aneurysm formation. J Am Coll Cardiol 1988; 12:19–24.

8

Issues in Thrombolysis: Insights from the GUSTO Trials on Studies of Coronary Reperfusion

ROBERT M. CALIFF

The GUSTO organization started as a group of investigators interested in improving outcomes in patients with acute myocardial infarction. Initially, it sought to develop a better understanding of coronary artery reperfusion and the relationship between reperfusion and subsequent clinical benefit. Over time, the complexity of this relationship has become increasingly apparent. The fundamental hypothesis that restoring coronary perfusion improves clinical outcomes has, however, been upheld. The magnitude of the effect is moderate, because it is not only the initial perfusion status of the artery that matters, but also its sustained perfusion. Intermittent reocclusion, as well as definitive reocclusion, also plays an important role in outcome. The picture becomes even more cloudy when we consider the impact of other factors on clinical outcome beyond simply the perfusion status of the infarct-related artery. Stroke, both hemorrhagic and nonhemorrhagic, may be more common with agents that achieve more prompt coronary reperfusion or with better anticoagulation. The appropriate use of other therapies that improve the healing of the myocardium and prevent arrhythmias is also important. Indeed, a recent GUSTO analysis demonstrated that simply using other proven therapies appropriately would have the same impact on mortality as reperfusion therapy itself (1).

The choice of coronary perfusion as the "surrogate" endpoint for the GUSTO group may have been fortunate for another reason. In this era of proliferating therapies, clinicians would like to believe that a surrogate endpoint can be used instead of clinical outcome to determine the relative merits of various therapeutic approaches. The use of surrogates would allow more rapid and less costly evaluation of therapeutic strategies. Coronary reperfusion is probably one of the most solidly supported surrogate endpoints in medical history, but the series of GUSTO trials points out that while surrogates can be used to screen for potentially useful therapies, it is risky to use them to distinguish ultimate clinical effectiveness. This finding with one of the most easily believable surrogates in medicine provides strong evidence that we must measure clinical outcomes to understand what these therapies are, in fact, accomplishing.

GUSTO-I

The fundamental finding of GUSTO-I was that early and sustained reperfusion of the infarct-related coronary artery improved clinical outcome in patients with ST-segment elevation acute myocardial infarction (MI) (2). Simply stated, the primary hypothesis was proven in the experiment. Accelerated alteplase and heparin administration resulted in an increase in early TIMI grade 3 flow, saving one life per 100 patients treated or preventing one death out of every seven that would have occurred with streptokinase treatment. An early publication from the angiographic substudy confirmed the link between infarct artery perfusion, left ventricular function, and clinical outcome (3).

An important finding of the angiographic study that is seldom referred to is the lack of a difference in reocclusion rates among the regimens. This observation was surprising, as a higher reocclusion rate was expected with alteplase. As attention has been focused on the early perfusion differences, it must be remembered that if the reocclusion rates had been different, the differences in clinical outcomes may not have been so highly correlated with differences in early perfusion. Furthermore, due to the later opening of vessels with streptokinase, perfusion rates beyond the first 90 minutes were not statistically significantly different among the regimens.

The one year follow-up data demonstrated that the survival advantage of accelerated alteplase was maintained but not enhanced over the first year (4). Indeed, the survival curves appeared to be parallel after the first 30 days. Parallel survival curves have been observed in all thrombolytic trials to date after the first 30 days.

The 2-year follow-up from the angiographic substudy found a strong relationship between perfusion at 90 minutes and a variety of clinical and functional status measures (5). Patients with perfusion of the infarct-related artery at 90 minutes had better survival, less heart failure, and less impaired functional status. The relative benefit of perfusion seemed to be amplified over time, and the benefit was not a function of the thrombolytic regimen but rather of the perfusion status achieved by that agent. The parallel nature of the survival curves and the diverging measures of left ventricular function and functional status have not been explained, although it is likely that more high-risk patients survived in the alteplase-treated population due to the benefits of the treatment, leaving a higher-risk population in the alteplase group at risk during longer-term follow-up.

Heparin was given intravenously in three of the four regimens used in GUSTO-I; in one of the streptokinase regimens, it was given subcutaneously. There was no difference in outcome between patients treated with streptokinase and subcutaneous or intravenous heparin. When patients treated with intravenous heparin were evaluated in detail, regardless of the thrombolytic agent, there was a strong relationship observed between the aPTT during treatment and subsequent outcome (Fig. 1) (6). As expected, the risk of bleeding increased directly as the aPTT increased, although patients with either a low aPTT or a high aPTT had worse clinical outcomes than patients with an aPTT between 50 and 70 seconds. Furthermore, the risk of both reinfarction and nonhemorrhagic stroke increased as the aPTT rose above 70 seconds.

A clustering of reinfarction events was observed shortly after discontinuation of the heparin. This surprising result requires consideration of unanticipated mechanisms. Perhaps the increased risk of death, stroke, and reinfarction occurred because of bleeding-associated hypotension following discontinuation of the heparin. Another possibility is that the excessive anticoagulation could lead to hemorrhage into the plaque with vascular occlusion against the opposite wall from the hemorrhage. Finally, higher doses of heparin have been shown to increase platelet aggregability (7–9), perhaps engendering a paradoxical hypercoagulable state.

GUSTO-II

One of the major messages from GUSTO-I was concern that heparin did not appear to adequately neutralize the procoagulant effects of thrombin. Just as the trial was ending, interesting pilot studies with the direct antithrombin hirudin were being conducted. Compared with the disadvantages of heparin—requiring antithrombin III for its activity, being too large to effectively neutralize clot-bound thrombin, and producing heparin-induced thrombocytopenia—hirudin appeared attractive. Furthermore, heparin is inactivated by platelet factor 4 and other plasma proteins, while hirudin is not. This recombinant protein derived from leech saliva displayed an impressive ability to maintain a predictable, steady aPTT when given as a weight-adjusted dose.

Pilot studies with hirudin in both unstable angina (10) and ST-elevation acute MI (11) showed a trend towards clinical benefit and favorable effects on surrogate markers. Angiographic studies demonstrated a higher rate of TIMI grade-3 flow in the first 90 minutes with hirudin than with heparin. The populations chosen for these phase II trials tended to be young and otherwise healthy, perhaps producing an overly optimistic picture of the potential toxicity.

Simultaneously with two other large trials (TIMI-IX and HIT 3), the GUSTO group began a large trial to examine the effects of hirudin versus heparin in the spectrum of patients with acute coronary syndromes. A factorial design was included in a subpopulation to determine whether direct coronary angioplasty or alteplase would lead to better clinical outcomes. All three major trials had to be stopped early by their safety committees because of an increased incidence of intracranial hemorrhage in the hirudin-treated patients (12–14). A review of the information indicated that the dose chosen had been too high and that the most likely reason problems had not been observed in the pilot studies was that the phase II studies did not include enough elderly patients or patients with comorbidities to uncover the bleeding risk that would be encountered in a broader population.

Both GUSTO-II and TIMI-IX were reconfigured with a lower dose of hirudin. The basic result of GUSTO-II was a small reduction in the incidence of death and myocardial infarction as a composite at 30 days that fell just short of statistical significance. The result was homogeneous in subgroups, and in the first 24–48 hours the event reduction was highly statistically significant (Fig. 2) (16). After 48 hours there was no increase in events in the hirudin group compared with the heparin group. Rather, the curves remained parallel after that time as events accrued equally in each group. The TIMI-IX trial showed a similar result in the first 24–48 hours, but beyond that time showed no benefit of hirudin (17).

A particularly interesting subgroup was the patients treated with streptokinase as the thrombolytic agent (18). In this population hirudin had a marked benefit compared with heparin. Combined with several other studies evaluating the combination of streptokinase and hirulog (19), another direct thrombin inhibitor, these results raise the possibility that hirudin adds more to streptokinase than to alteplase.

In an effort to understand the results of the trials of direct thrombin inhibitors, it may be worthwhile to review the coagulation cascade (Fig. 3) (20). After arterial injury the tissue factor complex is thought to be critical in leading to the activation of Factor X through a complex series of steps, which then eventually leads to the conversion of prothrombin to thrombin. If one simply inhibits thrombin that has already been produced, but does nothing about the ongoing coagulation cascade proximal to thrombin production,

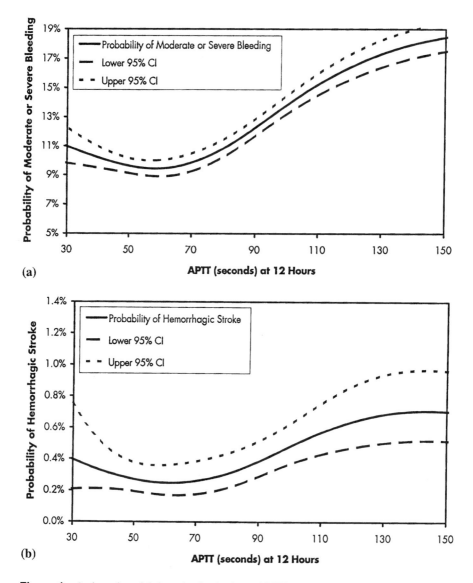

Figure 1 Activated partial thromboplastin times (aPTT) versus probability of moderate or severe bleeding (a), hemorrhagic stroke (b), nonhemorrhagic stroke (c), and reinfarction (d) 12 hours after enrollment in GUSTO-I. Dotted lines represent 95% confidence intervals. (From Ref. 6.)

when the therapy is stopped, the coagulation system may be poised to produce a prothrombotic state because of the activation of factors proximal to the production of thrombin.

Initial evidence for this problem of reactivation was generated from clinical observations by Theroux and colleagues in trials of heparin therapy in patients treated with and without aspirin (21). Later, Granger and colleagues observed that when intravenous heparin was stopped, markers of thrombin activation increased significantly (22). Fibrinopeptide A rose from 9.5 to 16.9 ng/ml, while prothrombin fragment F1.2 increased from 0.34 to 0.51 nmol/liter, and activated protein C also rose significantly. Analysis of the coagula-

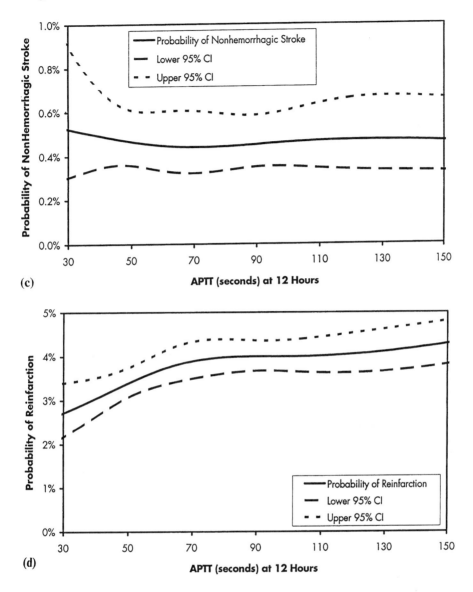

Figure 1 Continued

tion data from GUSTO-II confirms that thrombin inhibition alone does not suppress thrombin formation (23). Suppressing thrombin activity thus appears to have a clinical benefit that is limited if thrombin generation is not suppressed.

Thus, although pilot studies demonstrated a beneficial effect on TIMI grade 3 flow with hirudin, the total story with regard to clinical outcome became much more complicated. The heterogeneous population with acute coronary syndromes, coupled with the failure of hirudin to suppress thrombin formation, produced a clinical outcome difference less than expected in the study.

The outcomes of GUSTO-II and TIMI-IX bring up a critical issue in clinical trial

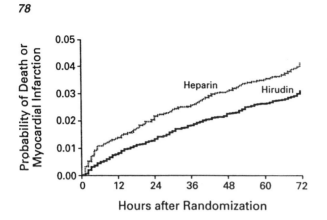

Figure 2 Kaplan-Meier estimate of the probability of death or myocardial infarction or reinfarction during the first 72 hours after randomization in GUSTO-IIb, according to treatment assignment. (From Ref. 15.)

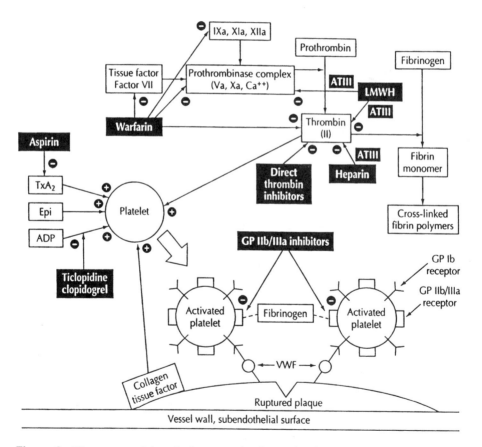

Figure 3 The process of thrombosis, a complex interaction between the vessel wall, platelets, and circulating clotting factors. (From Ref. 20.)

design and therapeutic development. If hirudin had been developed a decade ago, it would have been studied in the limited populations studied in the pilot trials, and it would probably have been deemed beneficial by surrogate endpoints. It would then have been placed on the market and physicians would have had to guess how to use it in the more complex situations they encountered in everyday practice. By doing the phase III clinical trials in broad populations, a more generalizable result was achieved, although the magnitude of the clinical benefit looks less positive than it would have in a carefully chosen population under ideal circumstances.

GUSTO-III

The basis for the GUSTO-III trial was the development of reteplase, a mutant form of tissue plasminogen activator. Because it lacks the finger, epidermal growth factor, and kringle-1 domains of wild-type tPA, the molecule has a longer half-life and somewhat less fibrin specificity. The longer half-life makes it well suited for bolus administration.

Pilot and phase II studies demonstrated great promise in terms of earlier and more complete perfusion. Substantially higher rates of TIMI 3 flow were demonstrated in comparison with previous experience with streptokinase. In a direct comparison with a 3-hour infusion of tPA, a significantly higher rate of TIMI 3 flow with reteplase was demonstrated in the first 60 and 90 minutes (24). In a comparison with front-loaded tPA administration, a higher rate of TIMI 3 flow at 90 minutes was also demonstrated (25). Based on these studies it was reasonable to postulate that the higher rate of early TIMI 3 flow with reteplase would lead to a lower mortality than with other thrombolytic agents.

An initial trial, INJECT, compared reteplase with streptokinase (26). No difference was found in mortality, although there was a strong trend towards a lower mortality with reteplase of approximately 0.5% at 30 days of follow-up. This nonsignificant difference was maintained at 6 months, at which time it approached 1%. The confidence intervals were consistent with a true effect of 1% at 30 days.

The GUSTO-III trial was designed to determine whether the higher early perfusion with reteplase would translate into survival benefit compared with accelerated tPA. Fifteen thousand patients were randomized in a 2:1 fashion to reteplase compared with alteplase. At 30 days of follow-up the mortality was 7.47% with reteplase compared with 7.24% with alteplase, and the composite of death and disabling stroke was 7.89% with reteplase compared with 7.91% with alteplase. No major differences in secondary endpoints were observed (16).

Why did the differences in 60- and 90-minute TIMI grade 3 rates not translate into better survival for reteplase? Several possible explanations must be considered. Scrutiny of the RAPID 2 results demonstrates that the 30-minute data actually show a benefit for alteplase with a 39% rate of TIMI grade 3 flow versus 27% with reteplase (25). These results are not definitive, however, as they were obtained in only a small proportion of patients enrolled in the study. The RAPID 2 study was not large enough to establish whether the reocclusion rates were the same or different with reteplase and alteplase.

Perhaps the most important aspect of GUSTO-III is the insight it provides into the issue of therapeutic equivalence. The estimates for the difference in death alone and death and various stroke outcomes are shown in Figure 4. Although each demonstrates a point estimate clearly in the territory that would be considered therapeutically equivalent, the

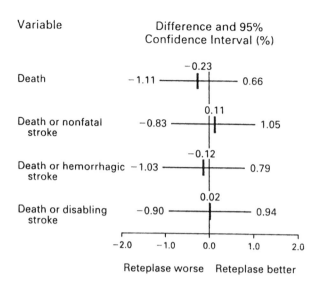

Figure 4 Kaplan-Meier estimate of mortality at 30 days in GUSTO-III, according to treatment group. (From Ref. 16.)

confidence intervals encompass estimates for the difference that are consistent with a difference in outcome that would influence that choice of therapy.

The GUSTO-III Steering Committee felt that the precedent for a clinically meaningful difference in thrombolytic agents was set by GUSTO-I, which was designed with power to demonstrate a 1% absolute difference or a 14% relative difference, whichever was smaller. Despite this confidence interval exceeding 1% for mortality with reteplase, many hospitals and practitioners have switched from alteplase to reteplase in clinical practice.

PERSPECTIVE

The GUSTO effort has yielded a variety of interesting insights into the treatment of acute coronary syndromes (Table 1). What started as a simple quest to determine the significance of improved coronary perfusion has evolved into a detailed evaluation of many other issues that arose as a result of this trial.

Antithrombotic Agents and Coronary Perfusion

Efforts to improve coronary perfusion with better fibrinolytic and antithrombotic agents are likely to produce only small incremental effects. Yet, the combination of multiple small incremental benefits yields significant survival advantages and protection from the debilitating outcomes of heart failure and reinfarction. The modest nature of the incremental benefit that is expected should not be discouraging. Rather the imperatives are to devise methods of doing trials of adequate size to know the impact of potential advances at a reasonable cost, to improve medical education and methods of health care delivery so that patients have access to the best therapies, and to constantly evaluate the intersection of science and practice to know which therapies should be tested.

Table 1 GUSTO/VIGOUR Trials

Trial name	Therapy tested	Patient population	Outcome
GUSTO-I(2)	Acc. tPA vs. SK	AMI: 41,021 at 1081 sites in 15 countries	Acc. tPA had survival benefit
GUSTO-IIb(15)	Hirudin vs. heparin	ACS: 12,142 at 373 sites in 13 countries	Hirudin had small advantage in reducing nonfatal MI
GUSTO-IIb PTCA(27)	Acc. tPA vs. PTCA	AMI: 1138 at 57 sites in 9 countries	PTCA has advantage, but smaller than expected
PARAGON A	Lamifiban vs. placebo	ACS: 2282 at 273 sites in 20 countries	Lamifiban reduced ischemic events but phase III study needed
PARADIGM	Lamifiban vs. placebo	AMI: 353 at 25 sites in 4 countries	Lamifiban appeared to be associated with more rapid and complete reperfusion
PURSUIT	Eptifibatide vs. placebo	ACS: 10,948 at 726 sites 28 countries	Eptifibatide reduced death of MI
GUSTO-III(16)	Reteplase vs. alteplase	AMI: 15,059 at 807 sites in 20 countries	Reteplase did not provide survival benefit over alteplase
GUSTO-IV ACS	Abciximab vs. placebo	ACS: 7500 at 400 sites in 15 countries	Ongoing
GUSTO-IV AMI	Abciximab with low-dose lytics vs. standard lytics	AMI: 15-20,000 at 800 sites in 20 countries	Pilot trial ongoing
ASSENT-II	TNK–tPA vs. alteplase	AMI: 16,500 at 1000 sites in 29 countries	Ongoing
HERO-II	Hirulog with SK vs. heparin with SK	AMI: 17,000 at 1000 sites in 32 countries	Ongoing
SYMPHONY	Sibrafiban vs. aspirin	Post-ACS: 6000 at 800 sites in 36 countries	Ongoing
PARAGON B	Lamifiban vs. placebo	ACS: 4000 at 400 sites in 21 countries	Ongoing

Acc. tPA = An accelerated regimen of tissue-plasminogen activator; ACS = acute coronary syndromes; AMI = acute myocardial infarction; ASSENT-II = assessment of the safety and efficacy of a new thrombolytic agent; HERO-II = hirulog early reperfusion/occlusion; GUSTO-I = global use of streptokinase and tPA for occluded coronary arteries; GUSTO-II, -III, -IV = global use of strategies to open occluded coronary arteries; PARADIGM = platelet aggregation receptor antagonist dose investigation and reperfusion gain in myocardial infarction trial; PARAGON = platelet IIb/IIIa antagonists for the reduction of acute coronary syndrome events in a global organization network; PTCA = percutaneous transluminal coronary angioplasty; PURSUIT = platelet glycoprotein IIb/IIIa in unstable angina: receptor suppression using Integrilin therapy; SK = streptokinase; SYMPHONY = Sibrafiban versus aspirin to yield maximum protection from ischemic heart events post–acute coronary syndromes.

In an effort to meet these imperatives, the VIGOUR organization has been developed to link coordinating centers for clinical trials using an efficient approach to addressing the right questions (28). The organization attempts to assess therapeutic developments to select the most promising ones for evaluation. In the next several years the group will be evaluating intravenous glycoprotein IIb/IIIa inhibitors combined with fibrinolytic agents (GUSTO-IV), "third-generation" fibrinolytics that can be given as a single bolus (ASSENT-II), the combination of hirulog with streptokinase (an important issue particularly for countries with great financial constraints) (HERO-II), and the use of adenosine to reduce infarct size.

Principles of Determining Therapeutic Benefit and Surrogate Endpoints

We are faced with a fascinating societal dilemma driven by two rapidly evolving areas of science—molecular biology and clinical trials. Molecular biology is producing a rapidly expanding array of therapeutic alternatives; potential new therapies far outnumber those that can be properly evaluated. At the same time, clinical science has much more effectively defined the criteria for an appropriate therapeutic evaluation. In the arena of acute coronary syndromes, after preliminary studies to verify that the biology is relevant and that the therapy indeed affects the biology, only clinical outcome studies can determine whether a therapy is effective. Since death is a major and common outcome in acute coronary syndromes, knowledge of the effect of a proposed therapy on death is necessary, which raises the necessary sample size for a relevant study to thousands of patients.

Perfusion of the culprit coronary vessel would seem to be the best possible "surrogate" endpoint. Substantial evidence exists that better perfusion is associated with better survival, and the GUSTO-I trial demonstrated a very close relationship between differences in early perfusion rates and differences in mortality. GUSTO-II and GUSTO-III, however, pointed out the frailty of perfusion as a surrogate. As nicely shown by Fleming and DeMets (Fig. 5), surrogates can be derailed by alternate pathways affecting the relevant clinical endpoints (29). In GUSTO-II, either the surrogate measurement in carefully selected populations did not carry over into broader populations or the failure to inhibit thrombin activation translated into no significant clinical benefit. In the direct angioplasty substudy, although the direction of the benefit was as expected, the magnitude may have been reduced by less than expected angiographic results of the angioplasty procedure. In GUSTO-III the failure of reteplase to produce a mortality benefit remains enigmatic.

The bottom line on trial methodology from the GUSTO studies is that anything less than adequately sized clinical trials with clinical outcomes as the primary endpoint has a significant risk of getting the wrong answer. Within the GUSTO trials, use of surrogates would have led to the following erroneous results: an overestimate of the benefit of alteplase, an incorrect dosing scheme for heparin, an overdose of hirudin in clinical practice and an overestimate of its potential benefit, an overestimate of the benefit of direct coronary angioplasty, and an incorrect assumption that reteplase lowers mortality compared with alteplase.

Equivalence

As our therapies continue to improve, the incremental benefit of each new advance is likely to be, on average, smaller. As discussed above, the sample size needed to demonstrate a small incremental benefit is large and expands more than linearly. This raises the important

Table 4 Baseline Characteristics of Patient Population

Characteristics	Thrombolysis	Angioplasty
No. of patients	56	47
Sex (M/F)	40/16	37/10
Age (yr)	62 ± 13	60 ± 11
ST elevation/depression	54/2	46/1
Infarct location		
Anterior	22	15
Inferior	30	31
Other	4	1
Hours from chest pain to randomization		
<4	43	35
≥4	13	12
Minutes to treatment[a]		
All patients	232 ± 174	277 ± 144
Randomized in <4 hr[b]	158 ± 56	210 ± 76
Randomized in ≥4 hr	477 ± 208	461 ± 128

[a] Defined as the start of intravenous thrombolysis in the thrombolysis group and the first balloon inflation in the angioplasty group. Plus-minus values are means ± SD.

[b] $p < 0.001$ for the difference between groups.

Of the 45 patients assigned to PTCA, 7 (15%) had recurrent ischemia, which required intervention (repeat PTCA 1, coronary bypass surgery 6) (Table 5). Of the 51 patients assigned to thrombolysis, 20 (36%) ($p < 0.01$ vs. PTCA group) developed recurrent ischemia requiring treatment with angioplasty in 16 and or surgery in 7 (3 patients had both attempted PTCA and surgery). There were no strokes in either of the treatment groups.

There were no significant differences in sestamibi measurements including myocardium at risk, final infarct size, or myocardial salvage for patients treated with primary dilatation compared with thrombolysis irrespective of the location of the infarction (Table 6, Figs. 2 and 3). On the whole there was greater myocardial salvage with anterior infarctions, but within each group there was substantial variability, with some patients having almost complete salvage and others minimal or no salvage. Both initial therapies resulted in salvage of approximately one-half of the myocardium at risk. Two patients (one in each group) had markedly negative salvage values, suggesting infarct extension. There was no significant difference in secondary endpoints of ejection fraction, recurrent infarction, or death during the initial and 6-month follow up duration (Table 7).

Table 5 In-Hospital Therapy and Outcome

	Thrombolysis	PTCA
Randomized	56	47
Received randomized therapy	51	45
Protocol PTCA successful	—	42
PTCA in hospital	16	1
CABG in hospital	7	6
Hospital deaths	2	2
Stroke	0	0

Table 6 Measurements with Sestamibi in 103 Randomized Patients for Whom Data on the Primary Endpoint Were Available

Measure	All patients			Patients with anterior MI			Patients with nonanterior MI		
	Thrombolysis	PTCA	p value	Thrombolysis	PTCA	p value	Thrombolysis	PTCA	p value
Myocardium at risk	31 ± 20	27 ± 21	0.25	47 ± 19	49 ± 16	0.74	21 ± 12	15 ± 11	0.05
Final infarct size	15 ± 17	13 ± 16	0.48	20 ± 22	18 ± 20	0.83	12 ± 10	10 ± 14	0.53
Myocardial salvage	15 ± 19	13 ± 19	0.64	27 ± 21	31 ± 21	0.61	7 ± 13	5 ± 10	0.47
95% confidence interval	10–20	8–18	—	18–36	20–42	—	3–11	2–9	—

All measurements are given as percentages of the left ventricle. Plus-minus values are means ± SD. MI denotes myocardial infarction.

21. Laster SB, O'Keefe JH Jr., Gibbons RJ. Incidence and importance of thrombolysis in myocardial infarction grade 3 flow after primary percutaneous transluminal coronary angioplasty for acute myocardial infarction. Am J Cardiol 1996; 78(6):623–626.

22. Collaborative Organization for RheothRx Evaluation (CORE). Effects of RheothRx on mortality, morbidity, left ventricular function, and infarct size in patients with acute myocardial infarction. Circulation 1997; 96(1):192–201.

23. Schaer GL, Spaccavento LJ, Browne KF, Krueger KA, Krichbaum D, Phelan JM, et al. Beneficial effects of RheothRx injection in patients receiving thrombolytic therapy for acute myocardial infarction. Results of a randomized, double-blind, placebo-controlled trial. Circulation 1996; 94(3):298–307.

24. O'Keefe JH, Grines Catheterization Laboratory, DeWood MA, Schaer GL, et al. Poloxamer-188 as an adjunct to primary percutaneous transluminal coronary angioplasty for acute myocardial infarction. Am J Cardiol 1996; 78(7):747–750.

25. Bateman TM, O'Keefe JH Jr., Williams ME. Design and implementation of a nuclear cardiology testing facility in a private-practice cardiology office setting. J Nucl Cardiol 1997; 4(2 Pt 1):156–163.

10

The Zwolle Primary PTCA Trial

FELIX ZIJLSTRA

Zijlstra F, de Boer MJ, Hoorntje JCA, Reiffers S, Reiber JHC, Suryapranata H. A comparison of immediate coronary angioplasty with intravenous streptokinase in acute myocardial infarction. N Engl J Med 1993; 328: 680–684.

Over the past decades, great efforts have been made to assess the optimal approach to patients with acute myocardial infarction. Attention has been focused on the restoration of normal blood flow through the infarct-related coronary artery. Coronary artery bypass grafting was the only accepted revascularization therapy in the 1970s. Although data from small studies suggested promising results of early reperfusion by means of bypass grafting (1,2), this approach was never tested in large-scale studies. In the 1980s, intravenous thrombolytic therapy became widely used (3–5), but all thrombolytic agents are hampered by modest reperfusion rates.

The Zwolle trial compared primary coronary angioplasty (angioplasty without prior or concomitant thrombolysis) with thrombolysis for acute myocardial infarction.

GENERAL OUTLINE OF THE TRIAL

Patient Selection

The research protocol was approved by the institutional review board of the Weezenlanden Hospital. Enrollment began on August 20, 1990, and ended on April 26, 1993. Inclusion criteria were: (1) symptoms compatible with acute myocardial infarction persisting for more than 30 minutes accompanied by an ECG with more than 0.1 mV ST-segment elevation in two or more contiguous leads; (2) presentation within 6 hours after symptom onset or between 6 and 24 hours if there was evidence of continuing ischemia; (3) age less than 76 years; and (4) no contraindication to thrombolytic therapy, including prior stroke or other known intracranial diseases, recent trauma or surgery, refractory hypertension, active bleeding, or prolonged cardiopulmonary resuscitation. Prior coronary artery bypass grafting, prior Q-wave or non–Q-wave infarction, and cardiogenic shock were not exclusion criteria. After informed consent was obtained, patients were randomly assigned to one of the two treatment modalities using a closed envelope system.

Treatment Protocol

All patients received 300 mg of aspirin IV followed by 80 mg/day PO and IV nitroglycerin in a dosage aimed at a systolic blood pressure of 110 mmHg. Intravenous heparin was given in a bolus of 10,000 U and thereafter as a continuous infusion adjusted to maintain the activated partial thromboplastin time between two and three times the normal value for at least 2 days. Other drugs such as β-adrenergic blockers, lidocaine, or calcium antagonists were given as indicated. Patients randomized to streptokinase received 1.5 million U IV in 1 hour. Patients randomized to coronary angioplasty were immediately transported to the catheterization laboratory and underwent coronary angiography followed by immediate coronary angioplasty if their coronary anatomy was deemed suitable. Both coronary arteries were visualized, and left ventriculography was not performed. The angioplasty was considered to be technically successful if there was a residual stenosis of less than 50% on visual estimation and a flow of TIMI grade 2 or 3. Time from admission to therapy was calculated as time from admission to the first balloon inflation or to the start of the streptokinase infusion.

Methods

Flow through the infarct-related vessel was scored according to the thrombolysis in myocardial infarction (TIMI) classification (6). Reocclusion was defined as a reduction in TIMI perfusion grade 2 or 3 to TIMI grades 0 and 1. To assess the restenosis rate and arterial patency in the angioplasty group, these patients underwent repeat coronary angiography after 3 months. Restenosis was defined as a more than 50% diameter stenosis measured quantitatively, following an initially less than 50% stenosis after primary coronary angioplasty. Patients in the angioplasty assigned group, who underwent coronary artery bypass surgery, who had an unsuccessful angioplasty or no procedure at all, did not have routine repeat angiography. Data from the coronary angiography and angioplasty procedures were collected and graded by two of the investigators. As blinding to angioplasty procedures was not possible, all angiograms were subsequently reviewed by an independent and experienced investigator, not involved in other aspects of the trial. Consensus on collateral flow, procedural success, TIMI flow before and after the angioplasty procedure, identification of the infarct-related vessel, and extent of coronary artery disease was reached in all cases. TIMI flow before angioplasty was judged at first injection of contrast material. Collaterals to the infarct-related vessel were classified as:

> Grade 0: no visible filling of any collateral channels
> Grade 1: filling of side branches of the vessel by means of collateral channels without
>   any dye reaching the epicardial segment of that vessel
> Grade 2: partial filling via collateral channels of the epicardial segment of the vessel
> Grade 3: complete filling of the vessel

Follow-up coronary angiography in the streptokinase-assigned patient group was also performed after 3 months. In both groups, however, this procedure was allowed to be performed earlier or later at the discretion of the attending physicians. In the angioplasty-assigned patient group, all catheterization laboratory events were scored carefully during and immediately after the emergency procedure. Major and minor in-laboratory events were defined as new events not present before arrival in the catheterization room. Catheterization laboratory events with primary coronary angioplasty were assessed according to the following classifications. Major catheterization laboratory events include death, cardiopulmonary resuscitation, ventricular fibrillation or tachycardia treated with electrical cardioversion, sustained hypotension defined as a systolic blood pressure ≤80 mmHg requiring continuous intravenous vasopressor support, the insertion of an intraaortic balloon pump, or both; and urgent surgery. Minor catheterization laboratory events include transient hypotension defined as a systolic blood pressure ≤80 mmHg requiring intravenous therapy; and bradycardia or atrioventricular conduction abnormalities requiring bolus of intravenous therapy, a temporary pacemaker, or both.

All infarct-related vessels were analyzed objectively with a personal computer–based quantitative coronary angiography (QCA) system (CMS: Cardiovascular Measurement System, Software version 2.0, Medis Medical Imaging Systems, Nuenen, The Netherlands). The basic algorithms have been described elsewhere (7). The system uses a high-quality cine-to-video converter that allowed a selected cine frame to be projected onto a digital video camera through an optical zoom lens. The video signal of the magnified region of interest was subsequently digitized. For calibration, the boundaries of a non-tapering part of the catheter were determined automatically over a length of approximately 2 cm. To determine the contours of the vessel, the user had only to indicate the beginning and end of the coronary segment to be analyzed. Thereafter the procedure runs automatically.

Creatine kinase (CK) and lactate dehydrogenase (LDH) were determined enzymatically on a Hitachi 717 automatic analyzer according to the International Federation of Clinical Chemistry (IFCC) recommendation at 30°C (8). Reference values for LDH are <320 U/liter (adults) and for CK are <110 U/liter (females) and <130 U/liter (males). Infarct size was estimated by measurements of enzyme activities using LDH as the reference enzyme. This method is equal to estimation of infarct size from α-hydroxybutyrate dehydrogenase (HBDH) and has been described in detail (9–11). Cumulative enzyme release from five to seven serial measurements up to 72 hours after symptom onset (LDH Q_{72}) was calculated by the Cardiovascular Research Institute Maastricht (W.Th.H.) with blinding to all data other than hospital registration number and date of birth.

Left ventricular ejection fraction was measured before discharge by radionuclide ventriculography using the multiple-gated equilibrium method following the labeling of red blood cells of the patient with ^{99m}Tc-pertechnetate (7). A General Electric 300 gamma camera with a low-energy all-purpose parallel-hole collimator was used. Global ejection fraction was calculated by a General Electric Star View computer using the fully automatic PAGE program. The use of this software program protects against operator bias. The reproducibility of this method is excellent, with a mean difference (±SD) between first and second values of duplicate measurements of 1.2 ± 1.1% (7).

Charges were calculated using estimates of unit charges concerning all aspects of medical care (12). These included hospital days (distinguishing between normal care, coronary care, and postoperative intensive care), diagnostic or therapeutic procedures, and medication (including the thrombolytic drugs given). Data were registered during the initial admission, during readmissions, and during visits to the outpatient clinic. By general survey of patients (mostly by telephone interview) and of the referring physicians, readmissions to other hospitals could be traced, and these data were added to the database. All patients were scheduled for follow-up angiography, and the charges for this procedure were included in the calculations. Unit charges for this procedures and hospital days were calculated on the basis of hospital administration data of 1992. These included the professional charges and were adjusted for the increased charges of procedures during the night or the weekend. The exchange rate for American dollars versus Dutch guilders of 1992 was used to convert to dollar amounts. Charges applied for a diagnostic catheterization were $900, angioplasty $4800, bypass surgery $10,800, one day in the coronary care unit $930, one day in the postoperative intensive care unit $1300, and one day on a general ward $300. Charges for streptokinase and tPA were $240 and $1200, respectively. The charges of additional pharmacological treatment were based on the average treatment charges of the various drugs according to their prices in 1992, including charges for prescription administration. Charges per month were estimated as aspirin $6, nitrates $12, diuretics $18, coumadin $20 (including coagulation tests), antiarrhythmic agents $21, beta-blockers $36, calcium blockers $42, angiotensin-converting enzyme inhibitors $63, and cholesterol-lowering drugs $81.

Statistical Analysis

All endpoints were analyzed according to the "intention-to-treat" principle. Differences between group means were tested by two-tailed Student's *t*-test. A chi-square method or Fisher's exact test was used to test differences between proportions. Statistical significance was defined as a *p* value of less than 0.05. Survival functions were calculated using the Kaplan-Meier product limit method (13). The Mantel-Cox (or log-rank) test was applied to evaluate the differences between survival functions. Odds ratios were calculated, which may be interpreted as relative risks with 95% confidence intervals (CI) (14).

In-Hospital Clinical Course

Baseline clinical characteristics and clinical course are shown in Table 1. In the angioplasty-assigned patient group, immediate angiography was performed in 151 patients; one patient died before angiography could be performed. He had severe three-vessel coronary artery disease at postmortem examination. Four patients did not have a significant coronary artery narrowing. Two of them, however, suffered a myocardial infarction, one of them showing residual thrombi in a large left circumflex artery. Coronary angioplasty was performed in 140 patients. Five patients with an open or small infarct-related artery were treated conservatively. Six patients with severe multivessel disease or left main stenosis had emergency coronary artery bypass grafting after insertion of an intraaortic counterpulsation balloon. Primary angioplasty of the infarct-related vessel was successful in 136 patients (97%), resulting in a less than 50% residual stenosis and a TIMI grade 2 or 3 flow at the end of the procedure. In four patients the infarct-related vessel could not be reopened. Three of these patients underwent immediate coronary artery bypass grafting; one was treated conservatively.

Of the 149 patients assigned to streptokinase therapy, one died before infusion could be started. Sixteen patients underwent a "rescue" coronary angioplasty because there was clinical evidence of failed reperfusion or hemodynamic collapse. In 15 patients the proce-

Table 1 Baseline Characteristics and Clinical Data

	Streptokinase (n = 149)	p-value	Angioplasty (n = 152)
Age (yr)	61 ± 9	0.06	59 ± 10
Male sex	121 (81%)	0.59	127 (84%)
Anterior infarction	68 (46%)	0.27	79 (52%)
Previous infarction	21 (14%)	0.11	32 (21%)
Time from onset to admission (min)	176 ± 172	0.43	195 ± 227
Killip class on admission			
I	122 (82%)	0.22	116 (76%)
II	15 (10%)	0.26	22 (14%)
III	9 (6%)	0.41	6 (4%)
IV	3 (2%)	0.14	8 (5%)
Multivessel disease	88 (59%)	0.63	95 (63%)
Hospital stay (days)	14.4 ± 6.8	0.003	12.3 ± 5.3
Stroke	3 (2%)	0.37	1 (1%)
Vascular repair	0 (0%)	1.0	1 (1%)
Mechanical ventilation	3 (2%)	0.68	2 (1%)
Heart failure	17 (11%)	0.03	7 (5%)
Bleeding	9 (6%)	0.97	8 (5%)
IABP	12 (8%)	0.28	19 (13%)
Peak CK (U/liter)	1,403 ± 1,276	0.33	1,268 ± 1,088

Values presented are mean value ± SD or number (%). Bleeding = bleeding requiring a blood transfusion or intracranial bleeding; CK = creatine kinase; heart failure = signs of heart failure requiring therapy with diuretic agents and angiotensin-converting enzyme inhibitors < 24 hours after admission; IABP = intra-aortic balloon pump; vascular repair = surgical repair of the femoral artery.

dure was successful; one underwent emergency coronary artery bypass grafting and was discharged alive after an otherwise uneventful in-hospital stay.

ANGIOGRAPHIC FINDINGS AND CATHETERIZATION LABORATORY EVENTS

Baseline angiographic data are shown in Table 2. All in-laboratory events are shown in Table 3.

Technical Details of Angioplasty Procedures

Technical characteristics of the actual primary angioplasty procedures are as follows: one balloon was used in 97 patients, two balloons in 33 patients, three balloons in 9 patients, and four balloons in 1 patient. The average number of balloons used per procedure thus was 1.41, whereas the mean number of balloons used in elective procedures in our institution is 1.28. The mean maximum balloon pressure was 9.9 atm (range 3–16), the number of inflations 3.2 (range 1–10), with a mean total inflation time of 530 seconds (range 90–

Table 2 Angiographic Data of Patients Assigned to Primary Coronary Angioplasty

	Grade	Baseline	60 min	90 min	120 min
Collaterals[a]	0	85 (60%)			
(n = 141)	1	45 (32%)			
	2	11 (8%)			
	3	0			
TIMI[b]	0	109 (72%)	56 (37%)	19 (13%)	7 (5%)[c]
(n = 151)	1	15 (10%)	11 (7%)	3 (2%)	1 (1%)
	2	17 (11%)	7 (5%)	7 (5%)	4 (3%)
	3	10 (7%)	77 (51%)	122 (81%)	139 (92%)

[a] Collateral classification: grade 0, no visible filling of any collateral channels; grade 1, filling of side branches of the vessel by means of collateral channels without any dye reaching the epicardial segment of that vessel; grade 2, partial filling via collateral channels of the epicardial segment of the vessel; grade 3, complete filling of the vessel.

[b] Thrombolysis in Myocardial Infarction (TIMI) grade is flow grade through the infarct-related vessel according to the TIMI study flow classification (min indicates minutes after admission).

[c] In four patients the infarct-related vessel was opened successfully more than 120 minutes after admission.

Table 3 Catheterization-Laboratory Events in the Primary Coronary Angioplasty Group (n = 140)

	n	Percent
Major in-laboratory events	20	14
Involvement:		
Right coronary artery	8	6
Left anterior descending artery	8	6
Left circumflex artery	2	1
Graft	1	1
Left main coronary artery	1	1
Cardioversion	6	4
Cardiopulmonary resuscitation	6	4
Dopamine/adrenaline support	8	6
Intra-aortic balloon pump support for hypotension	6	4
Urgent surgery	3	2
Minor in-laboratory events:	29	18
Involvement		
Right coronary artery	16	11[a]
Left anterior descending artery	6	4
Left circumflex artery	7	5
Brief bolus atropin or pressor	23	16
Temporary pacemaker	9	6

[a] Risk of minor in-laboratory events of right coronary artery angioplasty significantly higher (p = 0.042) than for angioplasty of other vessels.

2400). After a successful procedure, the attending interventional cardiologist described angiographic evidence of dissection in 29 patients (21%).

Follow-Up Angiography

Coronary angiography was performed after 22 ± 38 days (range 0–304) in 139 of the 149 patients assigned to streptokinase therapy. Eight patients died before coronary angiography was performed; two patients refused angiography.

The results of the quantitative coronary angiography analysis are depicted in Table 4. The minimal luminal diameter (MLD) of the infarct-related vessel increased from 0.25 ± 0.62 mm before to 2.22 ± 0.62 mm immediately after the primary angioplasty procedure. If all patients in the streptokinase group with an occlusion of the infarct-related vessel were excluded, the mean diameter-stenosis of the infarct-related vessel was $64 \pm 13\%$ and the mean minimal luminal diameter was 1.05 ± 0.41 mm. Repeat angiography was performed after 92 ± 67 days (range 1–389) in 130 of the 136 patients in the angioplasty group who actually underwent a successful procedure. Reasons for not performing repeat angiography were death in two patients, early elective coronary artery bypass surgery because of concomitant left main coronary artery disease in two patients, malignancy detected after randomization in one patient, and refusal in one patient. The infarct-related vessel was patent in 66% of the patients (92 of 139) who received streptokinase and 95% of those assigned to angioplasty therapy (123 of 130) ($p < 0.001$; odds ratio (OR): 8.9; 95% CI 3.7–23). In the angioplasty group seven patients (5%) had an occluded infarct-related vessel at follow-up angiography: the right coronary artery in 3 patients, both the left anterior descending artery and left circumflex artery in 2 patients. Of these seven patients three had a TIMI grade 2 flow immediately after the angioplasty procedure compared with two patients in the group with a patent infarct-related vessel at follow-up angiography ($p = 0.001$). Among the patients assigned to angioplasty therapy, only 7% had patent infarct-related vessels (TIMI grade 3 flow) at baseline, and 92% of the patients had patent vessels by 120 minutes after admission. QCA data of the infarct-related vessels in

Table 4 Quantitative Angiographic Data[a]

Variable	Angioplasty group				Streptokinase group
	Before ($n = 151$)	After ($n = 140$)	Follow-up at 92 ± 67 days ($n = 130$)	$p = $ Value	at 22 ± 38 days ($n = 139$)
Projections analyzed (no.)	2.0 ± 0.5	2.2 ± 0.5	2.2 ± 0.5	—	2.1 ± 0.5
Stenosis (%)	92 ± 19	27 ± 15	35 ± 22	<0.001	77 ± 20
Minimal luminal diameter (mm)	0.25 ± 0.62	2.22 ± 0.62	1.99 ± 0.83	<0.001	0.69 ± 0.60
Reference diameter (mm)[b]	—	3.04 ± 0.62 ($1.89 - 5.03$)	3.00 ± 0.66 ($1.45 - 4.99$)	0.924	3.00 ± 0.56 ($1.72 - 4.82$)
Largest balloon (mm)	2.93 ± 0.39	—	—	—	

[a] Plus-minus values are mean $\pm$ SD.
[b] By the interpolated method.

the angioplasty-assigned patient group at repeat angiography are shown in Table 4. Restenosis, defined as stenosis of more than 50% in the dilated segment, was observed in 24 of 125 patients in the angioplasty group (20%). Although evidence has accumulated that the incidence of restenosis reaches a plateau at 3 months, the clinical implications of restenosis will become clear only after at least 6 months of follow-up. Excluding all angiography without evidence of restenosis performed within 3 months after angioplasty, the rate of restenosis was 28% (24 of 87).

MYOCARDIAL SALVAGE AS MEASURED BY ENZYMATIC INFARCT SIZE AND PREDISCHARGE RADIONUCLIDE LEFT VENTRICULAR EJECTION FRACTION

Enzymatic Infarct Size

Values for peak creatine kinase and LDH estimated infarct size (LDH Q_{72}) are given in Table 5. Peak CK values tended to be lower in the angioplasty-treated patient group, but this difference was not statistically significant. Cumulative enzyme release during the first 72 hours, with sufficient data from the sequential measurements and accurate timing of symptom onset, could be calculated in 92% of all patients, and the data are given in Table 5. For 10 patients in the angioplasty group and for 7 patients in the streptokinase group, data were insufficient for adequate analysis. Eight patients died within the first 48 hours, before serial enzyme release could be determined. Estimated infarct size using LDH Q_{72} was lower in the angioplasty-assigned patients compared with patients assigned to receive streptokinase, representing a reduction of estimated infarct size of 23% (95% CI 13–32%). The difference of the LDH Q_{72} value between the two groups was greater in patients with anterior wall myocardial infarction than in patients with a nonanterior wall infarction.

The relation between time from onset of symptoms to reperfusion therapy and

Table 5 Enzyme Measurements and Estimated Infarct Size Expressed as LDH Q_{72}: Relation of Enzyme Measurements to Infarct Location and Interval from Onset of Symptoms to Admission

	Angioplasty	p	Streptokinase
Peak CK (U/liter)	1268 ± 1088 ($n = 141$)	0.37	1404 ± 1276 ($n = 135$)
LDH Q_{72} All infarcts (U/liter)	1003 ± 784	0.012	1310 ± 1198
LDH Q_{72} Anterior MI (U/liter)	1158 ± 918 ($n = 71$)	0.022	1606 ± 1264 ($n = 62$)
LDH Q_{72} Nonanterior MI (U/liter)	853 ± 580 ($n = 70$)	0.135	1060 ± 1085 ($n = 73$)
Time from symptom onset to admission:			
<2 hours: LDH Q_{72}, (U/liter)	967 ± 730 ($n = 81$)	0.01	1403 ± 1157 ($n = 65$)
>2 hours: LDH Q_{72}, (U/liter)	1052 ± 855 ($n = 60$)	0.36	1224 ± 1237 ($n = 70$)

LDH Q_{72} is also shown in Table 5. In patients admitted to the hospital within 2 hours after the onset of symptoms, an even more pronounced difference was seen: LDH Q_{72} was 967 ± 730 U/liter in the angioplasty group versus 1403 ± 1157 U/liter in the streptokinase group ($p = 0.010$), representing a reduction of estimated infarct size of 31% (95% CI 20–43%).

Left Ventricular Function

In 149 patients in the angioplasty group (98%) and 140 patients in the streptokinase group (94%), resting ejection fraction values were obtained. Three patients in the angioplasty-treated group and nine patients in the streptokinase-treated group died before nuclear studies were performed. Global ejection fraction was measured in all 289 survivors, whereas regional wall motion could be obtained in 273 patients (91%). The interval between acute myocardial infarction and time of nuclear study was less in the angioplasty group than in the streptokinase group (14 ± 13 days and 17 ± 21 days, respectively; $p = 0.04$). In all subgroups studied, resting global ejection fraction was significantly greater in patients assigned to primary angioplasty than in patients assigned to streptokinase therapy (Table 6). This difference was mostly due to better wall motion in the infarct-related region, although a relatively small but significant difference for non–infarct-related areas was also found between the two groups.

MORTALITY, REINFARCTION, AND CHARGES DURING LONG-TERM FOLLOW-UP

All outpatient reports were reviewed, and general practitioners as well as patients were contacted by telephone. For patients who had died during follow-up, hospital records and autopsy data were reviewed. No patient was lost to follow-up. Information was collected

Table 6 Global Ejection Fraction and Regional Wall Motion (%)

	Angioplasty	p	Streptokinase
EF (all patients)	50 ± 9 ($n = 149$)	< 0.001	45 ± 11 ($n = 140$)
IR wall motion (all patients)	42 ± 14	< 0.001	34 ± 13
NIR wall motion (all patients)	55 ± 11	0.005	51 ± 12
EF anterior MI	46 ± 12	0.002	39 ± 12
EF nonanterior MI	53 ± 9	0.02	49 ± 9
EF one-vessel disease	51 ± 8 ($n = 57$)	0.002	46 ± 10 ($n = 59$)
EF multivessel disease	48 ± 12 ($n = 92$)	0.002	43 ± 12 ($n = 81$)
Time from symptom onset to admission:			
<2 hours: EF, %	51 ± 10 ($n = 83$)	< 0.001	45 ± 11 ($n = 70$)
>2 hours: EF, %	48 ± 12 ($n = 66$)	0.04	44 ± 12 ($n = 70$)

EF = ejection fraction; IR = infarct-related; NIR = non–infarct-related, MI = myocardial infarction.

on mortality, the cause of death, and nonfatal recurrent myocardial infarction, defined as previously described (7).

Mortality

The mean follow-up time was 31 months (SD ± 11 months). A total of 32 patients (11%) died. A noncardiac cause of death was confirmed in eight patients; five in the angioplasty group and three in the streptokinase group. Two patients died from strokes that were not related to a cardiac event during follow-up; both had CT scan confirmation of the diagnoses. Five patients died of lung cancer and one with liver carcinoma. All diagnoses of malignancy were confirmed by autopsy.

Seven patients (5%) randomized to angioplasty died from a cardiac cause: cardiogenic shock or heart failure in four and sudden death in three patients. Seventeen patients (11%) randomized to streptokinase died from a cardiac cause: stroke in 1 patient, cardiogenic shock or heart failure in 10 patients, and sudden death in 6 patients. Survival curves are shown in Figure 1. The relative risk of cardiac death of streptokinase patients compared to angioplasty patients was 2.5 (95% CI 1.1–6.1).

Reinfarction

Reinfarctions occurred in 29 patients (19%) randomized to streptokinase compared to 5 patients (3%) randomized to angioplasty ($p = 0.001$). In the streptokinase group 14 reinfarctions occurred prior to coronary angiography compared to 2 reinfarctions prior to follow-up angiography in the angioplasty group ($p = 0.002$). Many of these infarct-related vessels were found to be occluded at angiography. Following the coronary angiogram that was used to assess patency of the infarct-related vessel, the difference in reinfarction rate was also significant (15 vs. 3; $p = 0.003$) in angioplasty patients and streptokinase patients. Eleven patients randomized to angioplasty had a nonfatal reinfarction or cardiac death

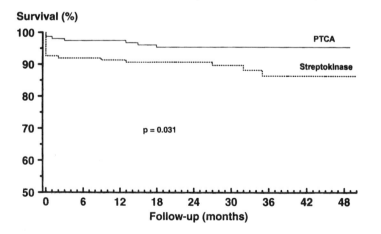

Figure 1   Incidence of cardiac death in 301 patients with acute myocardial infarction, randomized to treatment with streptokinase (----) or primary angioplasty (——) ($p < 0.031$).

Event-free Survival (%)

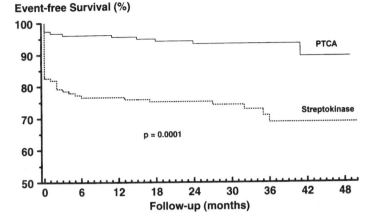

Figure 2   Incidence of cardiac death or nonfatal recurrent myocardial infarction in 301 patients with acute myocardial infarction, randomized to treatment with streptokinase (----) or primary angioplasty (——) ($p < 0.001$).

(7%) compared to 42 patients (28%) randomized to streptokinase ($p < 0.001$; see also Fig. 2). The relative risk of the combination of cardiac death and nonfatal reinfarction of streptokinase patients compared to angioplasty patients is 4.3 (95% CI 2.2–8.3).

Charges

The total medical charges including the initial hospital stay, readmissions, procedures such as angioplasty or bypass surgery, physician charges, and charges of pharmacological therapy were $18,402 per patient for the angioplasty-assigned patients and $18,229 per patient for the streptokinase patients. Recalculating the charges per survivor, the mean charges per patient amount to $19,979 per patient assigned to angioplasty and $21,055 per patient assigned to streptokinase. If charges were calculated for event-free survivors, the charges were $20,417 for patients assigned to angioplasty compared to $25,868 for patients assigned to streptokinase therapy.

DISCUSSION

This study shows that primary coronary angioplasty in patients with an acute myocardial infarction is associated with a higher patency rate of the infarct-related artery, less damage to the myocardium, and a lower incidence of cardiac death and recurrent infarction during follow-up, compared to thrombolytic therapy. Primary angioplasty did not result in an increase in medical charges. Patency of the infarct-related coronary artery is strongly related to clinical outcome, and this explains the improved clinical outcome after angioplasty compared to thrombolytic therapy.

The primary target of all reperfusion therapies is rapid and complete reopening of acutely occluded coronary arteries. This concept has recently been confirmed by the results of the GUSTO trial (Global Utilization of Streptokinase and Tissue plasminogen activator for Occluded coronary arteries) (15). Coronary patency, defined as the restoration of normal blood flow in the infarct-related vessel, results in myocardial salvage and improved survival. Patency rates achieved with primary angioplasty can currently not be obtained with thrombolytic agents (5,7,15,16). Indeed, our data indicate that a higher patency rate of angioplasty patients compared to streptokinase patients results in a higher left ventricular ejection fraction, a reduced incidence of reinfarction, and improved survival. This implies that thrombolytic agents or adjunctive therapies that would result in a higher rate of early and sustained TIMI 3 flow might offer similar benefit.

A second mechanism by which primary angioplasty results in a better long-term clinical outcome is the low incidence of reocclusion after successful angioplasty of less than 10%, compared to a reocclusion rate of 25–30% after successful reperfusion by thrombolytic agents (17,18).

The use of left ventricular ejection fraction as an endpoint in trials of acute myocardial infarction has been surrounded by controversies (19,20). Some investigators have shown relationships between early reperfusion (patency of the infarct-related artery) and limitation of infarct size and/or left ventricular function (21) and long-term survival (22). Our data strongly suggest that a higher, early, and sustained patency rate of the infarct-related vessel results in better left ventricular function. This is probably in part through the influence of successful reperfusion on left ventricular remodeling.

The impact of new therapeutic modalities on the financial burden of the health care system is becoming increasingly important. Therefore, it is reassuring that, although the initial charges of angioplasty were higher than those of thrombolytic therapy (12), after 31 ± 11 months primary angioplasty did not result in a further increase in the health care charges. In fact, the lower incidence of clinical events during follow-up probably results in an economic advantage of angioplasty over thrombolysis, as repeated loss of productive time can be avoided in a considerable number of patients.

It should be realized that our results were obtained in a hospital with an existing infrastructure for interventional cardiology including surgical back-up on a 24-hour per day basis. Our data clearly show that primary angioplasty is an excellent therapeutic option in hospitals with angioplasty facilities. Furthermore, this therapy can be used in many patients with an acute myocardial infarction who are not eligible for thrombolytic therapy. From a practical point of view, the most important remaining question is: Can and should we deliver primary angioplasty as a therapeutic option in patients with acute myocardial infarction who are admitted to hospitals without angioplasty facilities? Should small community hospitals start angioplasty programs? Probably not, as it would increase total medical costs and would result in low numbers of cases per hospital and per operator. This has been associated with a poorer outcome (23). Preliminary data show that in certain circumstances patients with acute myocardial infarction can be transported safely, and with limited time delay from a hospital without angioplasty facilities to an interventional cardiac catheterization laboratory (24). Further research into the implementation of primary angioplasty therapy into routine clinical practice should be one of our main goals for the coming years. Data from a German angioplasty registry with more than 60 participating hospitals show that the excellent results described in some of the randomized trials can be obtained in clinical practice (25).

Our study enrolled patients at a time when intracoronary stenting and new antiplatelet therapies were not yet incorporated into clinical practice, and the role of these important new developments during the acute phase of myocardial infarction has yet to be clarified (26,27).

CONCLUSIONS OF THE ZWOLLE TRIAL

The benefits of primary angioplasty compared to thrombolytic therapy with intravenous streptokinase are a higher patency rate of the infarct-related coronary artery, a better preserved myocardium as assessed by enzymatic infarct size and radionuclide left ventricular ejection fraction (in particular in patients presenting within 2 hours after symptom onset) and a lower rate of reinfarction and death during long-term follow-up, without an increase in total medical charges.

REFERENCES

1. Loop FD, Cheanvechai C, Sheldon WC, Taylor PC, Effler DB. Early myocardial revascularization during acute myocardial infarction. Chest 1974; 66:478–482.
2. DeWood MA, Spores J, Notske R, et al. Medical and surgical management of acute myocardial infarction. Am J Cardiol 1979; 44:1356–1364.
3. ISIS-2 Collaborative Group. Randomised trial of intravenous streptokinase, oral aspirin, both, or neither among 17, 187 cases of suspected acute myocardial infarction. Lancet 1988; 2:349–360.
4. Gruppo Italiano per lo Studio della Streptochinasi nell'Infarto Miocardico (GISSI). Effectiveness of intravenous thrombolytic treatment in acute myocardial infarction. Lancet 1986; 1: 397–402.
5. Granger CB, Califf RM, Topol EJ. Thrombolytic therapy for acute myocardial infarction. A review. Drugs 1992; 44:293–325.
6. TIMI Research Group. Immediate vs delayed catheterization and angioplasty following thrombolytic therapy for acute myocardial infarction. TIMI 2A results. JAMA 1988; 260:2849–2858.
7. Zijlstra F, de Boer MJ, Hoorntje JCA, Reiffers S, Reiber JHC, Suryapranata H. A comparison of immediate coronary angioplasty with intravenous streptokinase in acute myocardial infarction. N Engl J Med 1993; 328:680–684.
8. van der Heiden C, Bootsma J, Cornelissen PJHC, Hafkenscheid JCM, Oosterom R, Smit EM. Aanpassing van de aanbevelingen (NVKC) voor het meten van katalytische activiteitsconcentraties van enzymen in serum of plasma. Tijdschr NVKC 1987; 12:231–236.
9. de Zwaan C, Willems GM, Vermeer F, et al. Enzyme tests in the evaluation of thrombolysis in acute myocardial infarction. Br Heart J 1988; 59:175–183.
10. de Boer MJ, Suryapranata H, Hoorntje JCA, et al. Limitation of infarct size and preservation of left ventricular function after primary coronary angioplasty compared with intravenous streptokinase in acute myocardial infarction. Circulation 1994; 90:753–761.
11. van der Laarse A, Hermens WT, Hollaar L, et al. Assessment of myocardial damage in patients with acute myocardial infarction by serial measurement of serum a-hydroxybutyrate dehydrogenase levels. Am Heart J 1984; 107:248–260.
12. de Boer MJ, van Hout BA, Liem AL, Suryapranata H, Hoorntje JCA, Zijlstra F. A cost-effective analysis of primary angioplasty versus thrombolysis for acute myocardial infarction. Am J Cardiol 1995; 76:830–833.
13. Kaplan EL, Meier P. Nonparametric estimation from incomplete observations. J Am Stat Assoc 1958; 53:457–481.
14. Cox DR. Regression models and life tables. J R Stat Soc 1972; 34:187–220.
15. The GUSTO Angiographic Investigators. The effects of tissue plasminogen activator, streptokinase, or both on coronary artery patency, ventricular function, and survival, after acute myocardial infarction. N Engl J Med 1993; 329:1615–1622.

16. Grines CL, Browne KF, Marco J, et al. for the Primary Angioplasty in Myocardial Infarction Study group. A comparison of immediate angioplasty with thrombolytic therapy for acute myocardial infarction. N Engl J Med 1993; 328:673–679.

17. Meijer A, Verheugt FWA, Werter CJPS, Lie KI, van der Pol JMJ, van Eenige MJ. Aspirin versus coumadin in the prevention of reocclusion and recurrent ischemia after successful thrombolysis: a prospective placebo-controlled angiographic study. Circulation 1993; 87: 1524–1530.

18. White HD, French JK, Hamer AW, et al. Frequent reocclusion of patent infarct-related arteries between 4 weeks and 1 year: effects of antiplatelet therapy. J Am Coll Cardiol 1995; 25:218–223.

19. Califf RM, Harrelson-Woodlief L, Topol EJ. Left ventricular ejection fraction may not be useful as an end point of thrombolytic therapy comparative trials. Circulation 1990; 82:1847–1853.

20. Morris RM, White HD. Therapeutic trials in coronary thrombosis should measure left ventricular function as primary end-point of treatment. Lancet 1988; 1:104–106.

21. Simoons ML, Serruys PW, van den Brand M, et al. Early thrombolysis in acute myocardial infarction: limitation of infarct size and improved survival. J Am Coll Cardiol 1986; 7:717–728.

22. Simoons ML, Vos J, Tijssen JGP, et al. Long-term benefit of early thrombolytic therapy in patients with acute myocardial infarction: 5 year follow-up of a trial conducted by the interuniversity Cardiology Institute of the Netherlands. J Am Coll Cardiol 1988; 14:1609–1615.

23. Hannan EL, Racz M, Ryan TJ, et al. Coronary angioplasty volume outcome relationships for hospitals and cardiologists. JAMA 1997; 279:892–898.

24. Zijlstra F, van 't Hof AWJ, Liem AL, Hoorntje JCA, Suryapranata H, de Boer MJ. Transferring patients for primary angioplasty. A retrospective analysis of 104 selected high risk patients with acute myocardial infarction. Heart 1997; 78:333–336.

25. Zahn R, Vogt A, Neuhaus KL, Schuster S, Senges J for the ALKK Study Group. Angioplasty in acute myocardial infarction in clinical practice: the ALKK angioplasty registry (abstr). J Am Coll Cardiol 1997; 29:15A.

26. Suryapranata H. Primary stenting in acute myocardial infarction. Main session, Aug 29 1996; 18th Congress of the European Society of Cardiology, Birmingham, UK.

27. The Capture Investigators. Randomised placebo-controlled trial of abciximab before and during coronary intervention in refractory unstable angina: the CAPTURE study. Lancet 1997; 349:1429–1435.

Section C
Aspirin

As Sleight notes, the evidence from ISIS-2 of a clinically important treatment benefit of aspirin in acute myocardial infarction is completely compelling. The additive effect of aspirin and thrombolysis, which was also clearly demonstrated in ISIS-2, along with aspirin's low cost, ease of administration, and high tolerability have made it an essential part of the early and chronic treatment of patients with acute infarction. Whether the routine use of aspirin alone will be displaced by its combination with newer antithrombotic agents awaits the results of ongoing clinical trials.

12

ISIS-2

PETER SLEIGHT

Second International Study of Infarct Survival Collaborative Group.
Randomized trial of intravenous streptokinase, oral aspirin, both or neither
among 17,187 cases of suspected acute myocardial infarction: ISIS–2.
Lancet 1988; ii: 349–360.

INTRODUCTION

Although the first Antiplatelet Trialists Collaboration (ATC) had shown the benefit of longer-term aspirin in an overview of 10 trials in patients postinfarction (1), there had been only one previous small trial of a single tablet of aspirin in acute myocardial infarction (MI) (2).

The ISIS-2 trial was therefore planned as a 2×2 factorial design comparison of streptokinase versus placebo and aspirin versus placebo in patients presenting within 24 hours of a suspected MI. Since the gastric absorption of aspirin might be delayed in the presence of MI and by the administration of opiates, the first tablet (162.5 mg, enteric-coated or placebo) was to be chewed, with a subsequent daily dose of one tablet of active aspirin or placebo for 28 days. The endpoints were determined at 35 days (when any aspirin effect would be mostly gone) and at subsequent later follow-up, determined from government records.

The trial was funded by Behringwerke AG, a subsidiary of Hoechst, but was designed, executed, and analyzed independently of the company. The factorial design enabled the large-scale testing of aspirin in acute MI, which otherwise might have been difficult or impossible to fund because of the low cost of aspirin. The inclusion of aspirin in combination with streptokinase in one quarter of the patients did present some initial difficulty because, due to the possible risk of bleeding, the package insert for Streptase® warned against the combination of streptokinase with aspirin. In the end, the combination was hugely beneficial.

The dose of aspirin chosen—about half a normal tablet—was arbitrary; a lower dose, although likely to be effective in continued use, might not have been rapidly effective at onset, whereas it seemed that a higher dose would not be any more effective and would be likely to give rise to greater gastrotoxicity (3). With the benefit of hindsight the dose chosen seems about right.

Simple trial procedures, such as telephone randomization and limited discharge information, enabled the randomization of 17,187 patients from 415 hospitals in 16 countries. Patients were eligible if thought by their physicians to be cases of suspected MI without clear indications for, or contraindications to, streptokinase or aspirin. The contra-indications were risk of bleeding from peptic ulcer, recent surgery, or allergy to streptoki-nase or aspirin. At discharge a prerandomization ECG and a single-sided discharge form were returned. This enabled subsequent follow-up through government records.

   The ECG was read blind to the treatment allocation.

RESULTS

During the first 5 weeks there were 804 (9.4%) deaths among the 8587 patients allocated active aspirin compared with 1016 (11.8%) in those allocated placebo ($p < 0.00001$)—a highly impressive 23% SD4 reduction in the odds of death (4) (Fig. 1a). The benefit of aspirin was seen both with active streptokinase and placebo streptokinase infusion (Fig. 2). Active streptokinase plus active aspirin reduced the mortality on double placebo from 13.2 to 8% (Fig. 1b). The early mortality benefit from aspirin seen at 35 days persisted to a median follow-up of 15 months in the original publication and to 10 years in a later follow-up (5) (Fig. 3). With aspirin, unlike streptokinase, there was no decrease in benefit with increasing time from onset to randomization.

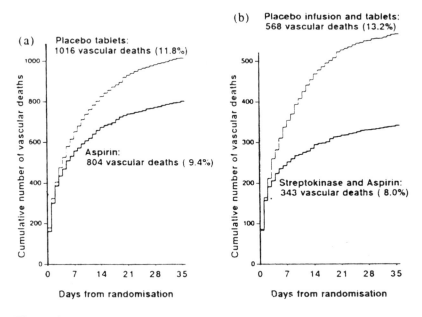

Figure 1 Cumulative vascular mortality in days 0-35. (a) All patients allocated active aspirin vs. all allocated placebo tablets; and (b) all patients allocated streptokinase + aspirin vs. all allocated neither. (Statistical tests to day 35—observed number of vascular deaths in active treatment group minus expected number, and the standard deviation of this difference: (a)–105.3 SD 20.2, (b)–112.1 SD 14.3). (From Ref. 4.)

Section D
Beta-Blockers: Early Use

The efficacy of early, intravenous use of beta-blockers in reducing mortality in patients with suspected acute myocardial infarction was established prior to the advent of acute reperfusion. The ISIS-1, Göteborg, and MIAMI trials all showed a mortality benefit to early treatment; ISIS-1 enrolled a sufficient number of patients to achieve clear statistical significance, even though entry criteria were not restrictive and the study population was at low risk (the 7-day mortality in the placebo arm was only about 4.5%).

The role of early beta blockade in the context of more ''modern'' infarction therapy with aspirin and thrombolysis was addressed by TIMI-IIB. Although there was no demonstrable mortality benefit (in a modest-sized trial not designed to detect one), early use of beta-blockers reduced the rate of recurrent ischemic events and was well tolerated.

Intravenous beta-blockers should be considered for all patients who do not have clear contraindications to their use within 12 hours of the onset of their infarction. These agents are likely to be especially beneficial in patients with tachycardia, hypertension, or ongoing ischemia.

13

ISIS-1

PETER SLEIGHT

Second International Study of Infarct Survival Collaboration Group.
Randomized trial of intravenous atenolol among 16,027 cases of
suspected acute myocardial infarction: ISIS-1. Lancet 1986; ii: 57–66.

INTRODUCTION

The ISIS-1 trial developed as a result of several converging strands. The first and initiating stimulus was the thesis work of Salim Yusuf, which examined two rival methods of measuring infarct size in humans (1). Sobel and Shell (2) favored the serial measurement of enzyme release from necrotic myocardial cells, whereas Braunwald and Maroko favored serial ECG maps of the precordium to determine infarct size (3). Yusuf, a newly qualified Indian Rhodes scholar to Oxford, set out to compare the two methods in a large number of consecutive patients presenting to the Radcliffe Infirmary in Oxford with acute myocardial infarction (AMI). By modification of both methods he was able to show a reasonable correlation between these measures and the severity of myocardial necrosis (1,4).

This seemed a good starting point to investigate whether treatment could reduce infarct size in humans. We therefore planned a study to evaluate the effects of beta-blockade. We began a randomized comparison of oral atenolol versus placebo but found that oral treatment only produced significant bradycardia after 24 hours or more, perhaps due to poor absorption of tablets in ill patients sedated by morphine, which delays gastric emptying (4). We therefore planned a trial using intravenous atenolol.

The second strand in the genesis of ISIS-1 was born in discussion with Richard Peto. Peto had been closely involved in the U.K. Medical Research Council trials of leukemia and had experience of the benefits of multicenter collaboration in order to recruit adequate numbers for statistical validity (5). He was also convinced of the need to have trials large enough to detect modest benefits rather than the overoptimistic hopes of individual investigators. This preliminary discussion led to a publication explaining the need for trials of adequate size (6). Peto pointed out that we would need several thousand patients randomized between beta-blockade and placebo or control to detect modest benefits, which would nevertheless be of great clinical importance in common diseases such as AMI. At that time this was a novel concept to cardiologists, but to their credit they joined in with great enthusiasm. In order to demonstrate that this was a practical and safe concept, we carried out a pilot survey (4).

This was very important, since at that time clinicians were understandably concerned and fearful that patients might be harmed by blockade of seemingly beneficial reflex responses to left ventricular (LV) damage. However, as Harris earlier pointed out (7), these primitive baroreflex and renin-angiotensin responses were probably initially designed to combat hypotension resulting from trauma or bleeding, leading to preservation of blood volume and of the supply pressure to vital organs such as the brain. They thus led to inappropriate responses, such as vasoconstriction and fluid retention, in patients with AMI. Even after the pilot trial clinicians were still fearful of precipitating heart failure and so were reluctant to randomize patients at higher risk of death.

A third strand was an overview of the use of beta-blockade in patients after myocardial infarction (8), which showed that beta-blockers were particularly beneficial in reducing sudden death and in preventing further myocardial infarction. At the time of this overview we speculated (on the basis of retrospective analysis) that beta-blockers with intrinsic sympathomimetic activity (ISA) might not be as effective as those without ISA. However, our caveat at the time (that this might be merely the result of data dredging) turned out to be justified, since a more recent French trial using acebutolol (which has moderate ISA) gave the most impressive result to date (9).

All three strands led to the genesis of the first mega trial in cardiovascular disease—ISIS-1.

ISIS-1 DESIGN

ISIS-1 was designed to detect a modest benefit from intravenous beta-blockade in AMI—a reduction of one death for every 200 patients treated. Peto calculated that we would need to recruit about 15,000 patients, a formidable prospect in those days.

We chose intravenous atenolol because a pilot study with oral atenolol showed no significant reduction in heart rate during the first 19–24 hours (10). A similar trial design was adopted in the MIAMI study, which began later and finished earlier after randomizing about 5500 patients to metoprolol or placebo. The results of MIAMI, although broadly similar to ISIS-1, did not achieve statistical significance, probably because of the smaller sample size (11).

In order to achieve randomization of around 15,000 patients, we strove to simplify the normal trial procedures and severely restrict the data collected (12). The data entry and discharge forms were reduced to single pages. Entry and randomization was by telephone (at the price of a local call). This eliminated the well-known manipulation of envelope-based randomization, since treatment allocation was not disclosed until all entry data identifiers [age, sex, blood pressure, heart rate (HR), diabetes, previous MI history, and hours from onset of pain] had been recorded.

Since the effect of intravenous beta-blockade on pulse rate is readily seen, we conducted an open trial with no placebo. Active treatment consisted of an immediate intravenous injection of atenolol 5 mg over 5 minutes followed by a further 5-mg injection 10 minutes later if undue bradycardia (HR < 40) had not occurred. This was followed by oral atenolol (50 mg b.d. or 100 mg o.d.) for one week.

In ISIS-1 we asked also for a prerandomization ECG to be sent for central reading. This revealed the problems inherent in such demands because some ECGs sent were clearly post treatment, rather than prerandomization. As a result later ISIS trials required the local physician to report the entry ECG by telephone.

The patients recruited were eligible if in the opinion of the responsible physician they were thought to be within 12 hours of the onset of an AMI. Follow-up after discharge was only of mortality, obtained through central government records.

The prerandomization ECG was read blind to treatment allocation and allotted (in order) to bundle branch block (R or L—age not determined) and coded otherwise as probable or possible infarction on the ECG depending on the degree of ST elevation. ST depression, Q-waves, or ST elevation were recorded separately.

RESULTS

In the event 16,027 patients with suspected AMI were randomized from 245 hospitals over 3½ years (June 1981 to January 1985). Baseline data were, as expected, highly com-

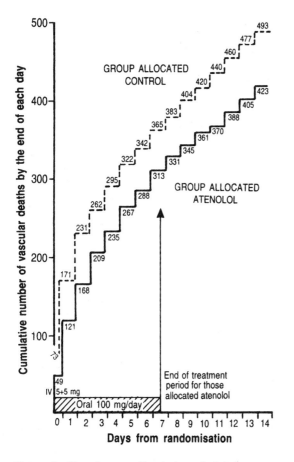

Figure 1 Vascular mortality during scheduled treatment period (days 0–7) and immediately after (to day 14). In both groups combined life-table analysis indicates vascular mortality of 4% at 1 week, 7% at 1 month, and 11, 14, and 16 at 1, 2, and 3 years, respectively. No ''rebound'' increase is apparent after the scheduled end of trial treatment on day 7. There happened to be slightly more patients allocated atenolol (8037) than control (7990): correction for this would effectively involve adding about two extra deaths to the control group. (From Ref. 12.)

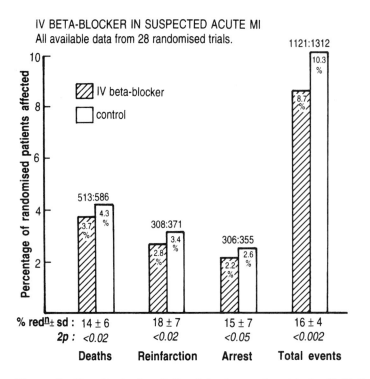

Figure 2 Mortality in days 0–7, reinfarction, and ventricular fibrillation in hospital from all available randomized trials of early IV beta-blockade in acute myocardial infarction. Total events are the sum of percentages for cardiac arrest, for reinfarction, and for deaths in days 0–7. (This total is about 10% greater than the percentages suffering at least one event, for a few suffered more than one type of event.) Percentages relate only to those with relevant data (certain information, particularly on reinfarction, was not recorded for a few studies). (From Ref. 12.)

parable. Mean baseline BP was approximately 145/79 mmHg; 38% were randomized within 4 hours of onset; mean age was 59 years. Only 7% did not continue to the oral atenolol phase. The mean dose of intravenous atenolol was 8.1 mg. The main endpoint was vascular mortality.

During the 7-day treatment period, there were 313 deaths with atenolol and 365 in the controls (3.89 vs. 4.57% ca. 15% reduction, $p = 0.04$). This placebo mortality rate is low because of the then fear of this treatment among the randomizing physicians. Later studies (9,11) suggest greater benefit in sicker patients.

Contrary to the opinion at the time, the benefit was seen even in the first 24–36 hours (121 atenolol vs. 171 control deaths; $p < 0.003$) (Fig. 1), i.e., the time when shock or heart block was most feared. There was a very small, though significant, 1.5% excess of inotrope use in patients given atenolol and a small excess of complete heart block, largely in patients with a prolonged P-R interval on the entry ECG. The results in ISIS-1 were reinforced by the data from MIAMI and from 26 small trials of intravenous beta-blockade in AMI (Fig. 2).

DISCUSSION

Retrospective analysis of the data suggested that the benefit was greatest in those with entry systolic blood pressures (SBP) > 110–120 mmHg. Overall the overview of all the evidence at the time of publication suggested that early intravenous blockade in selected patients with AMI might result in the avoidance of one death, one early reinfarction, and one early cardiac arrest for every 200 patients treated, with further gains from continuation long term.

A later audit of the causes of death in ISIS-1 for U.K. and Scandinavian patients showed that the treatment was particularly likely to reduce cardiac rupture and sudden death (13). Since cardiac rupture occurs particularly early in patients receiving thrombolysis (14), intravenous beta-blockade may be even more beneficial in conjunction with thrombolytic treatment than it was in ISIS-1, in the prethrombolytic era.

CONCLUSION

Perhaps because of the greater dramatic impact of thrombolysis, intravenous beta-blockade is now neglected in many countries (e.g., the United Kingdom), while being well used in others (e.g., the United States, Australia). At present, interest is reviving after promising results with carvedilol (15).

REFERENCES

1. Yusuf S. Thesis. Beta adrenergic blockade in myocardial infarction. University of Oxford, 1980.
2. Shell WE, Sobel BE. Biochemical markers of ischemic injury. Circulation 1976; 53:I98–I106.
3. Braunwald E, Maroko PR. ST-segment mapping. Realistic and unrealistic expectations. Circulation 1976; 54:529–532.
4. Yusuf S, Sleight P, Rossi P, Ramsdale D, Peto R, Furze L, Sterry H, Pearson M, Motwani R Parish S, Gray R, Bennett D, Bray C. Reduction in infarct size, arrhythmias, chest pain and morbidity by early intravenous beta blockade in suspected acute myocardial infarction. Circulation 1983; 67:32–41.
5. Peto R, Pike MC, Armitage P, Breslow NE, Cox DR, Howard SV, Mantel N, McPherson K, Peto J, Smith PG. Design and analysis of randomised clinical trials requiring prologed observation of each patient: 1. Introduction and design. Br J Cancer 1976; 34:585–612.
6. Yusuf S, Collins R, Peto R. Why do we need some large, simple randomised trials? Stat Med 1984; 3:409–420.
7. Harris P. Congestive cardiac failure: central role of the arterial blood pressure. Br Heart J 1987; 59:190–203.
8. Yusuf S, Peto R, Lewis J, Collins R, Sleight P. Beta blockade during and after myocardial infarction: an overview of the randomised trials. Prog Card Dis 1985; 27:335–371.
9. Boissel J-P, Leizorovicz A, Picolet H, Peyrieux JC. APSI (Acebutolol et Prévention Secondaire de l'Infarctus). Secondary prevention after high risk acute myocardial infarction with low dose acebutolol. Am J Cardiol 1990; 66:251–260.
10. Rossi PR, Yusuf S, Ramsdale D, Furze L, Sleight P. Reduction of ventricular arrhythmias by early intravenous atenolol in suspected acute myocardial infarction. Br Med J 1983; 286:506–510.

11. The MIAMI Trial Research Group: Metoprolol in acute myocardial infarction (MIAMI). A randomised placebo-controlled international trial. Eur Heart J 1985; 6:199–226.

12. ISIS-1 (International Studies of Infarct Survival) Collaborative Group. Randomised trial of intravenous atenolol among 16,027 cases of suspected acute myocardial infarction: ISIS-1. Lancet 1986; ii:57–66.

13. ISIS-1 (First International Study of Infarct Survival) Collaborative Group. Mechanisms for the early mortality reduction produced by beta blockade started early in acute myocardial infarction: ISIS-1. Lancet 1988; i:921–923.

14. Honan MB, Harrell FE, Reimer KA, Califf RM, Mark DB, Pryor DB, Hlatky MA. Cardiac rupture, mortality and the timing of thrombolytic therapy: a meta-analysis. J Am Coll Cardiol 1990; 16:359–367.

15. Basu S, Senior R, Raftery EB, Lahiri A. The association between cardiac events and myocardial ischaemia following thrombolysis in acute myocardial infarction and the impact of carvedilol. Eur Heart J 1996; 17:43–47.

sponding to an estimated 3200 patients with definite MI. The Steering Committee acted upon this option in September 1983, and by extending the recruitment period, a total number of 5778 patients was finally included.

Statistical Methods

The 15-day mortality was statistically assessed with Fisher's exact test in fourfold tables. Mantel-Haenszel's method was used to test differences in survival curves. p-Values are in general only given for analyses stated to be made according to the project protocol. A two-tailed test with a p-value of <0.05 was regarded as significant.

RESULTS

Mortality

There were 142 deaths in the placebo group and 123 deaths in the metoprolol group. The cumulative mortality for the trial period of 15 days was 4.9% in the placebo group and 4.3% in the metoprolol group, a difference of 13%, with 95% confidence interval of -8 to 33% (Fig. 1) (7,8).

Table 4 shows total mortality in all patients and in various baseline subgroups. In subgroups with the higher placebo mortality, the effect of metoprolol tended to be more marked than in the entire study population. Thus, patients with a clinical history of cardio-vascular disease or diabetes had a markedly higher placebo mortality, and the mortality reduction with metoprolol was between 24 and 49%. Time to treatment (above or below the median) did not influence placebo mortality, and there was no indication that very early start of treatment was better than later. All patients received their treatment within 24 hours of the onset of symptoms. Patients with a previous history of chronic treatment with cardiac glycosides and diuretics or given diuretics in hospital before randomization also had a markedly higher placebo mortality and a better reduction with metoprolol than the total study population.

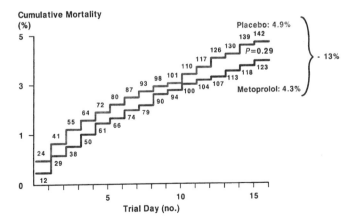

Figure 1 Cumulative mortality and number of deaths in the Metoprolol in Acute Myocardial Infarction Trial (5778 patients). (From Ref. 7.)

Table 4 Total Mortality in All Patients and in Various Baseline Subgroups

Group	Percent mortality (no. of deaths/pts)				Difference (%)
	Placebo		Metoprolol		
All patients	4.9	(142/2901)	4.3	(123/2877)	13
Clinical history					
Myocardial infarction	7.7	(36/467)	4.6	(21/459)	41
Angina pectoris	6.0	(51/855)	4.5	(36/798)	24
Congestive heart failure	9.5	(10/105)	6.3	(7/112)	34
Hypertension	7.6	(31/410)	4.9	(19/390)	36
Diabetes	11.3	(25/221)	5.7	(11/192)	49
Delay time					
≤6.7 hr (median)	4.9	(72/1477)	4.8	(68/1415)	1
>6.7 hr	4.9	(70/1424)	3.8	(55/1462)	24
Chronic treatment					
Cardiac glycosides	9.3	(17/182)	3.3	(5/152)	65
Diuretics	7.4	(32/430)	4.4	(18/406)	40
Treatment in hospital before randomization					
Diuretics	9.1	(31/341)	7.4	(24/326)	19

Source: Adapted from Ref. 7.

In a retrospective multivariate analysis the placebo patients could be classified into categories of increasing mortality risk. The major predictors of mortality among the baseline variables were age > 60 years (median), abnormal ECG at entry, history of MI, angina pectoris, congestive heart failure, hypertension, or diabetes, and chronic or acute treatment with diuretics and/or cardiac glycosides before randomization. Baseline characteristics for the placebo- and metoprolol-treated groups were comparable within the low-risk (≤2 risk predictors) and the high-risk (≥3 risk predictors) groups, respectively. As can be seen from Figure 2, metoprolol was associated with 29% lower mortality in the high mortality risk group (2038 patients), while there was no apparent effect in the low mortality risk group (3740 patients). For comparison, a similar analysis was performed from the Göteborg Metoprolol trial, from which it was found that mortality within 15 days after randomization was reduced by 45% in the high-risk group (780 patients) while no apparent effect was seen in the low mortality risk group (615 patients) (7–9). The difference between the treatment groups of the whole study population was maintained after 1 year of follow-up (10). In the MIAMI trial as well as the Göteborg Metoprolol trial, it was found that in subgroups with a high mortality, metoprolol had a more marked reduction. This has been reported in separate studies regarding diabetes (11) and hypertension (12).

Classification of deaths is seen in Table 5 (8). Most of the deaths occurred in hospital. Of those who died, about half had clinical congestive heart failure prior to death. A rather high proportion of the patients died by rupture of ventricular wall. Autopsy was very often performed to confirm a clinical suspicion of ventricular wall rupture. Analysis of death in subgroups according to type and site of infarction must be interpreted very cautiously. Since treatment was started during the phase of myocardial infarction evolution, the treatment has influenced a proportion of patients with definite infarctions of various types and sites. The majority of deaths occurred among patients with a definite myocardial infarction (137 deaths in the placebo group, $n = 2099$ patients, and 120 in the metoprolol group, lol in patients admitted for a suspected acute myocardial infarction. Acta Med Scand 1984; suppl 680:40–49.

6. The Göteborg Metoprolol Trial in Acute Myocardial Infarction. Am J Cardiol 1984; 53(13): 1D–50D.

7. The MIAMI Trial Research Group. Metoprolol in acute myocardial infarction (MIAMI). A randomised placebo-controlled international trial. Eur Heart J 1985; 6:199–226.

8. The MIAMI Trial Research Group. MIAMI:Metoprolol in Acute Myocardial Infarction. Am J Cardiol 1985; 56(14):IG–57G.

9. Hjalmarson Å. International beta-blocker review in acute and postmyocardial infarction. Am J Cardiol 1988; 61:26B–29B.

10. Herlitz J, Karlson BW, Hjalmarson Å. Mortality and morbidity during one year of follow-up in suspected acute myocardial infarction in relation to early diagnosis: experiences from the MIAMI trial. J Intern Med 1990; 228(2):125–131.

11. Malmberg K, Herlitz J, Hjalmarson Å, Rydén L. Effects of metoprolol on mortality and late infarction in diabetics with suspected acute myocardial infarction. Retrospective data from two large studies. Eur Heart J 1989; 10:423–428.

12. Herlitz J, Hjalmarson Å. Effects of metoprolol among hypertensives with suspected acute myocardial infarction. World Report 1990; 3:40–43.

13. Herlitz J, Waldenström J, Hjalmarson Å, for the MIAMI Trial Research Group. Infarct size limitation after early intervention with metoprolol in the MIAMI trial. Cardiology 1988; 75: 117–122.

14. ISIS-1 Collaborative Group. Randomised trial of intravenous atenolol among 16,027 cases of suspected acute myocardial infarction: first international study of Infarct Survival Collaborative Group: ISIS-1. Lancet 1986; 2:57–66.

16

TIMI-IIB

ROBERT ROBERTS and EUGENE BRAUNWALD

Roberts R, Rogers WJ, Mueller HS, Lambrew CT, Diver DJ, Smith HC, Willerson JT, Knatterud GL, Forman S, Passamani E, Zaret BL, Wackers FJT, Braunwald E for the TIMI Investigators. Immediate versus deferred β-blockade following thrombolytic therapy in patients with acute myocardial infarction. Results of the thrombolysis in myocardial infarction (TIMI) II-B study. Circulation 1991; 83: 422–437.

INTRODUCTION

Thrombolytic therapy represents a major development in the management of patients with acute myocardial infarction (AMI), reducing the mortality in such patients admitted to the hospital from about 14% in the 1980s (1) to about 7% (2). Nevertheless, early coronary artery reocclusion following thrombolytic therapy occurs in 10–20% and reinfarction is seen in at least 5% of patients receiving such therapy (3). Indeed, it is estimated that about 40% of the early deaths that occur following thrombolytic therapy are due to reinfarction (4). The TIMI-II trial, completed in 1988, was designed to determine whether these sequelae would be minimized by the routine performance, after thrombolytic therapy, of coronary arteriography and, if appropriate, percutaneous transluminal coronary angioplasty 18–48 hours after thrombolytic therapy (5,6). Within this trial, the effects of immediate versus deferred beta adrenoreceptor blocker (beta-blocker) therapy were also assessed in the beta-blocker substudy (7).

RATIONALE FOR BETA-BLOCKERS AS ADJUNCTIVE THERAPY IN REPERFUSION

In the prethrombolytic era, beta-blockers were widely used in patients with MI. Thus, oral beta-blockers begun days or weeks following AMI and administered chronically had been shown to improve survival (8,9). Also in the early hours of an evolving AMI, beta-blockers administered intravenously reduced early mortality (10). Since beta-blockers are used routinely in the treatment of hypertension and angina, many patients are already receiving these drugs at the time they develop AMI. Since antiarrhythmic drugs have been shown to be ineffective or deleterious as routine prophylactic measures in AMI, beta-blocker therapy has for a number of years been the initial choice for the prevention and treatment of many arrhythmias in patients with evolving myocardial infarction.

Prior to the thrombolytic era, patients surviving acute myocardial infarction exhibited a period of 6–12 weeks during which they are at especially high risk of recurrent ischemic and arrhythmic events which are amenable to beta-blocker therapy (11,12). However, after reperfusion treatment this period is shortened to 10–12 days and begins within hours of reperfusion (13). Thus, the need for immediate therapy and the potential for benefit exists. Accordingly, the beta-blockade substudy of the TIMI-IIB trial was designed to compare the safety and efficacy of beta-blockers given intravenously along with a thrombolytic agent and followed by oral beta-blockers with oral therapy begun 6 days after entry.

DESIGN OF TIMI-IIB

The 3534 patients with AMI enrolled in the TIMI-II trials were all treated with tissue plasminogen activator (tPA), heparin, and aspirin (5). The major inclusion criteria included: (1) age < 76 years; (2) chest discomfort suggestive of AMI ≥ 30 minutes; (3) ST segment elevation ≥ 0.1 mV in two contiguous leads; and (4) the feasibility of initiating thrombolytic therapy within 4 hours of the onset of the chest pain that precipitated hospital admission. The exclusion criteria included: (1) a history of cerebral vascular disease or of a bleeding disorder; (2) blood pressure > 180 mmHg systolic or 110 mmHg diastolic; (3) surgery within the previous 2 weeks; (4) recent prolonged cardiopulmonary resuscitation; (5) PTCA or severe trauma within 6 months; (6) previous coronary artery bypass surgery or prosthetic heart valve replacement; and (7) left bundle branch block, dilated cardiomyopathy, or other serious illness.

Thrombolytic therapy consisted of tPA administered in a dose not to exceed 100 mg starting with an initial 6 mg bolus followed by 54 mg in the first hour, 20 mg in the second hour, and 5 mg in each of the next 4 hours. Of the 2948 patients enrolled in TIMI-IIB, 1514 (51%) were excluded from the beta-blocker substudy because of the presence of the following contraindications to intravenous beta-blockade: (1) a ventricular rate < 55 bpm (27.1%); (2) systolic arterial pressure consistently < 100 mmHg (21.3%); (3) rales involving one-third or more of the lung fields or pulmonary edema on chest x-ray (16.4%); (4) significant first, second, or third degree arterio-ventricular block (12.4%); (5) asthma by history, wheezing on examination, or chronic obstructive lung disease (11.0%); and (6) an implanted pacemaker (0.3%). This left 1434 (49%) patients who were eligible for the beta-blocker substudy. Of these patients, 720 were randomized to the immediate intravenous therapy group and 714 to the deferred therapy group. These 1434 patients were also equally randomized to the invasive or conservative strategies of TIMI-IIB in a 2×2 factorial design.

Metoprolol was selected for this substudy since at the time of this trial it was the only beta-blocker approved for intravenous use during AMI. This agent is cardioselective and had been shown to be well tolerated in patients with evolving AMI. Three intravenous injections of 5 mg of metoprolol were given at 2-minute intervals for a total dose of 15 mg. Heart rate, rhythm, and systolic blood pressure were monitored at a minimum of

1-minute intervals during the intravenous administration of the drug and at 1- to 2-minute intervals for 15 minutes thereafter. Fifteen minutes after the administration of the third intravenous dose of metoprolol, patients were given 50 mg metoprolol orally, and this dose was repeated every 12 hours during the first 24 hours; 100 mg was given every 12 hours thereafter. In patients assigned to the deferred oral beta-blocker group, metoprolol was initiated on day 6 (50 mg every 12 hours for one day, and 100 mg every 12 hours thereafter.)

The primary endpoint of the substudy was the left ventricular ejection fraction measured at rest by radionuclide ventriculography prior to hospital discharge. Power calculations indicated that with the sample size of 340 patients in each of the four treatment groups [immediate and deferred beta-blockade, and the invasive (routine, early angiography) and conservative (angiography with ischemia) management strategy], it was possible to detect a 3 percentage point difference in the left ventricular ejection fraction at a significance level of 0.05 with a probability of 80%. Other endpoints included left ventricular ejection fraction at rest and, after exercise both at hospital discharge and at 6 weeks, total mortality, nonfatal reinfarction, and recurrent ischemic events at 6 and 42 days.

RESULTS

Myocardial infarction was confirmed by enzymatic or electrocardiographic evidence in 95% of the patients. No significant differences were observed in the baseline characteristics in the two beta-blocker groups.

Of the 720 patients assigned to immediate beta-blockers, intravenous metoprolol was initiated in 90%, and of these 95% received follow-up oral therapy as specified. The mean time interval from the onset of symptoms to the initiation of thrombolytic therapy was 2.6 hours and the mean interval between the latter and the intravenous administration of beta-blocker was 42 minutes. Of the 714 patients assigned to the deferred beta-blockade group, 82% were begun on oral metoprolol on day 6 as specified. Most of the remainder had developed a contraindication to beta-blockade between randomization and day 6.

The intravenous metoprolol was well tolerated by 90% of the patients in whom treatment was begun. The other 10% did not receive the full dose because of the transient development of adverse effects, usually bradycardia or hypotension. In the immediate beta-blockade group the systolic arterial pressure decreased by an average of 9.8% compared to 7.1% in the deferred beta-blockade group ($p < 0.01$). The diastolic arterial pressure did not differ significantly between the two groups. The mean heart rate decreased by an average of 6% in the immediate beta-blocker group compared to an increase in the deferred beta-blocker group ($p < 0.001$). The occurrence of accelerated idioventricular rhythm during tPA infusion was more common in the immediate than the deferred beta-blockade groups (36.5% vs. 31.1%; $p = 0.03$). Otherwise, neither the appearance nor resolution of dysrhythmias differed significantly between the two treatment arms.

There were no differences in the mean resting left ventricular ejection fractions at hospital discharge in the two treatment groups: 51.0% in the immediate and 50.1% in the deferred beta-blockade groups. Likewise, there were no significant differences in the left ventricular ejection fractions at 6 weeks (50.4% and 50.8%) (Table 1). The left ventricular ejection fractions during exercise at hospital discharge and at the 6-week follow-up were

Table 1 Resting and Exercise Radionuclide Left Ventricular Ejection Fraction at Discharge and at 6-Week Follow-Up

	Mean (%)		
	Immediate beta-blocker ($n = 720$)	Deferred beta-blocker ($n = 714$)	p
At discharge			
Resting EF	51.0	50.1	0.22
Invasive strategy	51.6	50.3	0.21
Conservative strategy	50.3	49.8	0.53
Baseline exercise EF	50.7	50.3	0.60
Peak exercise EF	54.3	54.1	0.81
Peak EF-baseline EF	3.6	3.8	0.66
Infarcted zone segmental EF (rest)	48.7	49.1	0.83
At 6 weeks			
Resting EF	50.4	50.8	0.56
Baseline exercise EF	50.5	51.2	0.38
Peak exercise EF	53.6	54.3	0.50
Peak EF-baseline EF	3.2	3.1	0.77
Infarcted zone segmental EF (rest)	50.8	51.4	0.68

EF = ejection fraction.

also similar in the immediate and the deferred groups. A similar lack of effect of immediate beta-blockade on ventricular function was observed both in patients assigned to the invasive and the conservative strategies.

Immediate beta-blocker therapy had no effect on mortality at 6 days or 6 weeks (Table 2). However, immediate beta-blockade reduced the incidence of reinfarction (2.7% vs. 5.1%, $p = 0.02$) and recurrent ischemic chest pain (18.8% vs. 24.1%, $p < 0.02$), and this benefit was maintained at 6 weeks, but not at 1 year.

Analysis of prespecified subgroups showed that patients in the immediate beta-blocker group treated within 2 hours of the onset of symptoms exhibited a reduced incidence of the combined endpoint of recurrent death or myocardial infarction (5.4% vs. 13.7%, $p = 0.007$). On the other hand, in the subgroup treated 2–4 hours after the onset of symptoms, the incidence of these clinical events in the immediate and deferred blockade were similar (7.8% vs. 8.2%). In a prespecified analysis, none of the 259 low-risk patients treated with beta-blockade had died at 6 weeks, while 7 of the 252 patients in whom beta-blocker therapy was deferred died within this time period ($p = 0.007$). This significant difference persisted at 1 year ($p = 0.009$).

DISCUSSION

Lack of Effect of Beta-Blockers on Ventricular Function

The expectation that intravenous beta-blockade administered with thrombolytic therapy to patients with AMI would preserve ventricular function to a greater extent than thrombolytic therapy alone was predicated on the hypothesis that beta-blockade would further

Table 2 Effect of Immediate Versus Deferred Therapy with Beta-Blockers on Secondary
Endpoints by Life-Table Estimates

	Percent of patients		
	Immediate beta-blocker ($n = 720$)	Deferred beta-blocker ($n = 714$)	p
At 6 days			
Death	2.4	2.4	0.98
Death or reinfarction	4.7	7.0	0.07
Fatal or nonfatal reinfarction	2.7	5.1	0.02
Nonfatal reinfarction	2.4	4.7	0.02
Fatal reinfarction	0.3	0.4	0.65
Recurrent chest pain	18.8	24.1	0.02
At 6 weeks			
Death	3.6	3.5	0.91
Death or reinfarction	7.2	9.7	0.10
Fatal or nonfatal reinfarction	4.5	7.3	0.03
Nonfatal reinfarction	4.0	6.6	0.03
Fatal reinfarction	0.7	1.0	0.55

limit infarct size. Since there were no differences in the ejection fraction at rest or with
exercise, either at hospital discharge or at 6 weeks, it may be reasonably concluded that
metoprolol did not limit infarct size *substantially* in the presence of thrombolytic therapy.
However, the possibility that beta-blockade effected a clinically significant, albeit smaller
difference in left ventricular function cannot be excluded

The initial experimental studies assessing the effect of beta-blockade on limitation
of infarct size were promising (14). However, studies to assess the effect of beta-blockade
on infarct size in patients have always been open to some criticism because of the lack
of an accurate, direct method to quantify the extent of myocardial damage. Three trials
in the prethrombolytic era addressed this question. In the Myocardial Infarction Limitation
Study (MILIS), infarct size was assessed using precordial ST-segment mapping, MB CK
enzymatic estimates, and pyrophosphate scintigraphy (15). Beta-blockade was initiated
from 4 to 18 hours (average 8.5 hr) after the onset of symptoms and did not limit infarct
size, nor did it improve left ventricular ejection fraction compared to placebo. In contrast,
the International Collaborative Study Group showed that intravenous timolol administered
an average of 3.4 hours after the onset of symptoms reduced infarct size as estimated by
cumulative release of CK (16). Similarly, in the MIAMI trial using intravenous metoprolol,
infarct size as reflected in maximum serum activity of aspartate amino transferase was
reduced (12).

Reinfarction Reduced by Beta-Blockers Following
Thrombolytic Therapy

In the TIMI-IIB beta-blocker substudy, the number of reinfarctions (fatal and nonfatal)
in the patients who received immediate beta-blockade was 19 (2.7%) compared to 36
(5.1%) in the deferred group over the 6-day period ($p = 0.02$), representing more than
a 40% relative reduction. Nonfatal reinfarction (2.4%) in the immediate beta-blocker group

was also about 40% lower than in the deferred group (2.4% vs. 4.7%, $p = 0.02$). At 6 weeks the incidence of reinfarction (fatal and nonfatal) was 4.5% in the immediate beta-blocker group and 7.2% in the deferred group ($p = 0.03$), and the incidence of nonfatal reinfarction was 4.0% vs. 6.6% ($p = 0.03$). Thus, it appears that the early intravenous administration of a beta-blocker along with thrombolytic therapy followed by oral administration effectively reduces the incidence of reinfarction and that this effect is maintained for at least 6 weeks.

The reduction in the frequency of reinfarction during the first 6 weeks in patients receiving immediate intravenous beta-blockade therapy is in keeping with observations made in the prethrombolytic era. Most of the large clinical trials performed in the pre-thrombolytic era were for secondary prevention, and beta-blockers were initiated as oral therapy most commonly 2–3 weeks following onset of infarction. Beta-blocker therapy was initiated intravenously within 24 hours followed by oral therapy in a number of trials, the largest of which was the First International Study of Infarction Survival (ISIS-1) trial (10,17), which included more than 16,000 patients admitted within 5 hours from the onset of symptoms. Treatment consisted of 5 mg of immediate intravenous atenolol followed by oral administration of 50 mg of atenolol every 12 hours for 7 days. In the ISIS-1 trial there was a nonsignificant trend towards a decreased incidence of reinfarction in the ateno-lol compared to the control group. In an attempt to resolve further this question, Yusuf pooled the data on 28 randomized trials that had utilized early intravenous beta-blockade and showed that the reinfarction rate was decreased by 18% ($p = 0.02$) (11) by early intravenous beta-blockade.

Effects on Arrhythmias, Chest Pain, and Recurrent Ischemia

No difference was observed in the incidence of ventricular arrhythmias between immediate and deferred beta-blocker therapy. By 6 days, recurrent chest pain had occurred in 18.8% of the patients randomized to the immediate beta-blocker group compared to 24.1% in the deferred beta-blocker group ($p = 0.02$). This reduction in recurrent ischemic pain was similar to that observed in previous beta-blocker trials carried out prior to the thrombolytic era (8–10,17–19).

Effect on Mortality

TIMI-IIB was underpowered to detect an effect of immediate, intravenous beta-blockers on mortality, and none was observed in the total population. However, the reduction of death in a prospectively identified low-risk subgroup of patients was significant ($p < 0.01$ at 6 weeks and 1 year). Although this observation is intriguing, because of the relatively small number of patients in this subgroup (511) it is not conclusive.

CONCLUSIONS

The results of the TIMI-IIB beta-blocker substudy indicate that intravenous beta-blockade is well tolerated in selected patients with early myocardial infarction undergoing reperfusion therapy. This intervention was not shown to improve ventricular function or reduce mortality in this modest-sized trial of 1434 patients. However, when added to thrombolytic therapy it was found to be effective in reducing the incidence of reinfarction and recurrent ischemia both at 6 days and at 6 weeks. It is therefore reasonable to administer intravenous beta-blockade for prevention of recurrent ischemia and reinfarction early in the course of myocardial infarction along with reperfusion therapy.

REFERENCES

1. May GS, Eberlein KA, Furberg CD, Passamani ER, DeMets DL. Secondary prevention after myocardial infarction: a review of long-term trials. Prog Cardiovasc Dis 1982; 24:331–352.
2. GUSTO Investigators. An international randomized trial comparing four thrombolytic strategies for acute myocardial infarction. N Engl J Med 1993; 329:673–682.
3. Ohman EM, Califf RM. Thrombolytic therapy: overview of clinical trials. Cor Artery Dis 1990; 1:223–233.
4. Ohman EM, Califf RM, Topol EJ, Candela RJ, Abbottsmith CW, Ellis SG, et al. Consequences of reocclusion after successful reperfusion therapy in acute myocardial infarction. Circulation 1990; 82:781–791.
5. TIMI Study Group. Comparison of invasive and conservative strategies after treatment with intravenous tissue plasminogen activator in acute myocardial infarction: results of the thrombolysis in myocardial infarction (TIMI) phase II trial. N Engl J Med 1989; 320:618–626.
6. Passamani E, Hodges M, Herman M, Grose R, Chaitman B, Rogers W, Forman S, Terrin M, Knatterud G, Robertson T, Braunwald E. The Thrombolysis in Myocardial Infarction (TIMI) Phase II Pilot Study: tissue plasminogen activator followed by percutaneous transluminal coronary angioplasty. J Am Coll Cardiol 1987; 10:51B–64B.
7. Roberts R, Rogers WJ, Mueller HS, Lambrew CT, Diver DJ, Smith HC, Willerson JT, Knatterud GL, Forman S, Passamani R, Zaret BL, Wackers FJT, Braunwald E for the TIMI Investigators. Immediate versus deferred beta-blockade following thrombolytic therapy in patients with acute myocardial infarction: Results of the Thrombolysis In Myocardial Infarction (TIMI) II-B subgroup analyses. Circulation 1991; 83:422–437.
8. The Norwegian Multicenter Study Group. Timolol-induced reduction in mortality and reinfarction in patients surviving acute myocardial infarction. N Engl J Med 1981; 304:801–807.
9. Beta-Blocker Heart Attack Trial Research Group. A randomized trial of propranolol in patients with acute myocardial infarction. Mortality results. JAMA 1982; 247:1707–1714.
10. ISIS-1 (First International Study of Infarct Survival) Collaborative Group. Mechanisms for the early mortality reduction produced by beta-blockade started early in acute myocardial infarction: ISIS-1. Lancet 1988; 1:921–923.
11. Yusuf S, Peto R, Lewis J, Collin R, Sleight P. Beta-blockade during and after myocardial infarction: an overview of the randomized trials. Prog Cardiovasc Dis 1985; 27:335–371.
12. The MIAMI Trial Research Group. Metoprolol in acute myocardial infarction (MIAMI): a randomized placebo-controlled international trial. Eur Heart J 1985; 6:199–226.
13. Schaer DH, Ross AM, Wasserman AG. Reinfarction, recurrent angina and reocclusion after thrombolytic therapy. Circulation 1987; 76:II–57.
14. Maroko PR, Kjekshus JK, Sobel BE, Watanabe T, Covell JW, Ross J Jr, Braunwald E. Factors influencing infarct size following experimental coronary artery occlusions. Circulation 1971; 43:67–82.
15. Roberts R, Croft C, Gold HK, Hartwell TD, Jaffe AS, Muller JE, Mullin SM, Parker C, Passamani ER, Poole WK, Raabe DS, Rude RE, Stone PH, Turi ZG, Sobel BE, Willerson JT, Braunwald E and the MILIS Study Group. Effect of propranolol on myocardial infarct size in a randomized, blinded, multicenter trial. N Engl J Med 1984; 311:218–225.
16. The International Collaborative Study Group. Reduction of infarct size with the early use of timolol in acute myocardial infarction. N Engl J Med 1984; 310:9.

17. ISIS-1 (First International Study of Infarct Survival) Collaborative Group. Randomized trial of intravenous atenolol among 16,027 cases of suspected acute myocardial infarction. ISIS-I. Lancet 1986; 2:57–66.

18. Yusuf S. Interventions that potentially limit myocardial infarct size: overview of clinical trials. Am J Cardiol 1987; 60:11A–17A.

19. Hjalmarson Å, Elmfeldt D, Herlitz J, Holmberg S, Malek I, Nyberg G, et al. Effect on mortality of metoprolol in acute myocardial infarction. Lancet 1981; 821:823–827.

Section E
Beta-Blockers: Delayed Use

As with early intravenous beta-blockade, the strongest evidence in favor of using these agents orally on a chronic basis comes from older studies performed before the use of reperfusion and antithrombotics. The Norwegian Multicenter Study and BHAT found the greatest benefit among high-risk patients—those with larger infarcts, advanced age, and ventricular arrhythmias. Although the magnitude of the treatment benefit is lower in patients without these poor prognostic markers, and may be lower still in patients who have had successful revascularization, the evidence still supports the broad use of these drugs in all infarct survivors. In low-risk individuals, therapy need not be continued indefinitely, but can probably be stopped after about 1 year.

17

The Norwegian Timolol Study

TERJE R. PEDERSEN

The Norwegian Multicenter Study Group. Timolol-induced reduction in
mortality and reinfarction in patients surviving acute myocardial
infarction. N Engl J Med 1981; 304: 801–807.

STUDY BACKGROUND AND OBJECTIVES

When the first beta-adrenergic blocking agent became available in the early 1960s (1),
its potential as an anti-ischemic drug was immediately recognized and tested in patients
with angina pectoris (2). During the next decade, several small clinical trials were carried
out using beta-blockers in the acute phase of myocardial infarction without convincing
results (3–12). In 1974, Wilhelmsson et al. (13) reported a significant reduction in sudden
death mortality using alprenolol compared with placebo in survivors of acute myocardial
infarction, starting treatment 4 weeks after infarction and continuing for 2 years. The study
comprised only 230 patients, and the difference in total mortality between the alprenolol
group and placebo was not statistically significant. Shortly afterwards a larger study reported reduction in mortality by practolol compared to placebo (14). However, a large
number of deaths occurring after withdrawal of the study drug had not been included in
the statistical analysis. When they were included, the difference in total mortality turned
out not to be statistically significant. In a subsequent study by Barber, practolol only
influenced prognosis favorably in a subset of patients (15).

These clinical trials were paralleled and followed by laboratory research indicating
several apparently favorable mechanisms of action of beta-blockers. In 1977, beta-blockers
had emerged as one of the most promising drugs in the prevention of ischemic heart
disease events. However, the clinical studies performed until then were inadequate in
either size or duration of follow-up, comprised mostly low-risk patients, had used low drug
dosages, faulty statistical methods, or had other deficiencies that rendered the results controversial. Therefore, a new study was undertaken with timolol. Screening for patients
started in January 1978, and the study was completed in October 1990. The main results
were published in April 1991 (16).

STUDY DESIGN

The methods were summarized in the first report and were published in detail in 1993 (16,17).

Design and Organization

The study was designed as a multicenter randomized, double-blind placebo-controlled trial with randomization in blocks within each center. Patients were recruited at 20 clinical centers in Norway. Each center had at least two investigators and a study nurse who coordinated follow-up. A steering committee of internists, cardiologists, a clinical epidemiologist, and a statistician was responsible for the study and reporting the results. This committee classified all deaths. The study was performed under the auspices of an ethical review committee who performed a total of three interim analyses of the study at predefined intervals.

Patients

Patients aged 20–75 years with a confirmed acute myocardial infarction admitted to the hospital within 48 hours of onset of symptoms were eligible for the study if they could be randomized 7–28 days after onset. Acute myocardial infarction was defined as the presence of at least two of the following three criteria:

1. Central chest pain of at least 15 minutes duration or acute pulmonary edema or cardiogenic shock if hypovolemia, intoxication, or cardiac valvular disease had been eliminated as a cause.
2. Electrocardiographic series with development of pathological Q-wave and/or transient T-inversion in at least two leads. A Q-wave was considered pathological if it had a width of ≥ 0.04 seconds and an amplitude of ≥ 0.4 mV or $\geq 25\%$ of the following R-wave. The ST-segment elevation had to be ≥ 0.1 mV in leads I, II, II, aVL, aVF, V_5, V_6 and/or ≥ 0.2 mV in leads V_2, V_3, and V_4. The T-inversion had to be ≥ 0.1 mV in amplitude.
3. Two separate serum aspartate aminotransferase (ASAT) values above the upper-normal limit or one such value accompanied by one elevated serum lactate dehydrogenase (LD) value. The change in enzyme value pattern had to be typical for acute myocardial infarction with the maximum value of ASAT within 36 hours and the LD value within 60 hours of onset of symptoms.

To qualify for the study, patients had to be in a clinically stable condition, be up and about, and all the following exclusion criteria had to be absent at the day of randomization:

1. Any contraindication for beta-blocker therapy:
    a. Uncontrolled cardiac failure defined as the presence of pulmonary rales or radiological evidence of pulmonary congestion despite carefully adjusted treatment with digitals and diuretics
    b. Resting heart rate less than 50 beats per minute
    c. Second- or third-degree atrioventricular block (patients with transient block lasting more than 7 days were also excluded)
    d. Sinoatrial block

Table 5 Nonfatal Recurrent Myocardial Infarction in Selected Subgroups

Characteristic	No. of patients entered		Nonfatal infarction			
			Placebo		Timolol	
	Placebo	Timolol	No.	%	No.	%
All patients	939	945	131	14.0	90	9.5
Sex						
Male	732	752	104	14.2	72	9.6
Female	207	193	27	13.0	18	9.3
Diabetes	46	53	10	21.7	2	3.8
Never smoked	212	195	31	14.6	15	7.7
Ex-smoker	234	238	38	16.2	22	9.2
Smoker	493	512	62	12.6	53	10.4
Q-waves in ECG						
New Q-wave	592	567	78	13.2	48	8.5
Only old Q-wave, uncertain Q or LBBB	128	157	27	21.1	20	12.7
No or normal Q-wave	219	221	26	11.9	22	10.0
Number of study risk factors						
0	255	263	38	14.9	31	11.8
1	253	272	35	13.8	18	6.6
2 or more	431	410	58	13.5	41	10.0
Blood pressure, standing systolic						
100–110	192	196	14	7.3	20	10.2
111–130	393	400	59	15.0	35	8.8
131–150	225	233	29	12.9	28	12.0
151 or more	123	112	26	21.1	7	6.3

LBBB = Left bundle branch block.

Table 6 Number of Patients with Confirmed and Suspected (Nonwitnessed) Primary Cardiac Arrest During Administration of Study Medication or Within 28 Days of Withdrawal

Category	Placebo ($n = 939$)	Timolol ($n = 945$)
Sudden death, witnessed	38	11*
Resuscitated, later dead	6	3
Resuscitated, primary survival	7	5
Subtotal	51	19*
Nonwitnessed death	23	7**
Total	74	26*

* $p < 0.001$; ** $p < 0.01$.

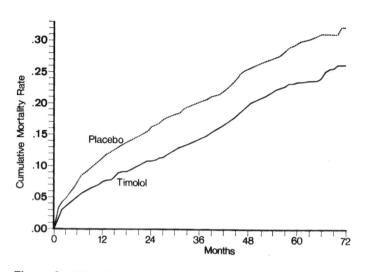

Figure 3   Life-table cumulative probability of death from all causes during 6 years extended follow-up after randomization (intention-to-treat). (From Ref. 19.)

DURATION OF EFFECT

The double-blind duration of the study was a maximum of 33 months. During this period the life-table curves for mortality continued to diverge for the first 24 months (Fig. 1); however, the estimate for the period of 24–33 months is uncertain because of smaller numbers of patients at risk. After completion of the double-blind period, most patients previously treated with timolol were prescribed timolol, whereas most patients in the placebo group were not. A 6-year extended follow-up study on all-cause mortality was carried out (19). The result is shown in Figure 3. The fact that the mortality curves of the two groups were parallel beginning 24 months after randomization does not suggest that continued timolol therapy is without value. Since more patients with large and complicated infarctions died earlier in the placebo group than in the timolol group, the latter contained more high-risk patients after 2 years. Only a convergence of the two curves would indicate loss of effect, but the gap achieved after 2 years of treatment persists, which indicate continued protection.

CONSEQUENCES OF THE TIMOLOL TRIAL

The Norwegian Timolol Study was the first randomized clinical trial that convincingly demonstrated that drug treatment for heart disease can improve survival. The study had a profound effect on how randomized clinical trials are considered by the medical community. The results, along with other beta-blocker trials that followed, changed medical practice.

The results indicate that most patients surviving an acute myocardial infarction should be treated with a beta-blocker. It is noteworthy that only 4% of all 3647 consecutively evaluated patients were excluded because of uncontrolled heart failure. When the trial was conducted, ACE inhibitors were not available. Today, many of the patients ex-

Table 1 Baseline Description of BHAT Treatment Groups

Baseline characteristic	Treatment group		p-value of difference
	Propranolol (n = 1916)	Placebo (n = 1921)	
Mean age (yr)	54.7	54.9	0.42
Male (%)	83.8	85.1	0.25
Mean systolic (mmHg)	112.3	111.7	0.10
Mean diastolic (mmHg)	72.5	72.3	0.34
Mean cholesterol (mg/dl)	212.7	213.6	0.52
Current smoker (%)	57.4	56.9	0.80
Medical history (%)			
Prior MI	13.9	13.2	0.52
Hypertension	41.4	40.1	0.41
Angina	35.8	36.5	0.63
Congestive heart failure	9.0	9.4	0.67
Diabetes	11.7	11.3	0.70
In-hospital events before randomization (%)			
Atrial fibrillation	6.8	5.7	0.14
Congestive heart failure	14.3	14.9	0.58
Ventricular tachycardia	23.0	23.2	0.88
Medications used at time of randomization (%)			
Antiarrhythmic	16.6	17.9	0.31
Anticoagulant	13.9	15.1	0.31
Antiplatelet	7.1	6.8	0.69
Diuretic	16.1	18.0	0.11
Vasodilator	36.0	36.3	0.83
Digitalis	12.5	13.0	0.62
Oral hypoglycemic	2.2	1.8	0.35
Anteriorly located MI (%)	27.8	25.7	0.14
Number of days between hospitalization and randomization			
Mean	13.9	13.7	0.62
Median	9	9	
Prevalence of ventricular arrhythmia on 24-hour ambulatory ECG[a] (%)	40.7	40.6	0.37

[a] Ventricular arrhythmia is defined as having an average of ≥ 10 ventricular premature beats (VPBs)/hour *or* at least one pair/run of VPBs *or* a multiform VPB. Data restricted to the 3290 patients with 24-hour ambulatory ECG.

consistent with the overall result of the trial. In the table, propranolol is shown to reduce mortality in the young and the old, in men and women, and in those identified as being high- or low-risk patients. Separate subgroup papers expanded upon these results (21–23). The larger absolute reduction in deaths among patients 60–69 years of age was of particular interest (22). Contrary to the practolol trial (10,11), having had an anterior myo-

Table 2 Cause-Specific Mortality by Treatment Group

Cause of death	Propranolol (n = 1916)		Placebo (n = 1921)		Percent reduction in risk	Absolute risk	p-value
	Number of deaths	Rate/ 100	Number of deaths	Rate/ 100			
All-cause[a]	138	7.2	188	9.8	26	−2.6	0.004
Cardiovascular disease	127	6.6	171	8.9	26	−2.3	0.009
Coronary heart disease[b]	119	6.2	164	8.5	27	−2.3	0.006
Sudden (<1 hr)[b]	64	3.3	89	4.6	28	−1.3	0.04
Nonsudden	55	2.9	75	3.9	26	−1.0	0.08
Other cardiovascular disease	8	0.4	7	0.4	−15	0.1	0.80
Noncardiovascular disease	11	0.6	17	0.9	35	−0.3	0.26

[a] Primary BHAT outcome measure.
[b] Secondary BHAT outcome measure.

cardial infarction (a protocol-specified subgroup analysis in BHAT) did not result in a greater or lesser treatment benefit.

Six months before BHAT results were announced, the results from the Norwegian Multicentre Study Group trial of timolol were published (24). This was a study of 1884 acute post-MI patients followed for a mean of 17 months. The risk groups identified in Table 3 are based upon those used in the timolol trial. In BHAT, the high-risk group was comprised of patients who had had at least one infarction before the BHAT MI or who had experienced a complication during hospitalization (including cardiogenic shock, persistent hypotension, atrioventricular shock, atrial fibrillation, ventricular fibrillation, pulmonary edema, and/or congestive heart failure). The low risk was comprised of all remaining patients. Whereas the timolol investigators reported greater reductions in the risk of death in the lower-risk group, BHAT reported that the relative benefit of propranolol was similar in both groups (27% and 28%), although the absolute reduction was greater among the high-risk patients.

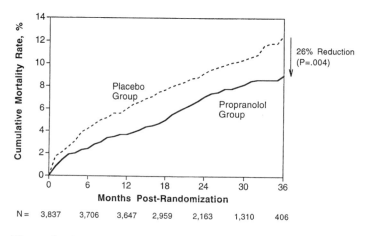

Figure 1 Cumulative life-table curves for all-cause mortality.

Table 3 All-Cause Mortality by Treatment Group and by Selected Baseline Characteristics

Baseline characteristic	Propranolol			Placebo			Percent reduction in risk	Absolute risk	p-value
	Deaths		Number in group	Deaths		Number in group			
	Number	Rate/100		Number	Rate/100				
Age									
30–59 years	78	6.0	1300	95	7.4	1288	19	−1.4	0.16
60–69 years	60	9.7	616	93	14.7	633	34	−5.0	0.008
Gender									
Male	116	7.2	1605	155	9.5	1635	24	−2.3	0.02
Female	22	7.1	311	33	11.5	286	39	−4.5	0.06
Risk group									
High	79	9.9	794	103	13.6	755	27	−3.7	0.02
Low	59	5.3	1122	85	7.3	1166	28	−2.0	0.05
Infarct location									
Anterior[a]	40	7.5	533	54	10.9	494	31	−3.4	0.06
Other	98	7.1	1383	134	9.4	1427	25	−2.3	0.03

[a] Prespecified BHAT subgroup hypothesis.

Cardiovascular Morbidity Results, Including Congestive Heart Failure

The incidence of definite nonfatal reinfarction during the mean 25.1-month follow-up period was 16% lower in the propranolol group (4.4% propranolol vs. 5.3% placebo), although this reduction in events was not statistically significant (25). Five patients in the propranolol group and seven in the placebo group had had two definite reinfarctions during follow-up. Of the 85 persons who had had at least one definite nonfatal reinfarction in the propranolol group, 12 (or 14.1%) subsequently died, as did 17 (16.8%) of the 101 patients in the placebo group who had had a reinfarction.

Coronary incidence (a prespecified secondary BHAT outcome measure) was defined as definite nonfatal reinfarction plus fatal coronary heart disease (i.e., total fatal and nonfatal coronary heart disease). In the propranolol group, 192 (10.0%) of the participants had experienced this outcome measure compared to 249 (13.0%) of the placebo participants. This 23% reduction in coronary incidence was statistically significant ($p < 0.01$).

When the coronary incidence rates and the rates of definite nonfatal reinfarction were stratified by age and risk group, the event rates for the propranolol group were always lower than the rates for the placebo group. Also, the relative reductions in risk were always greater in the older and higher-risk participants, suggesting a greater benefit in these patients.

The rates of new and recurrent definite congestive heart failure (CHF) were also examined and were stratified by prior history of CHF (25). Of the 345 patients in the propranolol group with a history of CHF, 14.8% experienced a recurrent episode. This contrasts with the 12.6% recurrence rate among the 365 placebo group patients with a history of CHF. Among the patients without a history of CHF, 5.0% of the propranolol group and 5.3% of the placebo group had experienced incident CHF. Overall, the rates of CHF between the two groups were identical (6.7%). When the rates of CHF are examined in the first 30 days post randomization (Fig. 2) (26), the incidence of CHF in patients without a history of CHF is noted to be almost identical between the two treatment groups (1.3% propranolol vs. 1.1% placebo). However, among the patients with a prior history of CHF, the incidence of recurrent CHF was 2.6 times greater among the propranolol patients (4.3% vs. 1.6%). It is noted, however, that the absolute difference in rates is small. The investigators also reported that the rate of study medication discontinuation due to perceived heart failure was only slightly higher among the propranolol patients (7.2% propranolol vs. 6.6% placebo).

Although the data showed that the incidence of CHF was greater in the subset of propranolol group patients with a history of failure (especially in the short-term), the question arose whether a history might truly be a contraindication for propranolol use. To address this issue, the trial investigators stratified the mortality and morbidity treatment analyses by CHF history (26). Remembering that patients with severe CHF were excluded from the trial, it is noted in Table 4 that propranolol actually had its greatest relative and absolute effects in patients with congestive heart failure, regardless of the outcome measure, and including a 47% reduction in sudden death.

Propranolol, Ventricular Arrhythmias, and Event Reduction

BHAT was conceived as a trial testing whether an agent with purported antiarrhythmic properties would reduce sudden death. During the planning phase, the investigators built

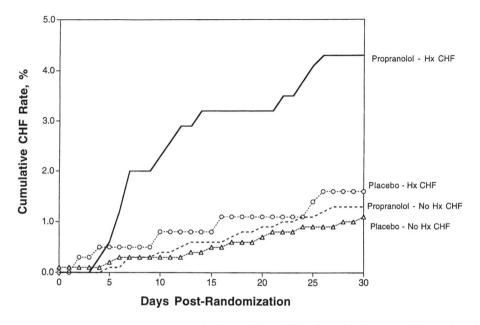

Figure 2 Cumulative rate of congestive heart failure (CHF) by prior history and by treatment group: First 30 days.

into the trial a number of activities designed to provide greater insight into how propranolol may work. To this end, 24-hour ambulatory ECG monitoring was performed at baseline on 3290 (86%) of the 3837 randomized participants and repeated 6 weeks postrandomization in a random sample of 840 patients (27,28). The protocol definition of ventricular arrhythmia (VA) was the presence of one or more of the following features on the 24-hour ambulatory ECG: an average of ≥10 ventricular premature beats (VPBs) per hour *or* at least one pair/run of VPBs *or* the presence of a multiform VPB (29).

It is noted in Table 5 that from baseline to the 6-week visit, propranolol was associated with a 15% overall reduction in the prevalence of VA compared to placebo ($p <$ 0.01). It is also noted that this reduction was essentially comparable for those with and without the arrhythmia at baseline. The effect of propranolol on clinical events (including mortality) in patients with and without VA at baseline was examined next (26). Table 6 presents all-cause and cause-specific mortality rates by treatment assignment and presence of VA from the 24-hour ECG. It is noted that for each outcome measure (1) patients with VA at baseline experienced higher event rates, regardless of treatment assignment; (2) patients assigned to the propranolol group experienced lower event rates, regardless of the outcome measure; and (3) the point estimates suggest that the patients with VA at baseline experienced greater absolute and relative reductions in mortality attributable to propranolol. The protocol-specified subgroup hypothesis that sudden death would be preferentially reduced in patients with complex ventricular arrhythmias was only suggested by the data: among patients with VA, propranolol was associated with a 28% reduction in sudden death, compared to a 16% reduction among the patients without VA. Employing a Mantel-Haenszel chi-square analysis of homogeneity (30), this difference in the relative reductions was not statistically significant. Both subgroups benefited from treatment, although it is noted that the higher event rate among patients with an arrhythmia translates

Table 4 Mortality and Morbidity by Treatment Group and by History of Congestive Heart Failure at Baseline

Outcome	Congestive heart failure at baseline	Propranolol			Placebo			Percent reduction in risk	Absolute risk	p-value
		Events		Number in group	Events		Number in group			
		Number	Rate/100		Number	Rate/100				
All-cause mortality	Yes	46	13.3	345	67	18.4	365	27	−5.0	0.07
	No	92	5.9	1571	121	7.8	1556	25	−1.9	0.03
Sudden death (<1 hr)	Yes	19	5.5	345	38	10.4	365	47	−4.9	0.02
	No	45	2.9	1571	51	3.3	1556	13	−0.4	0.50
Fatal/nonfatal coronary incidence	Yes	48	13.9	345	86	23.6	365	41	−9.6	0.001
	No	144	9.2	1571	163	10.5	1556	12	−1.3	0.22

Congestive Heart Failure at baseline is defined as having a history of CHF before the BHAT MI or having had CHF during hospitalization for the MI.

Table 5 Prevalence of Ventricular Arrhythmia at 6 Weeks by Treatment Group and Presence of Arrhythmia at Baseline[a]

Ventricular arrhythmia[b] at baseline	Propranolol			Placebo			Percent reduction in risk	Absolute risk	p-value
	VA at 6 weeks		Number in group	VA at 6 weeks		Number in group			
	Number	No. 100		Number	No. 100				
Present	118	69.4	170	132	79.5	166	13	−10.1	0.03
Absent	102	39.5	258	118	48.0	246	18	−8.4	0.06
Total	220	51.4	428	250	60.7	412	15	−9.3	0.007

[a] Subset of BHAT participants with a baseline and 6-week 24-hour ambulatory ECG.
[b] Ventricular arrhythmia (VA) is defined as having an average of ≥10 ventricular premature beats (VPBs) or at least one pair/run of VPBs or a multiform VPB.

Table 6 Cause-Specific Mortality by Treatment Group and by Presence of Ventricular Arrhythmia at Baseline[a]

		Propranolol			Placebo					
		Deaths		Number in group	Deaths		Number in group	Percent reduction in risk	Absolute risk	p-value
Outcome	Ventricular arrhythmia[b]	Number	rate/100		Number	rate/100				
All-cause	Present	70	10.4	672	101	15.2	666	31	−4.7	0.009
mortality	Absent	47	4.8	978	62	6.4	974	25	−1.6	0.13
CHD	Present	61	9.1	672	90	13.5	666	33	−4.4	0.01
mortality	Absent	40	4.1	978	52	5.3	974	23	−1.2	0.19
Sudden death	Present[c]	37	5.5	672	51	7.7	666	28	−2.2	0.11
(<1 hr)	Absent	21	2.1	978	25	2.6	974	16	−0.4	0.54

[a] Subset of BHAT participants with a 24-hour ambulatory ECG at baseline.
[b] Ventricular arrhythmia is defined as having an average of ≥10 ventricular premature beats (VPBs) or at least one pair/run of VPBs or a multiform VPB.
[c] Prespecified BHAT subgroup hypothesis.

to a greater absolute reduction in risk (i.e., more events are averted for every 100 high-risk patients treated).

Other analyses examining the effect of treatment on sudden death were also performed using the BHAT data. For example, using data recorded when a participant died, it was possible to examine the relationship between the diurnal timing of sudden death and use of propranolol (31). Of the 56 sudden deaths in the placebo group with this information, 38% occurred in the 6-hour period from 5 to 11 a.m., compared with 24% in the propranolol group. Excluding this period, there were nearly equal numbers of sudden deaths in the two groups, suggesting that propranolol prevented or blunted the previously reported midmorning rise in the occurrence of sudden death (32,33).

Significance of Propranolol-Induced Lipid Changes

It has long been documented that propranolol, like other beta-blockers without intrinsic sympathomimetic activity, increases serum triglyceride levels and decreases high-density lipoprotein (HDL) levels (34,35), both of which are associated with the development of coronary disease. For this reason, concern had been expressed about the long-term use of propranolol (36), regardless of the proven efficacy of the agent in postinfarction patients.

Lipids were analyzed in BHAT at baseline and throughout the follow-up period. In 1983, shortly after the publication of the main results, BHAT investigators reported that at the first annual follow-up visit, the propranolol patients had a mean HDL level 7% lower than the placebo group and a mean triglyceride level 14% higher (both $p < 0.001$) (37). Propranolol in these analyses had no effect on total cholesterol or on low-density lipoprotein, the most atherogenic lipoprotein fraction. It was later reported from BHAT that every 1-mg reduction in HDL in the propranolol group from baseline to 6 months was associated with only a 0.7% relative increase in all-cause mortality (38). Given that HDL was reduced in the propranolol group by 2.6 mg/dl during this time period, it was further estimated that the theoretical total increase in mortality due to the propranolol-induced decrease in HDL would thus be about 2%. However, even after multivariate adjustment for changes in HDL and triglyceride, the reduction in mortality associated with propranolol was still approximately 20%, or 10 times the estimated hazard. The analyses indicated that propranolol remained an effective prophylactic treatment in spite of its metabolic effects on HDL and triglycerides.

Side Effects, Compliance, and Use of Nonstudy Medications

BHAT demonstrated that propranolol was not only effective, but safe (18). All of the side effects detected in BHAT had been previously reported and were not unexpected. For example, the propranolol group reported significantly ($p < 0.05$) higher rates of tiredness (67% vs. 62%), bronchospasm (31% vs. 27%), diarrhea (6% vs. 4%), and cold hands and feet (10% vs. 8%). It is to be noted, however, that the absolute difference in rates for each complaint was no more than 5%. Some complaints usually identified with use of a beta-blocker were actually noted to be equally distributed between the two treatment groups: depression (41% propranolol vs. 40% placebo), nightmares (40% vs. 37%), and reduced sexual activity (43% vs. 42%). Survival analyses of these data also demonstrated that the incidence of many of these events changed over time and very often was linked to the precipitating myocardial infarction itself (39).

Compliance to study medication during the trial was good (18). About three-quarters of all participants in both treatment groups were still on their study medication at the last clinic visit. Furthermore, among the propranolol participants off study medication, 8% were on an open-labeled beta-blocker. Thus, 85% of the patients assigned to active treatment were on active treatment. Among the placebo patients, 13% were on an open-labeled beta-blocker. Thus, 87% of the patients assigned to placebo were not on active treatment.

During the course of follow-up, the use of most nonstudy medications was equal between the two treatment groups (18). Forty-one percent were on a diuretic, 12% were on another antihypertensive, 26% were on digitalis, 22% were on aspirin, and 18% were taking potassium. Not unexpectedly, antiarrhythmics were used more frequently among placebo patients (26% vs. 21%, $p < 0.001$).

BHAT AND RESULTS FROM OTHER CONCURRENT BETA-BLOCKER TRIALS

The results of two other large, double-blind, placebo-controlled, randomized clinical trials of beta-blockers in postinfarction patients were published the same year that the BHAT results were announced. The Norwegian Multicentre Study Group trial (24) (see Chap. 17) was designed to determine whether the beta-blocker timolol would reduce all-cause mortality in 1884 patients who had had an MI within the previous 7–28 days. Patients were followed for 12–33 months (mean = 17). All-cause mortality was reduced by 36% ($p < 0.001$), and sudden death was reduced by 44%(40). The other beta-blocker trial (see Chap. 14) was designed to determine whether metoprolol would reduce the 90-day mortality rate in 1395 patients who had had an MI within the previous 48 hours (41). This trial reported a 36% reduction in deaths during its short follow-up ($p < 0.03$).

Taken together, BHAT and the other two concurrent trials provided compelling evidence that beta-blockers do indeed reduce mortality and morbidity in patients who have suffered an acute MI.

LIMITATIONS AND EXTRAPOLATION OF RESULTS

Like all clinical trials, the questions BHAT was designed to answer precluded asking other questions. For example, whereas BHAT provided strong evidence that the use of propranolol was effective in reducing mortality and morbidity rates over 36 months of follow-up, because the trial ended it could not provide evidence for continued benefit beyond 36 months. Also, BHAT could not provide any evidence that the agent would be efficacious among patients who suffered an MI months or years earlier because participants were solely recruited within 3 weeks of their MI.

The impact of eligibility criteria must be considered in determining to whom the results can be generalized. Because patients with a severe contraindication to a beta-blocker (approximately 18% of age-eligible patients screened) were excluded from the trial, clearly the BHAT results cannot be extrapolated to them. It would, however, be reasonable to extrapolate the BHAT results to those patients who were excluded because they were already on or likely to be placed on a beta-blocker (another 18% of the patients screened). Similarly, it would also be reasonable to extrapolate the results to those patients who were excluded because of design challenges or because informed consent was not obtained (another 41%). Thus, it would be reasonable to expect that three-quarters of MI patients who survived at least 5 days and who were between 30 and 69 years of age would benefit from treatment with propranolol.

SUMMARY

The Beta-Blocker Heart Attack Trial was one of the first trials to demonstrate successfully the efficacy of an agent in decreasing mortality and morbidity in acute MI patients. The effects of propranolol on these outcomes were generally similar in all examined subgroups. Whereas the investigators expressed caution as to overinterpreting subgroup analyses, analyses of the BHAT data did suggest greater absolute benefit *among high-risk patients*, including those over 60 years of age (22) and those with evidence of ventricular arrhythmias (29). It was also demonstrated that the drug was safe and that compliance was high (18).

Given the BHAT results and the evidence accumulating from the other completed beta-blocker clinical trials, the BHAT investigators recommended in 1981 that propranolol be used for at least 3 years as a preventive treatment in patients who had recently survived a myocardial infarction and who had no contraindications for its use.

REFERENCES

1. Workshop on Chronic Antiarrhythmic Therapy and the Prevention of Sudden Death: Summary Report. Cardiac Diseases Branch, National Heart, Lung, and Blood Institute, National Institutes of Health, Bethesda, MD, 1976.
2. Maroko PR, Kjekshus JK, Sobel BE, Watanabe T, Covell JW, Ross Jr J, Braunwald E. Factors influencing infarct size following coronary occlusions. Circulation 1971; 43:67–82.
3. Reimer KA, Rasmussen MM, Jennings RB. Reduction by propranolol of myocardial necrosis following temporary coronary artery occlusion in dogs. Circ Res 1973; 33:353–363.
4. Reynolds JL, Whitlock RML. Effects of β-adrenergic receptor blocker in myocardial infarction treated for one year from onset. Br Heart J 1972; 34:252–259.
5. Wilhelmsson C, Vedin JA, Wilhelmsen L, Tibblin G, Werkö L. Reduction of sudden deaths after myocardial infarction by treatment with alprenolol: preliminary results. Lancet 1974; 2: 1157–1160.
6. Vedin A. Wilhelmsson C, Werkö L. Chronic alprenolol treatment of patients with acute myocardial infarction after discharge from hospital: effects on mortality and morbidity. Acta Med Scand 1975; 575(suppl):1–56.
7. Ahlmark G, Saetre H, Korsgren M. Reduction of sudden deaths after myocardial infarction. Lancet 1974; 2:1563.
8. Ahlmark G, Saetre H. Long-term treatment with β-blockers after myocardial infarction. Eur J Clin Pharmacol 1976; 10:77–83.
9. Barber JM, Boyle DM, Chaturvedi NC, Singh N, Walsh MJ. Practolol in acute myocardial infarction. Acta Med Scand 1975; 587(suppl):213–219.
10. Multicentre International Study. Improvement in prognosis of myocardial infarction by long-term beta-adrenoceptor blockade using practolol. Br Med J 1975; 3:735–740.
11. Multicentre International Study. Reduction in mortality after myocardial infarction with long-term β-adrenergic blockade using practolol. Br Med J 1977; 2:419–421.
12. Furberg CD, Friedewald WT. The effects of chronic administration of beta-blockade on long-

term survival following myocardial infarction. In: Braunwald E, ed. Beta-Adrenergic Blockade, A New Era in Cardiovascular Medicine. Amsterdam: Excerpta Medica, 1978:171–177.

13. The Beta-Blocker Heart Attack Research Group. Beta-Blocker Heart Attack Trial: design features. Cont Clin Trials 1981; 2:275–285.

14. Beta-Blocker Heart Attack Trial Research Group (monograph prepared by Robert P. Byington). Beta-Blocker Heart Attack Trial: design, methods and baseline results. Cont Clin Trials 1984; 5:332–437.

15. Walle T, Byington RP, Furberg CD, Mcintyre KM, Vokonas PS. Biologic determinants of propranolol disposition: results from 1308 patients in the Beta-Blocker Heart Attack Trial. Clin Pharm Ther 1985; 38:509–518.

16. DeMets DL, Hardy RJ, Friedman LM, Lan KKG. Statistical aspects of early termination in the Beta-Blocker Heart Attack Trial. Cont Clin Trials 1984; 5:362–372.

17. β-Blocker Heart Attack Study Group. The β-Blocker Heart Attack Trial. JAMA 1981; 246:2073–2074.

18. β-Blocker Heart Attack Trial Research Group. A randomized trial of propranolol in patients with acute myocardial infarction. I. Mortality results. JAMA 1982; 247:1707–1714.

19. Cox DR. Regression models and lifetables. J R Stat Soc 1972; 34:187–202.

20. Peto R, Pike MC, Armitage P, Breslow NE, Cox DR, Howard SV, Mantel N, McPherson K, Peto J, Smith PG. Design and analysis of randomized clinical trials requiring prolonged observation of each patient: introduction and design. Br J Cancer 1976; 34:585–612.

21. Furberg CD, Byington RP, for the Beta-Blocker Heart Attack Trial Research Group. What do subgroup analyses reveal about differential response to beta-blocker therapy? The Beta-Blocker Heart Attack Trial experience. Circulation 1983; 67(suppl 1):I-98–I-101.

22. Hawkins CM, Richardson DW, Vokonas PS, for the Beta-Blocker Heart Attack Trial Research Group. Effect of propranolol in reducing mortality in older myocardial infarction patients—The Beta-Blocker Heart Attack Trial experience. Circulation 1983; 67(suppl I):I-94–I-97.

23. Furberg CD, Hawkins CM, Lichstein E, for the Beta-Blocker Heart Attack Trial Study Group. Effect of propranolol in post-infarction patients with mechanical or electrical complications. Circulation 1984; 69:761–765.

24. Norwegian Multcenter Study Group. Timolol-induced reduction in mortality and reinfarction in patients surviving acute myocardial infarction. N Engl J Med 1981; 304:801–807.

25. Beta-Blocker Heart Attack Trial Research Group. A randomized trial of propranolol in patients with acute myocardial infarction. II. Morbidity results. JAMA 1983; 250:2814–2819.

26. Chadda K, Goldstein S, Byington R, Curb JD. Effect of propranolol after acute myocardial infarction in patients with congestive heart failure. Circulation 1986; 73:503–510.

27. Lichstein E, Morganroth J, Harrist R, Hubble E, for the BHAT Study Group. Effect of propranolol on ventricular arrhythmia: The Beta-Blocker Heart Attack Trial experience. Circulation 1983; 67(suppl I):I-5–I-10.

28. Morganroth J, Lichstein E, Byington RP, for the BHAT Study Group. Beta-Blocker Heart Attack Trial—impact of propranolol therapy on ventricular arrhythmias. Prev Med 1985; 14:346–357.

29. Friedman LM, Byington RP, Capone RJ, Furberg CD, Goldstein S, Lichstein E (writing group for the Beta-Blocker Heart Attack Trial Research Group). Effect of propranolol in patients with myocardial infarction and ventricular arrhythmia. J Am Coll Cardiol 1986; 7:1–8.

30. Mantel N, Haenszel W. Statistical aspects of the analysis of data from retrospective studies of disease. J Natl Cancer Inst 1959; 22:719–748.

31. Peters RW, Muller JE, Goldstein S, Byington R, Friedman LM. Propranolol and the morning increase in the frequency of sudden cardiac death (BHAT study). Am J Cardiol 1989; 63:1518–1520.

32. Willich SN, Levy D, Rocco MB, Tofler GH, Stone PH, Muller JE. Circadian variation in the incidence of sudden cardiac death in the Framingham Heart Study population. Am J Cardiol 1987; 60:801–806.

33. Muller JE, Ludmer PL, Willich SN, Tofler GH, Aylmer G, Klangos I, Stone PH. Circadian variation in the frequency of sudden cardiac death. Circulation 1987; 75:131–138.

34. Northcote RJ, Todd IC, Ballantyne D. Beta blockers and lipoproteins: a review of current knowledge. Scott Med J 1986; 31:220–228.

35. Van Brummelen P. The relevance of intrinsic sympathomimetic activity for β-blocker-induced changes in plasma lipids. J Cardiovasc Pharmacol 1983; 5:S51–S55.

36. Northcote RJ. β-Blockers, lipids, and coronary atherosclerosis: fact or fiction? Br Med J 1988; 296:731–732.

37. Shulman RS, Herbert PN, Capone RJ, McClure D, Hawkins CM, Henderson LO, Saritelli A, Campbell J. Effects of propranolol on blood lipids and lipoproteins in myocardial infarction. Circulation 1983; 67(suppl I):I-19–I-21.

38. Byington RP, Worthy J, Craven T, Furberg CD. Propranolol-induced lipid changes and their prognostic significance after a myocardial infarction—The Beta-Blocker Heart Attack Trial experience. Am J Cardiol 1990; 65:1287–1291.

39. Davis BR, Furberg C, Williams CB. Survival analysis of adverse effects data in the Beta-Blocker Heart Attack Trial. Clin Pharm Ther 1987; 41:611–615.

40. Lund-Johansen P. The Norwegian Multicenter Study on Timolol After Myocardial Infarction. Part II. Effect in different risk groups, causes of death, heart arrest, re-infarctions, re-hospitalizations and adverse experiences. Acta Med Scand 1981; 651(suppl):243–252.

41. Hjalmarson A, Herlitz J, Malék I, Rydén L, Vedin A, Waldenström A, Wedel H, Elmfeldt D, Holmburg S, Nyberg G, Swedberg K, Waagstein F, Waldenström J, Wilhelmsen L, Wilhelmsson C. Effect on mortality of metoprolol in acute myocardial infarction: a double-blind randomised trial. Lancet 1981; 2:823–827.

Section F
ACE Inhibitors: Early Use

Unlike beta-blockers, where early use is taken to mean immediate intravenous administration, the early use of angiotensin-converting enzyme (ACE) inhibitors generally refers to the oral use of these agents within 24 of hospitalization. This reflects the negative findings of the CONSENSUS-II trial, which found no benefit to very early, intravenous ACE inhibitor use, as well as the study design of the subsequent trials described in this section. Both large trials of early ACE inhibitor use in unselected patients (GISSI-3 and ISIS-4) found that higher-risk patients—those with anterior infarctions or with signs and symptoms of left ventricular dysfunction—derived more benefit from treatment than did those patients at lower risk. This concept was validated in the SMILE study. Nevertheless, a small but significant benefit occurs with the early use of these agents in all infarct patients. In the absence of clear contraindications (such as hypotension), these drugs should be considered as part of the early management of all patients with myocardial infarction. If subsequent evaluation finds no significant impairment of left ventricular systolic function, ACE inhibitors can be discontinued.

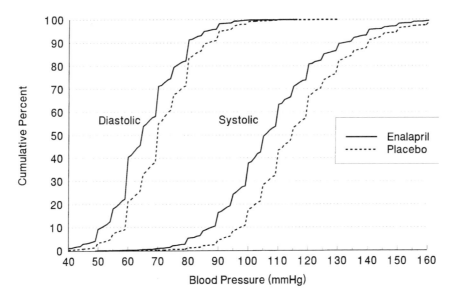

Figure 5 The lowest blood pressure after first dose of blinded treatment in the enalapril and placebo groups.

When all significant variables were tested for independent association with first-dose hypotension in a stepwise logistic regression procedure, a subset of variables were selected, all significantly associated with risk of a hypotensive reaction: age, prior history of hypertension, heart failure and/or peripheral atherosclerotic disease, inferior infarct location, low pretreatment systolic blood pressure, and pretreatment use of diuretics (10).

Hypotension remained a risk factor for mortality in the enalapril group even after adjustment for any of the independent variables. Because the hypotensive subgroup can only be defined after patients have been randomized and treated, we do not know if hypotension is causal to the increased mortality or only an epiphenomenon due to high-risk patients being particularly susceptible to first-dose hypotension when treated with enalapril.

In order to distinguish between these two alternatives, subgroups of patients based solely on baseline characteristics were identified. If first-dose hypotension was the cause of excess mortality, one would expect to see higher mortality with enalapril relative to placebo in the subgroup most likely to have first-dose hypotension with enalapril.

A discriminant analysis identified a score based on prestudy diastolic blood pressure and concomitant use of diuretics as best identifying patients likely to experience hypotension (10). Splitting the score into quartiles, first-dose hypotension was 10 times more frequent with enalapril than with placebo in the first quartile (highest risk). However, the ratio of enalapril to placebo mortality was similar in all quartiles (Table 6). This result strongly supports the conclusion that first-dose hypotension with enalaprilat in this setting merely identifies patients with high mortality risk regardless of therapy.

Among patients who entered the trial, 3467 received thrombolytic therapy. First-dose hypotension in patients treated with thrombolytics was associated with an overall mortality during follow-up of 12.8% compared to 6.8% without hypotension. Among patients not treated with thrombolytics, those who experienced first-dose hypotension had a mortality of 22.5% compared to 12.4% in patients without first-dose hypotension.

Table 6 Percent Occurrence of First-Dose Hypotension and Subsequent Mortality in Subgroups of Patients Identified by Baseline Risk of Hypotension

| | Percent of patients | | | |
| | Hypotension | | Mortality | |
Quartile	Enalapril	Placebo	Enalapril	Placebo
1	17.6	1.7	14.6	13.9
2	11.1	3.3	10.6	9.6
3	10.2	2.6	7.5	5.5
4	4.5	2.0	7.4	6.6

Source: Ref. 9.

Thrombolytics therefore reduced mortality proportionally in high-risk (first-dose hypotension) and low-risk (no hypotension) patients. First-dose hypotension was therefore not confounding the effect of thrombolytic treatment.

DISCUSSION

CONSENSUS-II was the first study to test whether early pharmacologic inhibition of the renin-angiotensin-aldosterone system is beneficial during acute myocardial infarction and the subsequent remodeling process. Previous studies in animals and patients had mostly suggested benefit in terms of smaller infarcts and less dilatation of the left ventricle (5,11), while a few were not supportive of benefit (12). However, the experience from CONSENSUS-I of marked short- and long-term benefit of treating patients with chronic heart failure prompted the design and planning of CONSENSUS-II. The study was stopped because of futility after a recommendation from the Data and Safety Monitoring Board, although there was also a major concern among the board members of a negative trend for mortality among patients aged >70 in the enalapril group (6). More recent studies have demonstrated benefit with ACE inhibitors started within day 1 of an acute myocardial infarction (13,14) as well as after day 3 (15,16). However, the effect in the nonselected patients appeared to be much smaller (13,14) than anticipated for the CONSENSUS-II and mostly restricted to the patients with anterior location of the infarcts, heart rates above 80 beats per minute, and among patients younger than 75 years.

CONSENSUS-II differs from other trials in that all patients were started on an intravenous dose of enalaprilat, the prodrug of enalapril, and a larger proportion of patients were older than 75 years and more often had a history of myocardial infarction. The mortality and the unfavorable effect of enalapril were largest among the elderly in CONSENSUS-II. Among patients younger than 60 years there was a trend in favor of benefit with enalapril relative to placebo (Table 3). The reason why the elderly do not seem to benefit from treatment is not defined. They were more likely to have a first-dose hypotension and more likely to use diuretics. First-dose hypotension was a transient phenomenon, but diuretics are known to potentiate the first-dose hypotension of intravenous ACE inhibitors (17,18) The low benefit of ACE inhibitors among the elderly is not restricted to the CONSENSUS-II. The elderly may be more dependent on the adaptive functions of the RAA system and suffer from more prolonged hypotension, which may cause myocardial

21

ISIS-4

PETER SLEIGHT

ISIS-4 (Fourth International Study of Infarct Survival) Collaborative
Group. ISIS-4: A randomized factorial trial assessing early oral captopril,
oral mononitrate, and intravenous magnesium sulfate in 58,050 patients
with suspected acute myocardial infarction. Lancet 1995; 345:669–685

INTRODUCTION

Several large randomized studies have shown the benefit of inhibition of angiotensin-
converting enzyme (ACE) in patients with left ventricular (LV) dysfunction (much of
which is on an ischemic basis) or in patients with LV dysfunction following a recent
myocardial infarction (1–7). These studies followed the seminal work of the Pfeffers and
their colleagues, which showed the prevention of LV dilatation (remodeling) by ACE
inhibition (captopril) in a rat model of moderate size infarction (8).

All of these studies showed the benefit of ACE inhibitors in reducing the progression
of LV dilatation (remodeling) and subsequent need for hospitalization, and finally reduction in mortality. However, these trials randomized patients whose infarction had occurred
months, weeks, or, at least, days earlier. Since most deaths from patients hospitalized with
acute myocardial infarction (AMI) occur in the first 48 hours, it seemed important to
assess the risks and benefits of ACE inhibitors in patients randomized during this very
early period after onset.

ISIS-4 (9) was one of several trials designed to examine this question; others are
separately addressed elsewhere, including other chapters of this volume (10–14).

ISIS-4 was more complex than the other studies in that it also tested (in a 3 × 2
factorial design) the use of captopril (Capoten® Bristol-Myers Squibb, BMS), oral mononitrate (Imdur® Astra), and magnesium. As in ISIS-2, where aspirin was studied along
with streptokinase, funding by BMS and Astra was used to test an ''orphan'' agent, magnesium.

This chapter will deal solely with the ACE inhibitor comparison with placebo in
ISIS-4. ACE inhibitors have complex effects on the circulation. They lower blood pressure
by several possible mechanisms. First, they reduce angiotensin II (AII) levels and hence
reduce vasoconstriction, blood pressure, and afterload. Reduction in peripheral AII also
reduces the release of noradrenaline from sympathetic nerve terminals (15), with the poten-

tial to reduce LV wall stress and arrhythmias (16). Reduction of brain AII, particularly in the medulla, increases baroreflex gain (17,18) and vagal tone (19), and also reduces reflex and nonreflex sympathetic tone. Several of the longer-term studies suggest that ACE inhibitors may reduce reinfarction by a number of mechanisms including enhanced fibrinolysis (20).

The main anxiety about very early ACE inhibition in ISIS-4 was the development of hypotension (21,22), particularly in patients receiving active nitrates and magnesium. Nevertheless, since many MI patients were already treated with nitrates and since, as a result of the LIMIT-2 study (see Chap. 36) (23,24) and other evidence (25), many physicians were considering the routine use of intravenous magnesium, we felt it important to test these together in a randomized study.

Because of the anxiety about possible harm from hypotension, the captopril dose was very carefully piloted over several years in around 1000 patients, beginning with 1-mg doses and gradually increasing (26,27); of course, blood pressure can fall quite rapidly in the acute phase of MI with no drug therapy.

The GISSI-3 pilot study (28) showed that the *excess* of hypotension caused by nitrates or ACE inhibition over placebo was only about 5 mmHg and that the fall with nitrates was more rapid than with lisinopril. In ISIS-4 we finally decided on an initial dose of 6.25 mg of captopril with rapid titration to 12.5 mg 2 hours later if the blood pressure fall was not worrisome. The dose could be increased to 25 mg 12 hours later and then to 50 mg b.i.d.

METHODS, PATIENT CHARACTERISTICS, AND TREATMENT

As in the previous ISIS studies, ISIS-4 used telephone randomization and simple procedures so that we were able to randomize 58,050 patients with suspected MI beginning 0–24 hours earlier from 1086 hospitals in 31 countries over a period of 2 years.

Around 80% of the patients had ST elevation on the initial EKG, 40% were within 6 hours of onset of symptoms, 28% were aged 70 years or over, and only 2% had SBP < 100 mmHg. Infarction was subsequently confirmed in 92% of randomized patients.

The trial drugs were started as soon as the patient's condition appeared stable, generally about an hour or so after thrombolysis (given to 70% of randomized patients) and aspirin (given to 94%); 5% received a nonstudy ACE inhibitor. There was good balance in the use of nonstudy treatments, except that slightly fewer patients on active captopril received nontrial ACE inhibition (4.7% vs. 6.0%).

At entry to the study, 17% had a history of a prior MI and 14% were in chronic heart failure; 12% were on prior diuretic treatment. Ninety-eight percent of patients started captopril or placebo tablets and were discharged on them in 81% and 85% of cases, respectively.

The analysis was on an intention-to-treat basis and involved comparisons between active captopril and placebo of 5-week total mortality, mode of death, and various nonfatal events, particularly reinfarction (since there was some concern that lower blood pressure might cause this), and cardiogenic shock.

Cardiogenic shock was uncommon (4%, compared with 7% in ISIS-3), perhaps because patients with low blood pressure (SBP < 100 mmHg) were excluded.

RESULTS

Oral Captopril Versus Placebo: Mortality

Five-week mortality was modestly but significantly reduced from 7.69% to 7.19% in the 29,022 placebo and 29,028 captopril-treated patients, respectively (Fig. 1). This 7% (SD3) proportional reduction had confidence intervals from 13 to 1% ($p < 0.02$) and corresponds to an absolute reduction of about five deaths per 1000 patients treated.

The proportional reduction in mortality was not statistically different among those

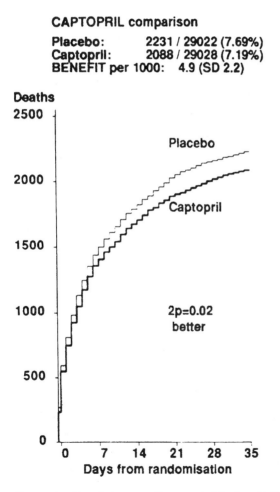

Figure 1 Cumulative mortality reported in days 0–35 in all patients allocated 28 days of oral captopril (thicker line) vs. placebo-allocated patients. (From Ref. 9.)

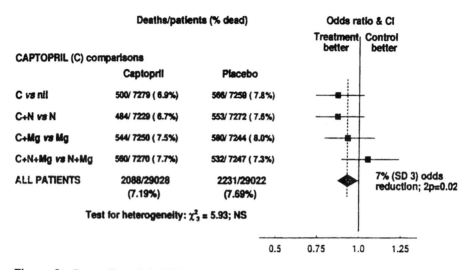

Figure 2 Captopril result in ISIS-4. Mortality in days 0–35 is subdivided by other randomly allocated study treatments. C = Captopril; N = mononitrate; Mg = magnesium. Odds ratios (ORs: black squares with areas proportional to the amount of "statistical information" in each subdivision) comparing the mortality among patients allocated the study treatment to that among patients allocated the relevant control are plotted for each of the treatment comparisons, subdivided by the other randomly allocated study treatments, along with their 99% confidence intervals (CIs: horizontal lines). For the overall treatment comparison, the result and its 95% CI is represented by a diamond, with the overall proportional reduction (or increase) and statistical significance given alongside. Squares or diamonds to the left of the solid vertical line indicate benefit (significant at $2p < 0.01$ when the entire horizontal line is to the left of the vertical line). Chi-square tests for evidence of heterogeneity of the sizes of the ORs in the subdivisions are also given. (From Ref. 9.)

allocated active captopril and active nitrate or magnesium (Fig. 2); although the point estimate for all three active agents versus control showed no benefit, the confidence limits overlap the overall result. In a trial that overall shows only a modestly significant result, such subgroup analyses need to be addressed cautiously.

Nevertheless, there has been anxiety about the use of ACE inhibitors in patients with hypotension, so it was somewhat reassuring that there was no excess mortality in captopril-allocated patients in days 0–1 among patients with low blood pressure at entry—a time when hypotension was most common.

Reinfarction—Other Clinical Events in Hospital

Despite concerns about the use of ACE inhibition early in MI, there was no significant increase in reinfarction. There was, however, an unexpected early excess of second- or third-degree heart block of 6 (SD2) per 1000 ($p < 0.001$) and a small excess of early cardiogenic shock. Again this excess was seen at a time when overall mortality was reduced. There was a larger increase in hypotension considered severe enough to stop treatment, 10% on captopril versus 4.8% on placebo ($p < 0.0001$), which was particularly large in patients with entry SPB < 100 mmHg (22% vs. 10.4%). There was also a small excess of renal dysfunction (1.1% vs. 0.6%), but this was not classified as severe.

DISCUSSION

In a trial such as ISIS-4 with only a moderately significant benefit, it is important to consider the result in light of other similar trials. Figure 3 shows the data available at the time of ISIS-4 publication. It can be seen that the 99% confidence limits of all the trials are compatible with the overall 6.5% reduction of short-term (4–5 week) mortality, although the CONSENSUS-II study was not encouraging. Although the CONSENSUS-II study was stopped early because of concerns about possible harm from enalapril, later analysis of all the data showed no evidence for this, although it also showed no benefit. It is not clear whether the unpromising result of the CONSENSUS-II study is due to bad luck, the use of an intravenous formulation, or possibly a sicker and more elderly population (see below).

The modest benefit seen in the early treatment/relatively unselective trials (Fig. 3) has been contrasted with the much more impressive results in trials such as SAVE, AIRE, and TRACE where treatment was (1) started later and (2) targeted at patients with identified LV dysfunction (see Sec. G). It must be pointed out that the benefit in these later trials was seen with longer-term treatment (of years rather than weeks). In ISIS-4 we did not think it desirable or practical in such a huge population to continue treatment beyond the time (4 weeks) when the patients would still be mainly under hospital supervision. If one compares the absolute benefit per month of treatment in the early versus the late/selective trials, they are quite comparable in cost-effectiveness.

Furthermore, it appears from the GISSI-3 trial that the early benefit, seen in the first

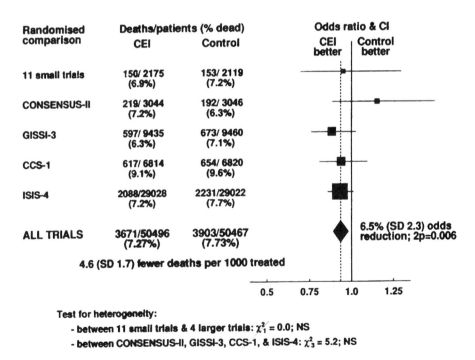

Figure 3 Systematic overview of effects on short-term mortality of starting converting enzyme inhibitors (CEI) early in acute myocardial infarction. There is no heterogeneity. Symbols are as in Figure 2. (From Ref. 9.)

few days, is not particularly from prevention of ventricular dilatation (as in the long-term selective trials), but rather from a substantial reduction in deaths due to cardiac rupture and from arrhythmia.

Proponents of the selective approach argue that some patients may be harmed by ACE inhibition treatment and that it is safer to be selective. However, it seems likely that cautiously titrated therapy will be more hazardous in the sicker patients who have more to gain and who, under the selective approach, would be treated anyway. Also, not all hospitals are able to carry out early assessment by echocardiography, as used in the TRACE study. A recent survey from a high proportion of all French coronary care units (29) showed that only 58% of patients underwent echocardiography before discharge, and so many fewer would receive this in the first 24 hours.

If one takes the AIRE criteria of a purely clinical definition of heart failure based on chest rales and x-ray congestion, then a good number of eligible patients would be missed. Furthermore, both the TRACE and AIRE studies enrolled patients well after a number of early hospital deaths had occurred, so comparison of these studies with the truly early trials is like comparing apples with oranges.

At this stage we should mention the recent speculation (31) based on a retrospective analysis of the SOLVD studies that ACE inhibition did not seem to benefit those patients who were also taking nontrial aspirin. This retrospective finding has not been confirmed by retrospective analysis of the other long-term ACE studies, where benefit of ACE was just as good in those taking aspirin as in those not on aspirin (S. Yusuf, personal communication).

What the early/relatively unselective trials have clearly shown is that ACE inhibition treatment is safe and saves lives provided that care is taken to avoid ACE inhibitors in patients who (1) are hypotensive, with an unstable hemodynamic state; (2) are not on a high dose of prior long-term diuretic treatment (e.g., 80 mg of furosemide daily) when angiotensin levels would be high; and (3) have no prior renal failure.

A later collaborative meta-analysis of all early ACE inhibition trials in MI has assembled individual patient data on approximately 100,000 randomized patients (30) aimed to gain more precise knowledge of the risks and benefits of this treatment and to identify subgroups of patients in whom the benefits or risks might be different. The results unsurprisingly are very similar to the ISIS-4 conclusions. As therein, the absolute benefits were particularly large in patients with anterior MI, Killip class 2-3, and heart rate > 100 bpm. However, the proportional benefits appeared similar in all age groups except that the risks appeared more and the benefits less in patents over age 75. In no subgroup did the treatment appear clearly harmful.

It is important to note that these benefits were seen on top of the other commonly recommended treatment for acute MI, namely, aspirin, thrombolytics, and beta-blockers. Equally important is that most of the mortality benefit in these early trials was seen during the first week, suggesting that the short-term benefit from early treatment involves different mechanisms, e.g., cardiac rupture and arrhythmic death, and so is complementary to the benefit seen from prevention of long-term LV dilatation.

Therefore, in public health terms, although one can see the appeal, especially to clinicians, of the targeted/selective approach, I believe that a strategy to treat most patients without contraindications will be the most effective approach, with a predischarge assessment of LV function for continuation of longer-term therapy.

If such a relatively unselective approach is taken, it need not be prohibitively expensive since it would seem reasonable to withdraw ACE inhibition before discharge in those patients with good LV function at this time. The previous longer-term trials suggest that if LV function is not normal at discharge, then treatment should be continued.

REFERENCES

1. The CONSENSUS Trial Group. Effects of enalapril on mortality in severe congestive heart failure: results of the Cooperative North Scandinavian Enalapril Survival Study (CONSEN-SUS). N Engl J Med 1987; 316:1429–1435.

2. Cohn JN, Johnson G, Ziesche S, Cobb F, Francis G, Tristani F, et al. A comparison of enalapril with hydralazine-isosorbide dinitrate in the treatment of chronic congestive heart failure. N Engl J Med 1991; 325:303–310.

3. The SOLVD Investigators. Effects of enalapril on survival in patients with reduced left ventricular ejection fractions and congestive heart failure. N Engl J Med 1991; 325:293–302.

4. The SOLVD Investigators. Effect of enalapril on mortality and the development of heart failure in asymptomatic patients with reduced left ventricular ejection fractions. N Engl J Med 1992; 327:685–691.

5. Pfeffer MA, Braunwald E, Moyé LA Basta L, Brown EJ, Cuddy TE, et al. Effect of captopril on mortality and morbidity in patients with left ventricular dysfunction after myocardial infarction. Results of the Survival and Ventricular Enlargement Trial (SAVE). N Engl J Med 1992; 327:669–677.

6. The Acute Infarction Ramipril Efficacy (AIRE) Study Investigators. Effect of ramipril on mortality and morbidity of survivors of acute myocardial infarction with clinical evidence of heart failure. Lancet 1993; 342:821–828.

7. Kober L, Torp-Pedersen C, Carlsen JE, Bagger H, Eliasen P, Lyngborg K, et al. A clinical trial of the angiotensin-converting enzyme inhibitor trandolapril in patients with left ventricular dysfunction after myocardial infarction. Trandolapril Cardiac Evaluation (TRACE) Study Group. N Engl J Med 1995; 333:1670–1676.

8. Pfeffer JM, Pfeffer MA, Braunwald E. Influence of chronic captopril therapy on the infarcted left ventricle of the rat. Circ Res 1985; 57:84–95.

9. ISIS-4 (Fourth International Study of Infarct Survival) Collaborative Group. ISIS-4: a randomised trial comparing oral captopril versus placebo, oral mononitrate versus placebo, and intravenous magnesium sulphate versus control among 58,050 patients with suspected acute myocardial infarction. Lancet 1995; 345:669–687.

10. Swedberg K, Held P, Kjekhus J, Rasmussen K, Rydén L, Wedel H. Effects of the early administration of enalapril on mortality in patients with acute myocardial infarction. Results of the Cooperative New Scandinavian Enalapril Survival Study II (CONSENSUS-II). N Engl J Med 1992; 327:678–684.

11. GISSI-3 (Gruppo Italiano per lo Studio della Streptochinasi nell'Infarto Miocardico). GISSI-3: effects of lisinopril and transdermal glyceryl trinitrate singly and together on 6-week mortality and ventricular function after myocardial infarction. Lancet 1994; 343:1115–1121.

12. Chinese Cardiac Study Collaborative Group. Oral captopril versus placebo among 13,634 patients with suspected acute myocardial infarction: interim report from the Chinese Cardiac Study (CCS-1). Lancet 1995; 345:686–687.

13. Kingma JH, Van Gilst WH, Peels CH, Dambrink JHE, Verheught FWA, Wielenga RP. Acute intervention with captopril during thrombolysis in patients with first anterior myocardial infarction: results from the Captopril and Thrombolysis Study (CATS). Eur Heart J 1994; 15: 898–907.

14. Ambrosioni E, Borghi C, Magnani B, for the Survival of Myocardial Infarction Long-term Evaluation (SMILE) Study Investigators. The effect of angiotensin-converting-enzyme inhibi-

tor zofenopril on mortality and morbidity after anterior myocardial infarction. N Engl J Med 1995; 332:80–85.

15. Ellis JL, Burnstock G. Angiotensin neuromodulation of adrenergic and purinergic co-transmission in the guinea-pig vas deferens. Br J Pharmacol 1989; 97:1157–1164.

16. James MA, Jones JV. Systolic wall stress and ventricular arrhythmia: the role of acute change in blood pressure in the isolated working rat heart. Clin Sci 1990; 79:499–504.

17. Ebert TJ. Captopril potentiates chronotropic baroreflex responses to carotid stimuli in humans. Hypertension 1985; 7:602–606.

18. Grassi G, Cattaneo BM, Seravalle G, Lanfranchi A, Pozzi M, Morganti A, et al. Effects of chronic ACE inhibition on sympathetic nerve traffic and baroreflex control of circulation in heart failure. Circulation 1997; 96:1173–1179.

19. Lumbers ER, McCloskey DI, Potter EK. Inhibition by angiotensin II of baroreceptor evoked activity in cardiac vagal efferent nerves. J Physiol 1979; 294:69–80.

20. Ridker PM, Gaboury CL, Conlin PR, Seely EW, Williams GH, Vaughan DE. Stimulation of plasminogen activator inhibitor in vivo by infusion of angiotensin II: evidence of a potential interaction between the renin angiotensin system and fibrinolytic activity. Circulation 1993; 87:1969–1973.

21. Sharpe N, Smith H, Murphy J, Greaves S, Hart H, Gamble G. Early prevention of left venticular dysfunction after myocardial infarction with angiotensin converting enzyme inhibition. Lancet 1991; 337:872–876.

22. Hall SA, Cooke GA, Tan LB. ACE inhibitors after myocardial infarction. Lancet 1994; 343: 1632–1633.

23. Woods KL, Fletcher S, Roffe C, Haider Y. Intravenous magnesium sulphate in suspected acute mycoardial infarction: results of the second Leicester Intravenous Magnesium Intervention Trial (LIMIT-2). Lancet 1992; 339:1553–1558.

24. Woods KL, Fletcher S. Long-term outcome after intravenous magnesium sulphate in suspected acute myocardial infarction: the second Leicester Intravenous Magnesium Intervention Trial (LIMIT-2). Lancet 1994; 343:816–819.

25. Roffe C, Fletcher S, Woods KL. Investigation of the effects of intravenous magnesium sulphate on cardiac rhythm in acute myocardial infarction. Br Heart J 1994; 71:141–145.

26. Conway M, Mohideen R, Adamopoulos S, Flather M, Collins R, Sleight P. A dose finding study for the initiation of captopril within 24 hours of acute myocardial infarction (pre-pilot study for ISIS-4). QJ Med 1989; 70–73:973–974.

27. ISIS-4 (Fourth International Study of Infarct Survival) Pilot Study Investigators. Randomized controlled trial of oral captopril, or oral isosorbide mononitrate and of intravenous magnesium sulphate started early in acute myocardial infarction: safety and haemodynamic effects. Eur Heart J 1994; 15:608–619.

28. Latini R, Avarzini F, De Nicolao A, Rocchetti M, and the GISSI-3 Investigators. Effects of lisinopril and nitroglycerin on blood pressure eary after myocardial infarction: the GISSI-3 pilot study. Clin Pharmacol Ther 1994; 56:680–692.

29. Danchin N, Vaur L, Genés N, Renault M, Ferriéres J, Etienne S, Cambou J-P. Management of acute myocardial infarction in intensive care units in 1995: a nationwide French survey of practice and early hospital results. J Am Coll Cardiol 1997; 30:1598–1605.

30. ACE-inhibitor Myocardial Infarction Collaborative Group. Indications for ACE-inhibitors in the early treatment of acute myocardial infarction: systematic overview of individual data from 100,000 patients in randomized trials. Circulation 1998; 97:2202–2212.

31. Cleland JGF. Anticoagulant and antiplatelet therapy in heart failure. Current Opinion in Cardiol 1997; 12:276–287.

22

SMILE

CLAUDIO BORGHI and ETTORE AMBROSIONI

Ambrosioni E, Borghi C, Magnani B for the Survival of Myocardial Infarction Long-Term Evaluation (SMILE) Study Investigators. The effect of the angiotensin-converting-enzyme inhibitor zofenopril on mortality and morbidity after anterior myocardial infarction. N Engl J Med 1995; 332:80–85.

INTRODUCTION

The prognosis for patients with acute myocardial infarction (AMI) has been drastically improved by the routine administration of drugs that prevent the onset and progression of left ventricular dysfunction following myocardial injury (1,2). Left ventricular dysfunction is a powerful predictor of mortality and the occurrence of congestive heart failure after myocardial infarction (3,4).

In particular, infarct expansion and left ventricular dysfunction can be limited by drugs that promote early myocardial reperfusion and/or myocardial salvage, such as thrombolytic agents, β-adrenergic blockers, and aspirin (1,5–7). However, the existence of a substantial proportion of patients who do not qualify for such therapeutic approach, because of a delayed hospital admission or the presence of individual contraindications to drugs (5–8), has created a strong rationale for the development of new therapeutic strategies to improve prognosis in patients with AMI, particularly when they cannot benefit from thrombolysis.

Since early activation of the renin-angiotensin-aldosterone system (RAAS) has been reported in patients with AMI (9–11) and has been associated with an increased risk of complications and a poorer prognosis (12), the blockade of this neurohumoral pathway has been identified as an effective therapeutic strategy for the treatment of patients with AMI (13). This was initially demonstrated in selected patients with symptomless ventricular dysfunction treated with angiotensin-converting enzyme (ACE) inhibitors some days after myocardial infarction (14,15). Subsequently some experimental and preliminary human data (2,16,17) also provided a strong rationale for the use of ACE inhibitors during the early phase of AMI, when the blockade of the RAAS could improve the hemodynamic profile and reduce the deleterious effects of neurohumoral activation.

237

We therefore planned a clinical trial aimed at evaluating the effects of ACE inhibitors started very early (<24 hr) during the clinical course of AMI in patients not eligible for thrombolytic treatment. Moreover, since anterior location of AMI is commonly associated with a greater degree of ventricular dysfunction (17) and the worst outcome in terms of mortality and occurrence of congestive heart failure (CHF) (18), it seemed a reasonable proposition to test the efficacy of early ACE inhibition in high-risk patients with anterior location of myocardial damage and independently on a prespecified level of ventricular dysfunction.

The Survival of Myocardial Infarction Long-term Evaluation (SMILE) trial was planned accordingly to test the hypothesis that oral administration of zofenopril calcium to patients with high-risk acute anterior myocardial infarction not undergoing thrombolysis would improve their clinical outcome by reducing the occurrence of major cardiovascular events.

STUDY ORGANIZATION AND METHODS

The SMILE trial was a randomized, multicenter, double-blind, placebo-controlled trial (19) in 1556 patients with an AMI of anterior location who were not eligible for thrombolytic treatment. The enrollment phase of the trial began in January 1991 and ended on November 1992. Patients of either sex aged 18–80 years were eligible for enrollment if they presented to the intensive care unit within 24 hours from onset of typical chest pain associated with electrocardiographic signs of definite anterior wall myocardial infarction and if they were not eligible for thrombolytic treatment because of late admission to intensive care unit or individual contraindications to systemic fibrinolysis (7,8). The principal exclusion criteria were Killip class IV on admission, supine systolic blood pressure less than 100 mmHg on admission, serum creatinine level greater than 2.5 mg/dl, history of CHF, current treatment with ACE inhibitors, contraindications to the use of ACE-inhibitors, and inability or refusal to give informed consent.

The SMILE study drug, zofenopril calcium, is a short-acting sulfhydryl-containing ACE inhibitor. It is a pro-drug ester analog of captopril with peculiar pharmacological and anti-ischemic properties (20–23). The initial dose of 7.5 mg of blinded medication was doubled every 12 hours to the final target dose of 30 mg b.i.d. if systolic blood pressure was >100 mmHg and no signs or symptoms of hypotension occurred. Concomitant treatment included analgesic agents, beta-blockers, nitrates, calcium-channel blockers, aspirin, inotropic drugs, diuretic agents, and anticoagulants as indicated.

Patients were seen during the in-hospital phase, after 4 weeks, and at the end of the follow-up period (6 weeks ± 3 days) to assess their clinical status, occurrence of adverse events, and compliance with treatment. Upon completion of the 6-week double-blind period, the treatment with zofenopril or placebo was stopped and patients were maintained on their other recommended therapy for 48 additional weeks and were then again blindly evaluated for survival status and occurrence of CHF.

STUDY ENDPOINTS

The primary objective of the SMILE study was the evaluation of the effect of zofenopril in addition to conventional treatment on the combined 6-week occurrence of death or severe congestive heart failure. Secondary prospectively defined endpoints included the effect of 6 weeks of treatment on (1) the occurrence of clinical signs of mild-to-moderate CHF, (2) the recurrence of myocardial infarction, and (3) the occurrence of angina. In addition we evaluated the effect of 6-week double-blind treatment on subsequent 1-year mortality.

All deaths occurring during the trial were classified as cardiac or noncardiac. Cardiac deaths included progressive heart failure, sudden death, recurrent MI, heart rupture, and electro-mechanical dissociation. Noncardiac deaths included cerebrovascular events, pulmonary embolism, and nonvascular causes of death. Progressive heart failure was classified by pump failure and cardiogenic shock. Sudden death was defined as a sudden, unexpected death that occurred within 1 hour of the onset of new symptoms.

Severe CHF included in the primary endpoint was defined by the presence after randomization of three out of four of the following clinical and radiological signs; 3° heart sound, bilateral pulmonary rales, radiological pulmonary congestion [> the grade II of Madsen et al. (24)] and peripheral edema despite the concomitant administration of positive inotropic drug, diuretics, and vasodilators other than ACE inhibitors and necessitating an open-label treatment with ACE inhibitors. Mild-to-moderate CHF during the follow-up phase was defined according to the New York Heart Association functional classification.

RESULTS

From January 1991 to November 1992 a population of 1556 patients were enrolled in the trial from a total of 154 Italian coronary care units. The distribution of baseline clinical characteristics was well balanced between the two treatment groups, as was the distribution of concomitant treatments (Table 1).

For the purposes of the present report, the results of the SMILE study (25) have been subdivided in two main sections summarizing separately the effects of treatment after 6 weeks (short-term) and 1 year (long-term). The reason for such an approach is the different availability of clinical data, which is complete for all randomized patients after 6 weeks. Conversely, after 1 year we have a complete set of data for mortality and CHF, whereas the rate of occurrence of other clinical events was available for only 80% of the whole population.

A third section will summarize the effects of zofenopril in the subgroups of patients without CHF on admission to the coronary care unit (26).

Short-Term Effects of Zofenopril Treatment in Patients with AMI

Mortality and Severe CHF

During the 6 weeks of double-blind treatment, death or CHF occurred in 83 of the 784 (10.6%) patients in the placebo group and 55 of the 772 (7.1%) of the patients undergoing zofenopril treatment (Fig. 1) with a risk reduction of 35% (95% CI 8–54%; $p = 0.016$). This reduction was mainly due to a decrease in the rate of severe CHF requiring open-label ACE inhibition (4.3% vs. 2.2%; risk reduction 49%; 95% CI 11–71%; $p = 0.018$). Sixty-five patients died in the placebo group (8.3%) compared with 50 in the zofenopril group (6.5%), with a reduction in the risk of death from all causes of 22% (95% CI −12–

Table 1 Compatibility of Study Groups at Baseline in the SMILE Study

Variable	Placebo (n = 784)	Zofenopril (n = 772)
Mean age (yr)	64.3	63.9
Age >70 yr (%)	31	29
Sex ratio, M/F (%)	73/27	72/28
Clinical history at admission (%)	21	20
Hypertension	40	39
Current smoker	41	41
Angina	33	32
Mean hours to hospitalization	9	9
Mean hours to randomization	15	15
Killip class I (%)	86	85
Killip class II–III (%)	14	15
Characterization of index MI (%)		
Q wave	52	53
ST elevation	65	67
Drugs < 24 hr of randomization (%)		
Antiplatelet agents	55	53
Beta-blockers	21	18
Calcium-channel blockers	10	10
Digoxin	6	7
Diuretics	19	17
Nitrates	44	43

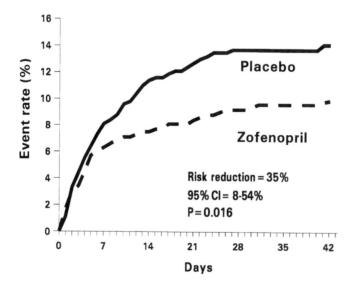

Figure 1 Combined occurrence of death and severe congestive heart failure after 6 weeks of treatment in the SMILE study.

48%; $p = 0.171$). Ninety-one percent of deaths (105/115) were due to cardiovascular causes (60 in the placebo group vs. 45 in the zofenopril group) with a risk reduction of 24% (95% CI -12–43%; $p = 0.171$) (Table 2). Among cardiovascular deaths there was a trend toward a reduction in mortality due to progressive heart failure (13 vs. 19 deaths) and sudden death (4 vs. 11 deaths) in the zofenopril group. Interestingly, we also observed a large reduction in the number of zofenopril-treated patients who died within 24 hours from randomization (1 vs. 8 deaths; $p < 0.01$). Deaths due to noncardiac causes (9%) were evenly distributed between the two treatment groups (Table 2).

Secondary Outcome Measures

The effects of 6-week treatment with zofenopril over the prospectively defined secondary endpoints of the study are summarized as follows. Clinical manifestation of stable or unstable angina occurred in 19.5% of the patients in the placebo group and in 16.6% of those treated with zofenopril with a risk reduction of 18% (95% CI -6 to 37%; $p = 0.082$). Reinfarction after randomization occurred in 23 patients with no difference between the two groups (12 placebo vs. 11 zofenopril). Clinical signs of mild-to-moderate CHF were observed in a total of 75 patients (11.7%) in the placebo group and in 52 patients (8.3%) treated with zofenopril with a risk reduction of 29% that reached a borderline statistical significance (95% CI -2 to 51%; $p = 0.054$). Interestingly, the extent of reduction was comparable among patients in NYHA class II (5.6% vs. 7.8%) and III (2.1% vs. 3.1%), thus suggesting a wide beneficial role of zofenopril treatment.

Effect of Treatment in Selected Clinical and Therapeutic Subgroups

The effects of zofenopril treatment in some high-risk subgroups of patients are reported in Table 3. The treatment with zofenopril reduced the combined occurrence of death and severe CHF in patients with (1) previous myocardial infarction (4.0% vs. 19.6%; $p = 0.0006$); (2) history of diabetes (7.2% vs. 16.5%; $p = 0.014$); (3) history of angina (7.4% vs. 16.3%; $p = 0.003$); and (4) history of hypertension (7.6% vs. 13.7%; $p = 0.021$).

The role of concomitant medication during the acute phase of AMI in the occurrence of combined endpoints is summarized in Table 3. Significant interactions were found among the use of zofenopril and the administration of calcium channel blockers, digoxin, and nitrates, whereas we were unable to find any significant interaction between zofenopril and aspirin or beta-blockers.

Table 2 Causes of Death in the SMILE Study

	No. of patients (%)	
Cause of death	Placebo ($n = 784$)	Zofenopril ($n = 772$)
Progressive heart failure	19 (2.4)	13 (1.7)
Sudden death	11 (1.4)	4 (0.5)
Myocardial rupture	10 (1.3)	8 (1.0)
Reinfarction	8 (1.0)	5 (0.6)
Other cardiac event	12 (1.5)	15 (2.0)
Cerebrovascular event	3 (0.4)	3 (0.4)
Noncardiac event	2 (0.3)	2 (0.3)
All causes	65 (8.3)	50 (6.5)

Table 3 Effects of Treatment on Primary Combined Endpoint in Some
Selected Subgroups of the SMILE Study

Variable	No. of events/ No. of patients (%)		RR (95% CI)	p-value
	Placebo	Zofenopril		
Sex				
Male	47/571 (8.2)	28/537 (5.0)	0.59 (0.36–0.95)	NS
Female	36/213 (16.9)	27/215 (12.5)	0.70 (0.40–1.21)	NS
Age (yr)				
<65	22/389 (5.6)	15/378 (3.9)	0.68 (0.35–1.34)	NS
>65	61/395 (15.4)	40/394 (10.1)	0.61 (0.40–0.93)	NS
Previous MI				
Yes	20/102 (19.6)	4/100 (4.0)	0.17 (0.05–0.52)	<0.006
No	63/682 (9.2)	51/672 (7.6)	0.84 (0.57–1.27)	0.38
History of diabetes				
Yes	27/164 (16.5)	10/139 (7.2)	0.39 (0.18–0.84)	0.014
No	56/620 (9.0)	45/633 (7.1)	0.77 (0.50–1.17)	NS
History of hypertension				
Yes	40/291 (13.7)	21/275 (7.6)	0.53 (0.30–0.91)	0.021
No	43/493 (8.7)	34/497 (6.8)	0.87 (0.52–1.45)	NS
Use of beta-blockers				
Yes	13/161 (8.0)	10/140 (7.1)	0.87 (0.37–2.04)	NS
No	70/623 (11.2)	45/632 (7.1)	0.60 (0.41–0.89)	NS
Use of calcium blockers				
Yes	13/82 (15.8)	2/74 (2.7)	0.14 (0.03–0.66)	0.005
No	70/702 (10.0)	53/698 (7.6)	0.74 (0.51–1.07)	0.12
Use of nitrates				
Yes	53/337 (15.7)	27/327 (8.2)	0.48 (0.29–0.79)	0.003
No	30/447 (6.7)	28/445 (6.3)	0.93 (0.54–1.58)	0.79
Use of aspirin				
Yes	35/431 (8.1)	26/409 (6.3)	0.77 (0.45–1.3)	NS
No	48/353 (13.5)	29/363 (8.0)	0.55 (0.33–0.89)	NS
Use of digoxin				
Yes	16/50 (32.0)	7/51 (13.7)	0.67 (0.9–0.88)	0.026
No	67/734 (9.1)	48/721 (6.7)	0.29 (0.52–1.03)	NS

NS = Not significant.

Blood Pressure Profile

A significant reduction of both systolic and diastolic blood pressure was observed after
24 hours and 1 week in both groups of patients. As expected, the decrease was significantly
enhanced in patients treated with zofenopril over the whole 24-hour period ($p < 0.005$).
The blood pressure values measured over the 6 weeks of follow-up showed a significant
decrease of systolic blood pressure in patients treated with zofenopril (week 1: −16.1 vs.
−12.9 mmHg; week 4: −14.5 vs. −11.9 mmHg; week 6: −10.1 vs. −6.2 mmHg; $p < 0.02$),
whereas diastolic blood pressure was not modified by ACE inhibition (week 1: −9.6 vs.
−8.6 mmHg; week 4: −8.9 vs. −7.9 mmHg; week 6: −6.1 vs. −5.2 mmHg; $p = 0.12$).

The overall incidence of hypotension, conservatively defined as a systolic blood
pressure value below 100 mmHg at any time during the study, was significantly increased

in patients treated with zofenopril (132 patients, 17.1%) when compared to patients treated with placebo (70 patients, 8.9%; $p < 0.0001$). However, the rate of discontinuation because of symptomatic or severe hypotension (systolic blood pressure < 90 mmHg) and the rate of first-dose hypotension were not increased in patients treated with zofenopril (3.8% vs. 2.7% and 0.6% vs. 0.3%, respectively).

Concomitant Pharmacological Treatment and Safety Profile

Upon discharge, no differences were reported in the use of beta-blockers, aspirin, diuretics, and nitrates between patients treated with zofenopril or placebo, whereas the use of digoxin was less among patients taking zofenopril (5.8% vs. 8.4%; $p = 0.04$), in agreement with the lesser occurrence of clinical manifestations of CHF.

During the 6 weeks of double-blind treatment, a small proportion of patients complained of side effects, and the proportion of those who permanently discontinued the treatment was 6.8% in the placebo group and 8.6% in the zofenopril group. The main cause of discontinuation in both groups was symptomatic or severe (systolic blood pressure < 90 mmHg) hypotension with no differences in the rate of withdrawal between patients treated with zofenopril (3.8%) or placebo (2.7%; p not significant). None of the common side effects of ACE inhibitors were significantly increased in patients treated with zofenopril, probably because of the marginal proportion of events and the short period of observation.

One-Year Effects of Zofenopril Treatment in Patients with AMI

Mortality

The 1-year actual mortality curves for all patients according to their original treatment allocation are depicted in Figure 2. Cumulative 1-year mortality was significantly reduced

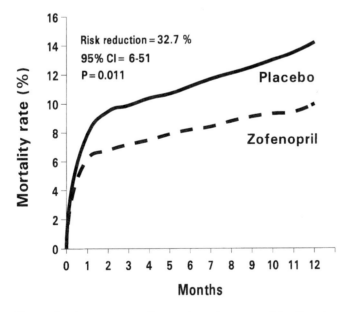

Figure 2 One-year mortality rate in patients treated for 6 weeks with zofenopril or placebo in the SMILE study.

in patients who underwent the 6-week treatment with zofenopril when compared with patients treated with placebo. In particular, cumulative mortality was 10.0% (77/772) in the zofenopril group and 14.1% (111/784) in the group of patients treated with placebo, with a 33% significant reduction in the risk of death (95% CI 6–51%; $p = 0.011$) that cannot be explained by differences in the concomitant pharmacological or surgical treatment (Table 4).

Long-term mortality was investigated in some subgroups of patients. In elderly patients (age > 70 years) the 1-year mortality was significantly reduced in patients treated with zofenopril (33/164; 20%) when compared to the group of patients taking placebo (61/19; 31.9%) with a risk reduction of 37.3% (95% CI 1–61%; $p = 0.024$). The effect of zofenopril treatment on long-term mortality seems to be prevalent in male patients where the administration of the ACE inhibitor resulted in a 39% reduction in the risk of death (95% CI 6–60%; $p = 0.026$), which was greater that that observed in the female counterpart (risk reduction: 24.6%; 95% CI −27/56%; $p = 0.288$). However, because of the higher death rate observed in women (23.4% vs. 11.8%), a simple evaluation of the benefit of zofenopril treatment based on the calculation of the relative risk of death does not completely define the role of sex. Indeed, if we consider the effects of zofenopril in terms of absolute risk reduction in men and women, the number of lives saved is 26 of 1000 and 28 of 1000 patients, respectively, without any difference between the two groups.

Among the most debated issues around the use of ACE inhibitors in patients with AMI is the importance of blood pressure before drug treatment. For this reason we have investigated the effects of zofenopril in patients with systolic blood pressure on admission of <130 mmHg. In this subgroup, the mortality rate was significantly reduced by active treatment with a risk reduction of 38.4% (95% CI 22–60%; $p = 0.01$), which was largely comparable with that observed in the general population.

As for the role of infarct size, categorized by CK, we have observed a greater beneficial effect of zofenopril in patients with the larger infarcts (Fig. 3). The reduction in the risk of death was 48.2% (95% CI 1–73%; $p = 0.049$) in patients with large MIs (peak CK above the upper hinge) and only 23% (95% CI = −58/63%; $p = 0.484$) in patients with small MIs (below the lower hinge), with a highly significant reduction in the absolute proportion of lives saved (40 of 1000 vs. 18 of 1000 patients; large vs. small MIs). Interest-

Table 4 Concurrent Treatments During 1-Year of Observation in the SMILE Study

Treatment	Placebo (%) ($n = 633$)	Zofenopril (%) ($n = 616$)	p-value
Digitalis	6.3	8.0	0.25
Diuretics	12.6	13.1	0.79
ACE inhibitors	25.8	26.1	0.20
Calcium blockers	15.9	21.1	0.024
Beta-blockers	13.1	10.4	0.06
Aspirin	79.5	82.7	0.08
Nitrates	32.6	34.3	0.53
Antiarrhythmic drugs	3.7	3.0	0.46
Lipid-lowering agents	4.5	3.0	0.14
Noncardiovascular drugs	9.6	11.0	0.19
PTCA	6.5	7.4	0.78
CABG	5.8	7.1	0.95

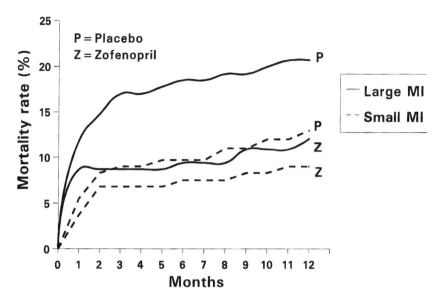

Figure 3   Effects of infarct size on 1-year mortality rate in the SMILE study.

ingly, the mortality rate observed in patients with larger infarct size and treated with zofenopril (12.1%) was superimposable on that observed in patients with small MIs and treated
with placebo (13.8%; Fig. 3), thereby suggesting the capacity of early zofenopril treatment
to interfere with the processes of infarct expansion during the acute phase of MI.

    Among the other possible determinants of prognosis in patients with AMI is whether
the infarct is transmural. The comparison between patients with Q-wave and non–Q-wave
MI (Fig. 4) clearly demonstrates that a significant drug effect can be observed only in

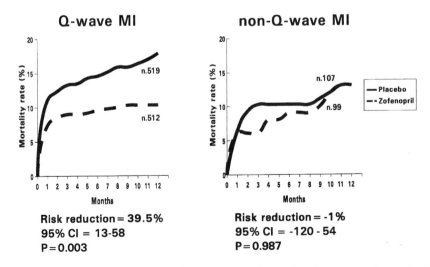

Figure 4   Effects of infarct type (Q-wave vs. non–Q-wave) on 1-year mortality rate in the SMILE
study.

patients with Q-wave MI, where the 6-week treatment with zofenopril was associated with a 39.5% reduction in the long-term risk of death (95% CI 13–58%; $p = 0.003$). In patients with non–Q-wave MI, zofenopril treatment did not produce any significant benefit in terms of survival.

Besides the above-mentioned subgroups of patients, all characterized by a specific prognostic profile that could be improved by the early administration of an ACE inhibitor, we have also examined the effect of zofenopril treatment in a small subgroup of subjects not taking any pharmacological treatment during the 12 months of follow-up. In this population we had the unique opportunity of evaluating the primary effect of zofenopril treatment without the confounding influence of the use of other concomitant cardiovascular drugs. Interestingly, even in this population of subjects, 6-week treatment with zofenopril significantly reduced the long-term risk of death by 29.5% (95% CI 6–68%; $p = 0.014$), and these data strongly suggest the capacity of early ACE inhibition per se of improving the prognosis of patients with AMI.

Secondary Outcome Measures

The effect of 6-week treatment with zofenopril over the 1-year incidence of major cardiovascular events was assessed in over 80% of the cumulative SMILE population. The findings, summarized in Table 5, do not show any significant difference among patients treated with zofenopril or placebo.

Effects of Treatment in Patients Without CHF

To evaluate the effects of ACE inhibitors on the onset and progression of congestive heart failure, we have separately investigated the clinical effects of early zofenopril administration in patients without a history or clinical signs of CHF on hospitalization (27). In this rather large subgroup of 1146 patients, we assessed the effects of zofenopril on the development of CHF according to the same criteria utilized in the main study. In particular, the prevalence of CHF, either mild to moderate or severe, was the main objective and was evaluated 6 weeks and 1 year after AMI.

The cumulative prevalence of CHF was not modified by zofenopril after both 6 weeks (13.2% vs. 13.6%; $p = $ NS zofenopril vs. placebo) and 12 months (14.3% vs. 15.3%; $p = $ NS zofenopril vs. placebo). Conversely, the prevalence of severe CHF was significantly reduced in patients treated with ACE inhibitors (1.6% vs. 2.6%; risk reduction 55.5%; 95% CI 9–63%; $p = 0.032$) as was the combined occurrence of death and severe CHF (4.8% vs. 8.2%; risk reduction 59%; 95% CI 11–71%; $p = 0.024$). Moreover, the

Table 5 Effect of 6 Weeks of Treatment with Zofenopril on the 1-Year Prevalence of Major Cardiovascular Events

Event	Placebo (%) ($n = 633$)	Zofenopril (%) ($n = 616$)	p-value
Angina	21.5	23.8	0.626
Re-IMA	3.7	3.4	0.802
Cumulative CHF	14.8	15.4	0.743
PTCA	2.1	2.6	0.780
CABG	5.8	7.2	0.958

percentage of patients experiencing a deterioration to severe CHF (Class IV NYHA) after 1 year was significantly reduced in the zofenopril-treated population (11% vs. 24.3%; *p* = 0.001). The lack of any difference in the incidence of mild-to-moderate CHF can be explained by the reduced mortality rate observed in the zofenopril-treated population, which probably included a greater proportion of patients with early LV dysfunction who were prone to the development of CHF. Interestingly, these findings strongly support the ability of zofenopril to prevent the progression of CHF toward the more severe stages and support the early use of ACE inhibitors even in patients where AMI is not complicated by clinical signs of CHF.

GENERAL CONSIDERATIONS

Acute myocardial infarction is a critical condition whose clinical outcome is strongly influenced by the complex interactions between the extent of initial myocardial injury, the concomitant neurohumoral activation, and the degree of hemodynamic failure. The extent of left ventricular dilatation has been identified as an important marker of prognosis after infarction and strictly correlates with mortality and development of symptomatic congestive heart failure (2–4). This is of particular importance in patients not undergoing thrombolysis (5) and in those with anterior myocardial infarctions who have a poorer prognosis in terms of mortality and onset of heart failure (17,18). The SMILE study, using a randomized, placebo-controlled, double-blind design, was able to demonstrate that the early administration of an ACE inhibitor can significantly improve the clinical prognosis of patients with high-risk acute anterior myocardial infarction not undergoing thrombolysis. In particular, the administration of zofenopril, given within 24 hours of the onset of symptoms and continued for 6 weeks in such a population of patients, resulted in a significant reduction in the combined proportion of subjects who died or developed clinical signs of severe CHF. Importantly, these results were obtained without pretrial selection of patients to exclude those who could not tolerate the drug, and this strategy could increase the relevance of the findings to normal clinical practice.

The results of the SMILE trial support some convincing therapeutic issues about ACE inhibitors and AMI:

1. The beneficial effects of early treatment with ACE inhibitors is confirmed for a population with a high degree of left ventricular dysfunction and renin-angiotensin activation (anterior AMI).
2. Treatment with ACE inhibitors is safe and beneficial in a clearly defined patient population that is clinically relevant and excluded from any aggressive treatment schedule.
3. The SMILE data do not support the existence of a negative influence of early ACE inhibition on coronary perfusion and/or recovery of cardiac function after acute anterior myocardial damage. Indeed, the benefits of zofenopril administration were achieved in a population of patients not undergoing pharmacological reperfusion, where the role of coronary perfusion pressure is critical.
4. The beneficial effects of ACE inhibitors cannot be attributed to the selection criteria since the two populations of SMILE patients were well balanced in terms of concomitant treatments and distribution of risk factors known to in-

fluence the prognosis of myocardial infarction (age, sex, diabetes, previous MI, Killip classification).

5. The beneficial effect of ACE inhibitors does not appear to result from a treatment effect of the drug on preexisting chronic CHF, since the study population did not include patients with preexisting CHF whose outcome could be improved by the treatment with ACE inhibitors (29,30).

6. The results of the SMILE study strongly suggest that an early treatment with an ACE inhibitor can have a significant beneficial effect on both short- and long-term prognosis in patients with AMI.

7. The risk reduction in terms of mortality appears to be distributed among different subgroups even though a greater benefit was seen in patients with large MI and Q-wave MI.

8. The results of the SMILE study suggest that the risk of severe hypotension can be largely prevented by a progressive increase of drug dosing during the acute phase of MI. Conversely, the occurrence of mild-to-moderate hypotension, which is significantly increased in patients undergoing ACE inhibition, does not directly influence prognosis. In the SMILE study a greater occurrence of mild hypotension was observed in the zofenopril group despite improved outcome.

9. The benefit of early administration of zofenopril can be clearly demonstrated even in patients without clinical signs of CHF on admission, thereby suggesting a preventive role of early ACE inhibition over the mechanisms responsible for the progressive development of CHF and related death rate.

10. Finally, the results of the SMILE study are in agreement with many available data and support the notion that early ACE inhibition started hours after the onset of symptoms of MI can induce beneficial hemodynamic and metabolic changes that prevent left ventricular remodeling and improve clinical outcome and survival in patients with acute myocardial infarction. The study provides a considerable demonstration that the benefit arising from the use of ACE inhibitors in AMI is mainly related to the existence of a baseline risk amenable to pharmacological treatment. We suggest that routine, early administration of ACE inhibitors in patients with myocardial infarction can be presently considered a reasonable strategy, particularly in high-risk subgroups and in patients with large anterior myocardial infarctions.

REFERENCES

1. Yusuf S, Sleight P, Held P, McMahon S. Routine medical management of acute myocardial infarction:Lessons from overviews of recent randomized controlled trials. Circulation 1990; 82(suppl II):117–134.

2. Pfeffer MA, Braunwald E. Ventricular remodeling after myocardial infarction: experimental observations and clinical implications. Circulation 1990; 31:1161–1172.

3. White HD, Norris RM, Brown MA, Brandt PWT, Withlock RML, Wild CJ. Left ventricular end-systolic volume as the major determinant of survival after recovery from myocardial infarction. Circulation 1987; 76:44–51.

4. Hammermeister KE, DeRouen TA, Dodge HT. Variables predictive of survival in patients with coronary disease: selection by univariate and multivariate analysis from clinical, electro-

cardiographic, exercise, arteriographic, and quantitative angiographic evaluation. Circulation 1979; 59:421–430.

5. Cairns JA, Collins R, Fuster V, Passamani ER. Coronary thrombolysis. Chest 1989; 95:73S–87S.

6. ISIS-1 (First International Study of Infarct Survival) Collaborative Group. Randomised trial of intravenous atenolol among 16027 cases of suspected acute myocardial infarction: ISIS-1. Lancet 1986; ii:57–66.

7. ISIS-2 (Second International Study of Infarct Survival) Collaborative Group. Randomised trial of intravenous streptokinase, oral aspirin, both, or neither among 17,187 cases of suspected acute myocardial infarction: ISIS-1. Lancet 1988; ii:349–360.

8. Gruppo Italiano per lo Studio della Streptochinasi nell'Infarto Miocardico (GISSI). Effectiveness of intravenous thrombolytic treatment in acute myocardial infarction. Lancet 1986; i: 397–402.

9. Dargie HJ, McAlpine HM, Morton JJ. Neuroendocrine activation in acute myocardial infarction. J Cardiovasc Pharmacol 1987; 9(suppl 2):S21–S24.

10. Santos RA, Brum JM, Brosnihan KB, Ferrario CM. The renin-angiotensin system during acute myocardial ischemia in dogs. Hypertension 1990; 15(suppl 1):121–127.

11. McAlpine HM, Morton JJ, Leckie B, Rumley A, Gillen G, Dargie HJ. Neuroendocrine activation after acute myocardial infarction. Br Heart J 1988; 60:117–124.

12. Vaney C, Waeber B, Turini G, Margalith D, Brunner HR, Perret C. Renin and the complications of acute myocardial infarction. Chest 1984; 86:40–44.

13. Ambrosioni E, Borghi C. Potential use of ACE-inhibitors after acute myocardial infarction. J Cardiovasc Pharmacol 1989; 14(suppl 9):S92–S94.

14. Pfeffer MA, Braunwald E, Moyè LA, et al. Effect of captopril on mortality and morbidity in patients with left ventricular dysfunction after myocardial infarction. N Engl J Med 1992; 327: 669–677.

15. Sharpe N, Smith H, Murphy J, Hannan S. Treatment of patients with symptomless left ventricular dysfunction after myocardial infarction. Lancet 1988; 1:255–259.

16. Ambrosioni E, Borghi C, Magnani B, for the SMILE Pilot Study Working Party. Early treatment of acute myocardial infarction with angiotensin-converting enzyme inhibition: safety considerations. Am J Cardiol 1991; 68:101D–110D.

17. Pye M, Oldroyd KG, Ray SG, Christie J, Ford I, Cobbe SM, Dargie HJ. Effects of early captopril administration on left ventricular dilatation after acute myocardial infarction. Circulation 1990; 82(suppl 3):III–674.

18. Stone PH, Raabe DS, Jaffe AS, et al. Prognostic significance of location and type of myocardial infarction: independent adverse outcome associated with anterior location. J Am Coll Cardiol 1988; 11:453.

19. Ambrosioni E, Borghi C, Magnani B. Survival of Myocardial Infarction Long-term Evaluation (SMILE) study: rationale, design, organization and outcome definitions. Controlled Clin Trials 1994; 15:201–210.

20. DeForrest JM, Waldron TL, Krapcho J, et al. Preclinical pharmacology of zofenopril, an inhibitor of angiotensin I converting enzyme. J Cardiovasc Pharmacol 1989; 13:887–894.

21. Cushman DW, Wang FL, Fung WC, et al. Differentiation of angiotensin converting enzyme (ACE) inhibitors by their selective inhibition of ACE in physiologically important target organs. Am J Hypertens 1989; 2:294–307.

22. Van Gilst WH, Scholtens E, De Graeff PA, De Langen CDJ, Wesseling H. Differential influences of angiotensin converting enzyme inhibitors on the coronary circulation. Circulation 1988; 77(suppl 1):1–24.

23. Westlin W, Mullane K. Does captopril attenuate reperfusion-induced myocardial dysfunction by scavenging free radicals? Circulation 1984; 71(suppl 1):30–39.

24. Madsen EB, Gilpin E, Slutsky RA, Ahnve S, Henning H, Ross J Jr. Usefulness of chest x-ray for predicting abnormal left ventricular function after acute myocardial infarction. Am Heart J 1984; 108:1431–1436.

25. Ambrosioni E, Borghi C, Magnani B, on behalf of the SMILE Study Investigators. The effect of the angiotensin-converting-enzyme inhibitor zofenopril on mortality and morbidity after anterior myocardial infarction. N Engl J Med 1995; 332:80–85.

26. Borghi C, Ambrosioni E, Magnani B, on behalf of SMILE Study Investigators. Effects of the early administration of zofenopril on onset and progression of congestive heart failure in patients with anterior wall acute myocardial infarction. Am J Cardiol 1996; 78:317–322.

Section G
ACE Inhibitors: Delayed Use

If patients are not already treated with ACE inhibitors early in their course, then institution of therapy can be more selective. The data supporting the chronic use of ACE inhibitors in patients with significant left ventricular impairment or clinical congestive heart failure are overwhelming. All infarct survivors with impaired ventricular function or clinical heart failure should receive ACE inhibitors at the final doses established by these trials for an indefinite period of time, unless they have a clear contraindication or a demonstrated intolerance to them.

23

SAVE

MARC A. PFEFFER and EUGENE BRAUNWALD

Pfeffer MA, Braunwald E, Moye LA, Basta L, Brown EJ, Cuddy TE, Davis BR, Geltman EM, Goldman S, Flaker GC, Klein M, Lamas GH, Packer M, Rouleau J, Rouleau JL, Rutherford J, Wertheimer JH, Hawkins CM, on behalf of the SAVE Investigators. Effect of captopril on mortality and morbidity in patients with left ventricular dysfunction after myocardial infarction. Results of the survival and ventricular enlargement trial. N Engl J Med 1992;327:669–677.

INTRODUCTION

The impressive strides in the management of patients with acute myocardial infarction and its chronic sequelae have been based on evidence derived from definitive clinical trials. These trials have demonstrated the relative benefits and adverse consequences of several therapies. Over the past decade, reperfusion strategies and antiplatelet therapies have made a major favorable impact on the management of patients with acute myocardial infarction. Simultaneous with these advances in the management of acute myocardial infarction has come the recognition of the clinical importance of treatment with angiotensin-converting enzyme (ACE) inhibitors. Administration of an ACE inhibitor after myocardial infarction has been demonstrated to prolong life whether or not a reperfusion strategy was utilized. The clinical benefits of ACE inhibitor therapy in the management of acute and chronic myocardial infarction are so well entrenched that use of this therapy is now endorsed by major international cardiology professional societies (1,2). Indeed, usage patterns of ACE inhibitors for patients with myocardial infarction are employed in guidelines to assess the quality of medical care.

The Survival and Ventricular Enlargement (SAVE) study was the first major clinical trial to test the hypothesis that the administration of an ACE inhibitor improves clinical outcome in patients who have experienced a myocardial infarction (3). The SAVE study was firmly rooted in mechanistic animal (4) and human studies (5), which indicated that a myocardial infarction may initiate further long-term unfavorable topographic changes of left ventricular size and shape (ventricular remodeling). The ability of ACE inhibitor therapy to favorably modify these structural changes and the strong association between the extent of ventricular enlargement and the risk of death provided the rationale to embark on a major trial of ACE inhibitor therapy with clinical outcomes. As suggested by the trial's acronym, the investigators sought to link the process of ventricular enlargement with survival. This chapter will review the rationale, design, and major findings of the SAVE trial.

Rationale

Interruption of coronary blood flow results in prompt regional systolic dysfunction—akinesis or dyskinesis. The extent of this abnormality in cardiac wall motion has been related quantitatively to the reduction in global ejection fraction. By use of the rat model of coronary ligation with its inherent wide range of histologic damage, the influence of infarct size on ventricular performance was readily quantitated (6). An interesting observation from this model of chronic myocardial infarction was that despite a reduced ejection fraction, resting cardiac output was generally maintained, except in the animals with extensive (greater than 40% of left ventricular surface) infarctions (6). In some respects, ventricular enlargement could be considered an important adaptive mechanism to maintain the stroke volume of the ventricle that had undergone infarction, since less fractional shortening is needed from the larger chamber to produce the same stroke volume (7). However, in a detailed analysis of the temporal course of ventricular enlargement following myocardial infarction in this model, it became apparent that ventricular remodeling tended to be progressive, continuing well beyond the early phase of hemodynamic improvement (4). The magnitude of ventricular enlargement is largely dependent on the extent of myocardial damage and on the time interval since the infarction.

Since this progressive enlargement was viewed as detrimental, it was considered to be an appropriate target for pharmacologic therapy. Dr. Janice Pfeffer conceived of the use of ACE inhibitor therapy to reduce wall stress, the intrinsic stimulus of this adverse cardiac remodeling, and thereby attenuate the process of progressive ventricular enlargement (8). Her detailed studies in the rat with coronary ligation demonstrated that chronic therapy with the ACE inhibitor captopril led to a reduction in the structural changes that occur in the left ventricle. When compared to untreated animals with comparable infarct sizes, the captopril-treated animals had lower ventricular end-diastolic pressures and operating volumes (8). In a separate series of studies, our laboratory demonstrated that these favorable alterations in ventricular volume and function produced by ACE inhibitor therapy also improved survival (9).

Clinical studies have underscored that a myocardial infarction can indeed initiate progressive deleterious changes in left ventricular size and shape that can be attenuated by ACE inhibitor therapy (10). Investigators at Johns Hopkins University (5,11) demonstrated that the infarcted region may thin and elongate during the early phase of an acute myocardial infarction. This process, termed infarct expansion, occurred in a subset of patients and was associated with a heightened risk for subsequent adverse cardiovascular events (12). Moreover, patients manifesting early infarct expansion had a predilection for late ventricular enlargement. Patients with the more extensive infarctions, especially anterior wall infarcts involving the ventricular apex, were at heightened risk for progressive ventricular enlargement. Several well-focused mechanistic studies demonstrated, as had earlier studies in animals, that ACE inhibitor therapy could reduce the extent of ventricular enlargement that occurs in the months and years following a myocardial infarction (13–15). Although these trials were too small and were not designed to test the clinical effectiveness of this new use for ACE inhibitors, they did provide strong rationale for employing these therapies to reduce ventricular enlargement and thus improve long-term clinical outcome. The SAVE study, therefore, was based on the preliminary animal and human studies demonstrating the benefit of captopril in attenuating ventricular enlargement after myocardial infarction. The trial was specifically designed to address the question of whether long-term administration of captopril after acute myocardial infarction would improve survival and reduce the proportion of patients who experience a marked deterioration in cardiac performance (3).

Design and Conduct

The SAVE study was a randomized, double-blind, placebo-controlled trial of 2231 patients (16). The trial was a cooperative venture involving investigators at 112 participating hospitals in the United States and Canada. Since the animal and preliminary clinical studies suggested less efficacy of ACE inhibitor in cases of minimal-to-small myocardial infarction, the entry criteria required objective evidence of left ventricular dysfunction. Therefore, the study enrolled patients identified as having an ejection fraction of 40% or less by radionuclide angiography. When the SAVE study started, the results of the initial Cooperative North Scandinavian Enalapril Survival Study (CONSENSUS) (17) demonstrating an improvement in survival with the use of an ACE inhibitor in patients with severe heart failure were available, and the Studies of Left Ventricular Dysfunction (SOLVD) (18) evaluating the use of the ACE inhibitor enalapril in patients with symptomatic heart failure were just beginning enrollment. The SAVE investigations made a major effort to define a unique population to test the protective role of an ACE inhibitor by identifying patients with left ventricular dysfunction who had not already clinically required use of an ACE inhibitor for the treatment of symptomatic heart failure.

Modern concurrent management of patients with acute infarct was encouraged. The goal was to determine whether this unique use of an ACE inhibitor provided any advantage when added to existing therapies. The trial was designed to permit the treating physicians to optimize individual therapies and procedures, except for the use of the ACE inhibitor, which was determined by protocol in a double-blind fashion. Coronary revascularization was required before randomization (3–16 days) in patients manifesting clinical ischemia. All eligible consenting patients received an open-label test dose of captopril (6.25 mg). In 19 of 2250 cases (<1%), either the study investigator or the patient then decided not to enter the randomized phase. The 2231 patients in the study cohort were then randomized to receive either captopril (6.25 mg) or placebo with a target of titrating to 25 mg t.i.d. during the hospitalization. The investigators were instructed to attempt to titrate to 50 mg t.i.d. on subsequent outpatient visits. The trial was designed to have long-term follow-up, so that the last patient enrolled would be followed for at least 2 years. The primary objective of the study was to determine whether this use of captopril would reduce the number of patients who either died or developed a marked deterioration of ventricular dysfunction, as defined by a nine-unit reduction from baseline to an end-of-study repeat radionuclide ejection fraction. The study was designed with other prespecified cardiovascular endpoints, such as development of heart failure and myocardial infarction.

RESULTS

Patient Demographics

Mean time to randomization was 11 days after myocardial infarction. The two treatment arms (placebo and captopril) were well matched in their baseline characteristics; the mean

Table 1   Total Mortality and Marked Deterioration in Left Ventricular Ejection Fraction

Outcome	Placebo (n = 1116)	Captopril (n = 1115)	Risk reduction	p-value
All-cause mortality	275 (24.6)	23 (20.4)	19%	0.019
Death or survival with reduction in EF by ≥9 units	400 (35.8)	34 (30.3)	15%	0.006

age was just over 59, and 82% were male. The average peak creatine kinase level was over 13 times the upper limit of normal for each laboratory; however, only 40% of the patients were Killip class II or greater. Fifty-five percent of the patients had anterior-lateral Q-waves, and the mean ejection fraction was 31%. With enrollment starting in 1987, it was of interest to note that at the randomization process, aspirin or other anti-platelet medications were used in 73% of the population, beta-blockers in 35%, calcium channel blockers in 42%, and digitalis in 26%.

The median follow-up was 42 months at completion of the trial. ACE inhibitor therapy resulted in a statistically significant, 19% reduction in all-cause mortality. As compared with placebo recipients, fewer ACE inhibitor–treated patients either died or had a reduction in left ventricular ejection fraction (Table 1). The significant difference in mortality was attributed to a 21% reduction in the risk of cardiovascular death (Fig. 1), since mortality due to noncardiovascular causes was quite similar in the two treatment groups (placebo group: 41/1116 [3.7%]; captopril group: 40/1115 [3.6%]).

Regardless of treatment assignment, the development of heart failure, whether de-fined as requiring augmentation or initiation of digitalis and diuretic therapy, symptoms requiring ACE inhibitor therapy, or hospitalization for management of heart failure each identified a patient group with a multifold higher risk of death compared to patients who did not manifest these findings (Table 2). Assignment to captopril therapy was associated with a marked reduction in the development of each of the definitions of heart failure and, importantly, with a reduction in subsequent deaths following the development of heart failure (Fig. 2). These findings strongly supported the prestudy rationale of the pre-

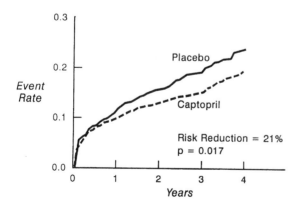

Figure 1   Cardiovascular mortality.

Table 2 Relative Risk of Death in Patients Experiencing Severe Heart Failure

Event	Incidence (%)	Risk of death (95% CI)
Severe heart failure		
ACE therapy	13	4.5 (3.6–5.6)
Hospitalization	15	6.4 (5.3–7.8)
Initiate or augment digitalis or diuretic	28	4.7 (3.9–5.7)

ventive role for this unique use of an ACE inhibitor in patients with asymptomatic left ventricular dysfunction following myocardial infarction.

In addition to lower mortality and fewer manifestations of heart failure, administration of captopril led to important reductions in the incidence of recurrent myocardial infarctions and other coronary vascular events. One hundred and seventy (15.3%) patients randomized to placebo, and only 133 (11.9%) of those randomized to captopril experienced another myocardial infarction during the 5 years after the qualifying event. This 25% risk reduction ($p = 0.015$) had an important impact on the overall results of the trial since patients experiencing a recurrent myocardial infarction were six times more likely than other SAVE patients to die during the follow-up period. This finding of a reduction in recurrent myocardial infarction with assignment to captopril was firmly supported by the observation that fewer patients in the captopril group underwent coronary revascularization. Indeed, the 24% reduction in revascularization procedures ($p = 0.014$) was of similar magnitude and time course as that observed for myocardial infarction. The risk of experiencing a major coronary event, defined as either a myocardial infarction or coronary revascularization, was reduced by 24% ($p = 0.0012$) in the captopril-treated group (Fig. 3). The decrease in the use of revascularization procedures was observed both with respect to percutaneous transluminal coronary angioplasty as well as coronary artery bypass graft-

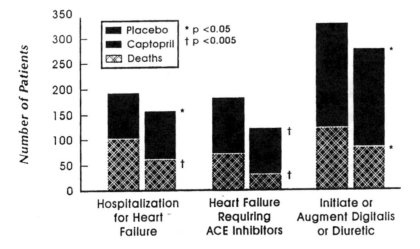

Figure 2 Mortality and CHF morbidity. The bars represent numbers of patients that develop this heart failure endpoint. The shaded areas are those who developed the endpoint and subsequently died.

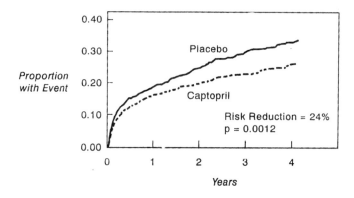

Figure 3 Cumulative events of clinical MI or coronary revascularization.

ing. Moreover, although there was a correspondingly lower proportion of revascularization procedures performed in the SAVE centers in Canada compared with those in the United States, the risk reduction for a postrandomization revascularization procedure with assignment to captopril was similar in the two countries (Fig. 4).

With the reductions in both heart failure as well as related myocardial ischemic events, it was not surprising that the total rates of hospitalization for cardiovascular events were significantly reduced by captopril therapy. Although only 28 patients (1.3%) in this trial of 2231 underwent a resection of a left ventricular aneurysm, it is of interest that the distribution was 8 captopril-treated patients (0.7%) versus 20 (1.8%) placebo recipients. This difference represents a 58% reduction ($p = 0.032$) and thus supports the prestudy rationale.

In regard to the prespecified endpoint of cardiovascular death and morbidity (devel-

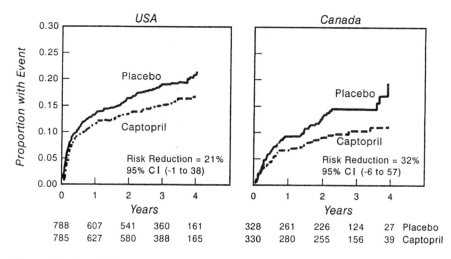

Figure 4 Cumulative curves for first revascularization (PTCA or CABG) by country.

opment of severe heart failure or recurrent myocardial infarction), the risk reduction attributed to captopril therapy was 24% ($p < 0.001$). This reduction from 40.1% in placebo-treated to 32.2% in captopril-treated patients on an intention-to-treat basis indicates that there will be 79 fewer major such cardiovascular events per 1000 patients treated by captopril. This translates into the need to treat only 13 patients to prevent one instance of either cardiovascular death, development of heart failure, or myocardial infarction in this selected myocardial infarction population.

Subgroups

The Cox multiple regression analysis of data from the SAVE trial demonstrated that advanced age, lower baseline ejection fraction, prior myocardial infarction, and history of hypertension or diabetes were each independently associated with an increased risk of death (Table 3). Of interest were findings that use of thrombolytic therapy, aspirin, or beta-blockers was independently associated with a significant reduction in the risk of death. Importantly, in this model the beneficial action of captopril therapy in prolonging survival was also shown to be significant and independent of these other risk factors and therapies (Table 3). ACE inhibitor use in this patient population should, therefore, be considered an important additional opportunity to reduce the risk of death and other cardiovascular sequelae following myocardial infarction.

Detailed subgroup analyses support the conclusion that the beneficial actions of captopril were relatively uniform among the SAVE population (19). No major subgroup experienced an excessive or minimal therapeutic effect. There were no significant interactions in multiple prespecified subgroups for either all-cause mortality or the combined fatal and nonfatal cardiovascular endpoints (19). Baseline left ventricular ejection fraction and Killip classification are two particularly illustrative examples of predefined subgroups that influence the clinical interpretation of the overall trial results. As would be anticipated, randomized patients whose ejection fraction was below the median of 32% had a much higher incidence of cardiovascular mortality and morbidity than did patients whose ejection fraction was above the median (Fig. 5). Comparable benefits of captopril therapy were observed in those with ejection fractions above and below the median (Fig. 5). These findings suggest that improvements in clinical outcomes may be obtained in patients with relatively well-preserved left ventricular function. Similarly, patients who developed pul-

Table 3 Total Mortality: Cox Multiple Regression Model

Endpoints	Adjusted risk ratio	95% CI	p-value
Age (yr)	1.03	(1.02, 1.04)	<0.001
Baseline EF (%)	0.94	(0.92, 0.95)	<0.001
Prior MI	1.36	(1.13, 1.65)	0.001
Gender (M)	0.90	(0.70, 1.16)	0.402
Systolic BP (mmHg)	1.01	(1.00, 1.01)	0.010
Thrombolytic use	0.73	(0.60, 0.92)	0.008
Aspirin use	0.84	(0.70, 1.01)	0.065
Beta-blocker use	0.74	(0.60, 0.92)	0.006
Captopril	0.80	(0.67, 0.96)	0.017

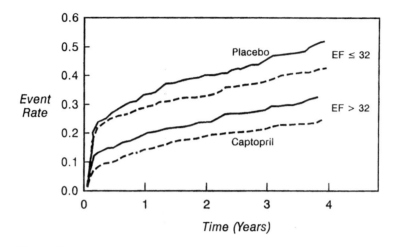

Figure 5 Cardiovascular mortality/morbidity in relation to baseline ejection fraction above and below median. The dashed line is captopril-treated, the solid line is placebo-treated.

monary congestion during the acute phase of their infarct (Killip class II or higher) were much more likely to experience an adverse cardiovascular event than those who were Killip class I. The reduction in incidence of cardiovascular events with the use of captopril therapy was again comparable in both of these subgroups (Fig. 6). It is important to note that despite the selection of SAVE participants using a depressed (≤40%) ejection fraction as a criterion for enrollment, 60% of the randomized patients did not manifest pulmonary congestion during the acute phase of their infarction (Killip class I). This subgroup analysis provides a strong justification for the identification and treatment of asymptomatic patients with left ventricular dysfunction.

Patients selected by their treating physician at the time of randomization into SAVE to receive a beta-blocker exhibited a more benign course than those not treated with these

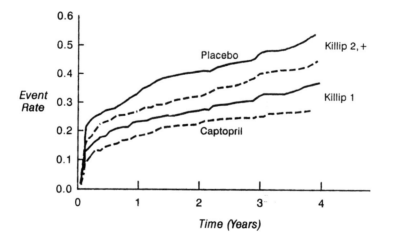

Figure 6 Cardiovascular mortality/morbidity in relation to prerandomization Killip classification. The dashed line is captopril-treated, the solid is placebo-treated.

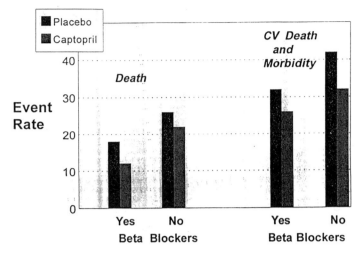

Figure 7   Event rate for patients in the SAVE trial according to therapy with captopril or placebo in the presence or absence of concomitant therapy with beta-blocking agents.

agents. Since the use of beta-blockade was not protocol controlled, it is likely that the physician's choice was influenced by other covariants that influenced outcome. However, the use of the ACE inhibitor was randomized, and, therefore, it can be concluded that the benefits observed in the subgroups both with and without beta-blockade use was a result of the ACE inhibitor. It is encouraging to note that the lowest rate of adverse cardiovascular events was achieved in the group given both therapies (Fig. 7). This observation supports the position that ACE inhibition does not supplant other proven therapies but provides additive benefits.

MECHANISTIC SUBSTUDIES

Quantitative Echocardiography

The quantitative echocardiographic substudy provided the most direct mechanistic evaluation of the rationale underlying SAVE. The objectives of this substudy were to determine whether quantitative two-dimensional echocardiographic evaluation of left ventricular size (cavity area) would provide predictive information regarding the risk of subsequent cardiovascular events and whether, as in previous studies, captopril therapy would alter the course of ventricular enlargement following myocardial infarction (20). Importantly, although not specifically statistically powered, the echocardiographic component also attempted to attain some linkage between captopril's effect on ventricular enlargement and clinical events. The Core Laboratory for the 2-D echocardiograms, under the direction of Dr. Martin St. John Sutton, approved the baseline studies for 512 of the 785 submissions as being technically adequate for the quantitative analysis. The demographics of the cohort selected for the echocardiographic substudy were similar to those of the total patient population. The information obtained from the baseline study was of prognostic significance and, indeed, added independent information to other key descriptors such as age, history of prior infarct, diabetes, hypertension, use of thrombolytic therapy, and, importantly, the left ventricular ejection fraction determined from a nuclear study. In essence, the echocar-

Table 4 Multivariate Regression Model for Predicting Total Mortality Systolic Cavity Area

	Relative risk	Confidence interval		Wald χ^2	p-value
		Lower bound	Upper bound		
Age	1.52	1.23	1.89	14.72	<0.001
Gender (M)	0.93	0.54	1.60	0.08	0.78
Prior myocardial infarction	1.57	1.05	2.37	4.78	0.028
Diabetes	1.19	0.75	1.87	0.55	0.46
Hypertension	1.33	0.89	2.00	1.92	0.166
Thrombolysis	0.70	0.43	1.13	2.17	0.141
LVEF	0.57	0.42	0.77	12.92	<0.001
Echo systolic area	1.12	1.04	1.21	9.06	0.003

The relative risk is computed for a change in 10 units for age and ejection fraction. It is computed for a change of 1.96 times the standard deviation of reproducibility for the echo measures (5.75 for systolic cavity area). LVEF indicates left ventricular ejection fraction.

diographic ventricular area, either systolic or diastolic, was one of the most important baseline descriptors for predicting mortality (Table 4).

From that baseline, the change in ventricular area over time was affected by captopril therapy, which resulted in a clear attenuation in enlargement (Fig. 8). The placebo group demonstrated time-dependent left ventricular enlargement, which was reduced in patients randomized to captopril therapy. Although this type of information regarding ventricular enlargement and the influence of an ACE inhibitor confirmed previous studies (10), the SAVE experience was the largest, and the combination of the number of patients studied with the duration of follow-up yielded a sufficient number of clinical events to show definitively that patients whose ventricle enlarged after enrollment were much more likely to experience an adverse cardiovascular event (Fig. 9). Randomization to captopril, as in the total study, resulted in fewer patients experiencing cardiovascular death, heart failure, or recurrent myocardial infarction (31.8% vs. 20.7%, $p = 0.01$). Thus, patients randomized to captopril were not only less likely to demonstrate ventricular enlargement but also less likely to have a clinical event.

This echocardiographic substudy therefore provided the critical mechanistic linkage between ventricular structural changes and clinical events in this population of patients who experienced a myocardial infarction. Thus, captopril was, as anticipated, beneficial in attenuating left ventricular enlargement, and those patients who did not demonstrate further ventricular enlargement after enrollment were more likely to have a benign course. In contrast, patients with enlargement were a high-risk group. While captopril reduced the proportion of patients who exhibited further enlargement, captopril-assigned patients who showed further ventricular enlargement were as likely as a placebo-assigned patients to have had ventricular enlargement (Fig. 10). One of the major actions of captopril therefore was to reduce the proportion of patients with progressive enlargement and thereby reduce the proportion at high risk for adverse cardiovascular events.

Neurohormones

At the outset of the trial, a major effort was made to determine the prognostic implications of neurohormone activation. Under the leadership of Dr. Jean-Lucien Rouleau, 522 pa-

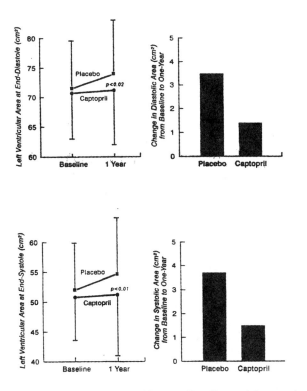

Figure 8 Echocardiographic area. Baseline and 1 year, placebo and captopril groups.

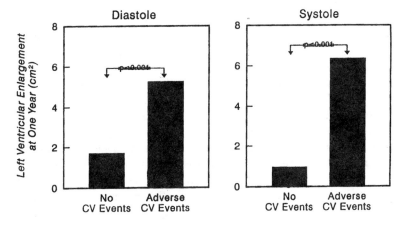

Figure 9 Overall change in left ventricular area of the patients in the echo cohort with respect to whether or not they experienced an adverse cardiovascular event.

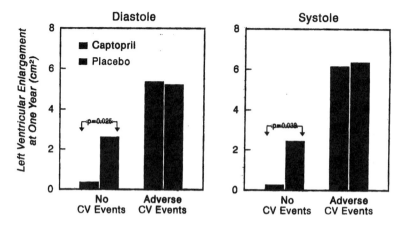

Figure 10   Change in left ventricular area with respect to development of an adverse cardiovascular event broken out by treatment assignment. Captopril-assigned patients were less likely to have a clinical event. However, if an adverse cardiovascular event occurred, the captopril-treated patient was as likely as a placebo to be an enlarger.

tients were enrolled in neurohormone substudies for baseline, 3-month, and 1-year determinations of norepinephrine, epinephrine, aldosterone, vasopressin, and renin activity (21); in a smaller subset ($n = 246$) of patients, atrial natriuretic peptide and pro-atrial natriuretic peptide were also measured (22). Detailed analyses of neurohormone profiles indicated that a proportion of the SAVE patients showed activation (greater than 2 standard deviations above normal controls) of one or another of these markers of neurohormonal activity (23). Activation in general was associated with higher risk for cardiovascular events, but in many cases this increased risk would have been detected by other patient characteristics such as ejection fraction and medication use (23). The prohormone for atrial natriuretic peptide, N-terminal proANF, appeared to be particularly useful as an independent marker for cardiovascular death and the risk of developing heart failure (22). As anticipated, N-terminal proANF was increased in patients who were Killip II or greater, those with prior infarct, and in those whose baseline medical therapy included a diuretic. However, in a Cox proportional hazard analysis, which included these predictors of adverse outcome as well as other important patient characteristics, higher N-terminal pro-ANF was one of the most important *independent* risk factors for cardiovascular death, second only to ejection fraction (22). Of the five neurohormones evaluated in this manner with a multivariate model, the N-terminal proANF provided the greatest information regarding risk of subsequent cardiovascular death and was even more predictive for the endpoint of cardiovascular death or the development of heart failure (22).

Although the neurohormones have been known to predict subsequent cardiovascular events, a separate series of studies within SAVE evaluated whether the baseline neurohormonal profile could be used to indicate the potential effectiveness of the ACE inhibitor therapy. Here the SAVE study provides an important negative finding. Specifically, the benefits of the randomization to the ACE inhibitor captopril did not reside only in those patients with activation of the renin-angiotensin system or any other specific neurohormone (23). Similarly, although elevated catecholamine levels are generally predictive of adverse events, the benefits of receiving beta-blocker at baseline could not be demonstrated to be a function of baseline catecholamine levels (24). Results of these ancillary studies on neurohormones underscore the complexity of the relationships with plasma markers of neurohormone activation, generally pointing to adverse prognosis but lacking sufficient specificity to direct the use of pharmacologic therapy.

Adverse Experience

During the 5 years of follow-up, a substantial proportion of patients on either captopril or placebo reported at least one episode of lightheadedness. In the captopril-treated group, 367 (32.9%) reported lightheadedness versus 318 (28.5%) in the placebo group. When one looks at the actual discontinuation of study drug related to a hypotensive event or symptom, only 48 (4.3%) of the active therapy versus 14 (1.3%) of the placebo patients discontinued therapy ($p < 0.001$). Other significant differences between placebo and captopril groups included rash, cough, and taste alteration (Table 5). Only 22 (2.0%) of the captopril and 18 (1.6%) of the placebo patients had a creatine level in excess of 2.5 mg/dl during treatment ($p = $ NS; Table 5).

Economic Implications

In addition to weighing the clinical effectiveness against the adverse drug-associated events, the cost required to obtain these clinical benefits is an additional major consideration. The SAVE study had an independent cost-effective analysis conducted, which used actual resource utilization data as well as quality of life to express cost/quality-adjusted year of life saved (25). This initial analysis demonstrated that the incremental cost-effectiveness ratio for quality-adjusted life-years utilizing captopril after myocardial infarction in the SAVE population was in the range of $3,700 to $10,400, depending on the assumptions used in the model. These figures place this use of captopril well within the range of other accepted proven therapies such as lipid lowering for secondary prevention, coronary bypass grafting for three-vessel or left main disease, and thrombolytic therapy in acute myocardial infarction. In the sensitivity analysis, an obvious factor that influences the cost of a quality-adjusted life-year saved is the actual expense of the therapy. In recent years, captopril has become available in generic formulations at a fraction of the cost used in the prior analysis. From an informal survey of several local pharmacies, it now appears

Table 5 Discontinuations Due to Adverse Experiences

Events	Discontinuations		
	Captopril	Placebo	*p*-value
Hypotension/related symptoms	48 (4.3)	14 (1.3)	≤0.001
Rash	35 (3.1)	12 (1.1)	≤0.001
Cough	29 (0.2)	2 (2.6)	≤0.001
Changes in renal function	15 (1.3)	6 (0.5)	NS
Taste alteration	8 (0.7)	1 (0.1)	≤0.05
Angioedema	3 (0.3)	0 (0.0)	NS

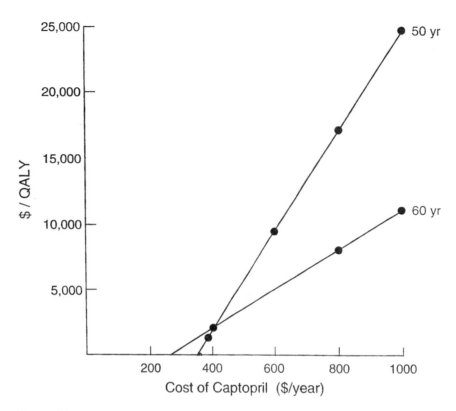

Figure 11   SAVE study: incremental cost-effectiveness of captopril therapy.

that captopril at a dose of 50 mg t.i.d. could be obtained for under $400.00 a year. In our model, this use of captopril therapy can be considered both life and cost-saving (Fig. 11).

SUMMARY

The SAVE study was the culmination of a ''bench-to-bedside'' investigative approach. The initial animal experiments that indicated that this new use of an angiotensin-converting enzyme inhibitor could prevent ventricular enlargement and improve survival following myocardial infarction were followed by small safety and mechanistic clinical studies supporting this concept. The SAVE study was a direct test of this hypothesis and clearly demonstrated the clinical utility of captopril in patients who experienced a myocardial infarction that resulted in left ventricular dysfunction. The reductions in deaths as well as the development of heart failure were in keeping with the animal experience. The reduction in the incidence of coronary events went beyond the insight provided from the animals and provides the rationale for an even broader use of this form of therapy in patients with coronary disease. Since the results of the SAVE study were reported, ACE inhibitors have been studied in a much broader population of patients with acute and chronic myocardial infarctions. The overall results from this international research effort clearly support the findings in SAVE and underscore the benefits of ACE-inhibition therapy following myocardial infarction.

REFERENCES

1. Ryan TJ, Anderson JL, Antman EM, Braniff BA, Brooks NH, Califf RM, Hillis LD, Hiratzka LF, Rapaport E, Riegel BJ, Russell RO, Smith EE, Jr., Weaver WD. ACC/AHA guidelines for the management of patients with acute myocardial infarction. A report of the American College of Cardiology/American Heart Association Task Force on Practice Guidelines (Committee on Management of Acute Myocardial Infarction). J Am Coll Cardiol 1996; 28:1328–1428.
2. The Task Force on the Management of Acute Myocardial Infarction of the European Society of Cardiology: Acute myocardial infarction: pre-hospital and in-hospital management. Eur Heart J 1996; 17:43–63.
3. Moyé LA, Pfeffer MA, Braunwald E, on behalf of SAVE study. Rationale, design and baseline characteristics of the survival and ventricular enlargement trial. Am J Cardiol 1991; 68:70D–79D.
4. Pfeffer JM, Pfeffer MA, Fletcher PJ, Braunwald E. Progressive ventricular remodeling in rat with myocardial infarction. Am J Physiol 1991; 260 (HCP 29):H1406–H1414.
5. Eaton LW, Weiss JL, Bulkley BH, Garrison JB, Weisfeldt ML. Regional cardiac dilatation after acute myocardial infarction. Recognition by two-dimensional echocardiography. N Engl J Med 1979; 300:57–62.
6. Pfeffer MA, Pfeffer JM, Fishbein MC, Fletcher PJ, Spadaro J, Kloner RA, Braunwald E. Myocardial infarct size and ventricular function in rats. Circ Res 1979; 44:503–512.
7. Fletcher PJ, Pfeffer JM, Pfeffer MA, Braunwald E. Left ventricular diastolic pressure-volume relations in rats with healed myocardial infarction: effects on systolic function. Circ Res 1981; 49:618–626.
8. Pfeffer JM, Pfeffer MA, Braunwald E. Influence of chronic captopril therapy on the infarcted left ventricle of the rat. Circ Res 1985; 57:84–95.
9. Pfeffer MA, Pfeffer JM, Steinberg C, Finn P. Survival after an experimental myocardial infarction: beneficial effects of long-term therapy with captopril. Circulation 1985; 72:406–412.
10. Pfeffer MA, Braunwald E. Ventricular remodeling after myocardial infarction. Experimental observations and clinical implications. Circulation 1990; 81:1161–1172.
11. Erlebacher JA, Weiss JL, Weisfeldt ML, Bulkley BH. Early dilation of the infarcted segment in acute transmural myocardial infarction: role of infarct expansion in acute left ventricular enlargement. J Am Coll Cardiol 1984; 4:201–208.
12. Jugdutt BI, Michorowski BL. Role of infarct expansion in rupture of the ventricular septum after acute myocardial infarction: a two-dimensional echocardiographic study. Clin Cardiol 1987; 10:641–652.
13. Pfeffer MA, Lamas GA, Vaughan DE, Parisi AF, Braunwald E. Effect of captopril on progressive ventricular dilatation after anterior myocardial infarction. N Engl J Med 1988; 319:80–86.
14. Sharpe N, Smith H, Murphy J, and Hannan S. Treatment of patients with symptomless left ventricular dysfunction after myocardial infarction. Lancet 1988; 1:255–259.
15. Sharpe N, Smith H, Murphy J, Greaves S, Hart H, and Gamble G. Early prevention of left ventricular dysfunction after myocardial infarction with angiotensin-converting-enzyme inhibition. Lancet 1991; 337:872–876.
16. Pfeffer MA, Braunwald E, Moyé LA, Basta L, Brown EJ, Jr., Cuddy TE, Davis BR, Geltman EM, Goldman S, Flaker GC, Klein M, Lamas GA, Packer M, Rouleau J, Rouleau JL, Rutherford J, Wertheimer JH, Hawkins CM, on behalf of the SAVE Investigators. Effect of captopril

on mortality and morbidity in patients with left ventricular dysfunction after myocardial infarction. Results of the Survival and Ventricular Enlargement Trial. N Engl J Med 1992; 327: 669–677.

17. The CONSENSUS Trial Study Group. Effects of enalapril on mortality in severe congestive heart failure. Results of the Cooperative North Scandinavian Enalapril Survival Study (CONSENSUS). N Engl J Med 1987; 316:1429–1435.

18. The SOLVD Investigators. Effect of enalapril on survival in patients with reduced left ventricular ejection fractions and congestive heart failure. N Engl J Med 1991; 325:293–302.

19. Moyé LA, Pfeffer MA, Wun C, Davis BR, Geltman E, Hayes D, Farnham DJ, Randall OS, Dinh H, Arnold M, Kupersmith J, Hager D, Glasser SP, Biddle T, Hawkins CM, Braunwald E. Uniformity of captopril benefit in the SAVE study: subgroup analysis. Eur Heart J 1994; 15(suppl B):2–8.

20. St. John Sutton M, Pfeffer MA, Plappert T, Rouleau JL, Moyé LA, Dagenais GR, Lamas GA, Klein M, Sussex B, Goldman S, Menapace FJ, Parker JO, Lewis S, Sestier F, Gordon DF, McEwan P, Bernstein V, Braunwald E, for the SAVE Investigators. Quantitative two-dimensional echocardiographic measurements are major predictors of adverse cardiovascular events after acute myocardial infarction: the protective effects of captopril. Circulation 1994; 89:68–75.

21. Rouleau J, Moye L, deChamplain J, Klein M, Bichet D, Packer M, Dagenais G, Sussex B, Arnold J, Sestier F, Parker J, McEwan M, Bernstein V, Cuddy T, Delage F, Nadeau C, Lamas G, Gottlieb S, McCans J, Pfeffer M. Activation of neurohumoral systems following actue myocardial infarction. Am J Cardiol 1991; 68:80D–86D.

22. Hall C, Rouleau JL, Moyé L, de Champlain J, Bichet D, Klein M, Sussex B, Packer M, Rouleau J, Arnold JMO, Lamas G, Sestier F, Gottlieb S, Wun CC, Pfeffer M. N-terminal proatrial natriuretic factor. An independent predictor of long-term prognosis after myocardial infarction. Circulation 1994; 89:1934–1942.

23. Rouleau JL, deChamplain J, Klein M, Bichet D, Moyé L, Packer M, Dagenais G, Sussex B, Arnold JM, Sestier F, Parker J, McEwan P, Bernstein V, Cuddy T, Lamas G, Gottlieb S, McCans J, Nadeau C, Delage F, Hamm P, Pfeffer M. Activation of neurohumoral systems in postinfarction left ventricular dysfunction. J Am Coll Cardiol 1993; 22:390–398.

24. Vantrimpont P, Rouleau JL, Wun CC, Ciampi A, Klein M, Sussex B, Arnold JMO, Moyé LA, Pfeffer MA, for the SAVE Investigators. Additive beneficial effects of beta-blockers to angiotensin-converting enzyme inhibitors in the Survival and Ventricular Enlargement (SAVE) study. J Am Coll Cardiol 1997; 29:229–236.

25. Tsevat J, Duke D, Goldman L, Pfeffer MA, Lamas G, Soukup JR, Kuntz KM, Lee TH. Cost-effectiveness of captopril therapy after myocardial infarction. J Am Coll Cardiol 1995; 26: 914–919.

24

AIRE

ALISTAIR S. HALL and STEPHEN G. BALL

The Acute Infarction Ramipril Efficacy (AIRE) Study Investigators. Effect of ramipril on mortality and morbidity of survivors of acute myocardial infarction with clinical evidence of heart failure. Lancet 1993;342:821–828.

The early clinical/scientific objectives carefully defined in the prospectively published AIRE study protocol (1) derived inspiration from a number of different sources. Three scientific papers were particularly influential. The first of these was the report of Swedberg and colleagues on behalf of the CONSENSUS-I investigators, as this demonstrated a major reduction in the mortality of patients with severe heart failure treated with the ACE inhibitor enalapril (2). Yusuf et al. are also credited for their instructive dissertation entitled "Why do we need some large, simple, randomized trials?" (3) as are Pfeffer and Pfeffer for their studies performed in rats with experimental myocardial infarction (4,5).

Other important influences resulted from the priorities and former experiences of principal authors Stephen Ball at the Glasgow MRC (Medical Research Council) Hypertension Unit and Alistair Hall at St. James's University Teaching Hospital in Leeds. Interestingly, a further significant influence on the design and consequent success of the AIRE study was the absence of prior experience in leading multinational clinical investigations. Consequently the AIRE study, conceived by clinicians with clinical priorities preeminent, was necessarily highly attentive to published scientific maxims, i.e., prospectively defined, independently conducted, multicenter, multinational, randomized, double-blind, placebo-controlled, intention-to-treat, and with a robust total mortality primary endpoint.

THE YORKSHIRE STUDY OF INFARCT SURVIVAL

The acronym AIRE (Acute Infarction Ramipril Efficacy) derived from a wish to identify the origins of the investigation. (Aire is the name of the river around which the city of Leeds was formed.) As we were first-time mortality trialists, we had major practical and resource constraints. Consequently, we attempted to optimize all practical aspects of the design with the dual objectives of minimizing the likelihood of treatment risks and maximizing the probability of treatment benefit. Immutable priorities included complete adherence to the Helsinki Declaration on Ethical Clinical Research.

In a size calculation document written in 1987, the need to investigate a minimum of 1815 patients was stated based on the following six assumptions:

1. Predicted average follow-up period of 15 months.
2. Predicted mortality of 20% at 15 months
3. "Relevant clinical improvement" defined as 25%, giving rise to an expected mortality of 15% in the treatment group at 15 months.
4. Statistical power of at least 80% at a significance level of 5% (two-tailed).
5. Log-rank test to be used to compare treatment groups.
6. Primary trial analysis of all-cause mortality to be conducted on the basis of intention-to-treat.

These key assumptions extensively define the thinking behind the AIRE study's unique design (1). Based on the medical literature published prior to 1987, extremely accurate predictions were made regarding the likely outcome of a trial not completed until 1993. Intentions were clearly and prospectively stated.

THE VALUE OF PRIOR KNOWLEDGE

The ISIS "mega-trial" philosophy (6) purposely assumes very little about the likely responses of subgroups of patients to an experimental therapy. A major premise of the "large and simple" trial approach is that subgroups of patients perceived to have a single condition (e.g., suspected acute myocardial infarction) can be expected to respond to a treatment intervention in a qualitatively similar way, albeit to a differing extent. Prior scientific data that suggest a basis for patient selection are considered to be either unreliable or excessively restrictive. In contrast, the Bayesian approach to clinical trials presupposes that prior knowledge can greatly instruct the design, conduct, and interpretation of an investigation. In designing AIRE we had prior information concerning the likely placebo group mortality and also the potential magnitude of beneficial effects that might result when treating patients with heart failure with angiotensin-converting enzyme (ACE) inhibitor therapy.

PREDICTED PLACEBO GROUP MORTALITY RATE

To prospectively predict the mortality of patients randomized to placebo, the following four assumptions were made:

1. A clinical diagnosis of cardiac failure subsequent to acute myocardial infarction (AMI) would form the basis for patient selection
2. The definition of cardiac failure be based on the classification of "mechanical complication" as used in the retrospective analysis of the BHAT (Beta-Blocker Heart Attack Trial) investigation (7)
3. Increasing severity of cardiac failure would be associated with increasing mortality
4. The average duration of follow-up for the study would be about 15 months

The precise definition of cardiac failure used in the BHAT post hoc subgroup analysis was "one of the following complications at the time of infarction, but before enrollment (average 13.48 days): pulmonary edema, cardiogenic shock, persistent hypotension, basilar rales or symptoms/signs of heart failure requiring therapy with digitalis and/or diuretics" (7). Most of these complications were reported to be mild or transitory, as persisting heart failure was considered to be a major contraindication to beta-blockade and hence to entry into the BHAT study. Patients selected for BHAT were therefore considered to have had less severe heart failure than those to be included in AIRE. Though the use of beta-blockade in AIRE was to be permitted, it was expected that overt heart failure would restrict use in many patients. The presence of cardiogenic shock was considered to be a contraindication to ACE inhibitor use and hence also to inclusion into AIRE.

The recorded mortality of BHAT patients with mechanical complications treated with placebo (other than cardiogenic shock and sustained hypotension) was 18.5% at an average follow-up period of 25 months. This figure provided an estimate of the expected mortality for AIRE. It was considered to be conservative for the following two reasons:

1. The average time of enrollment in BHAT was 13.8 days after AMI, whereas in AIRE it was expected to be nearer 6 days after AMI, causing hospital mortality to contribute to mortality rates.
2. Patients eligible for BHAT despite "mechanical complications" were considered to have a lower mortality than selected for AIRE based on the assumption that worse heart failure correlates with worse prognosis.

A second and potentially more realistic estimate of mortality was derived from the prospective study of Elmfeldt and Wilhelmsen (8), which was the quoted source of the BHAT definition of heart failure. One year after hospital discharge a mortality rate of 18% was observed for men and women aged 55 years or younger who had had a myocardial infarction complicated by clinical heart failure. Based on these observations, a 12-month mortality estimate for AIRE of <18% seemed likely due to exclusion of patients with severe heart failure. However, inclusion of patients of all ages and also allowing for deaths occurring during in-hospital follow-up suggested that a 12-month mortality of 18% was a realistic estimate. Interpolation to 15 months indicated a predicted placebo group mortality of about 20% (Fig. 1).

MEANINGFUL CLINICAL BENEFIT

In 1984 a relative risk reduction (RRR) of 25% was considered to be the maximum that might realistically be expected in a cardiovascular trial (3). Furthermore, it was suggested that a relative risk reduction of less than 25% was unlikely to be considered as "clinically useful," particularly if absolute mortality rates were low. However, in 1987 the CONSENSUS-I trial reported a RRR of 40% at 6 months and 31% at 12 months for patients with severe heart failure treated with enalapril (2). Furthermore, a systematic review of papers reporting mortality reductions resulting from ACE-inhibitor use in patients with heart failure reported a mean RRR of about 50% (16). Also, a survival study conducted in rats with experimentally induced heart failure (after coronary artery ligation) described benefit of a similar magnitude (5). Consequently, we conservatively predicted a RRR for AIRE

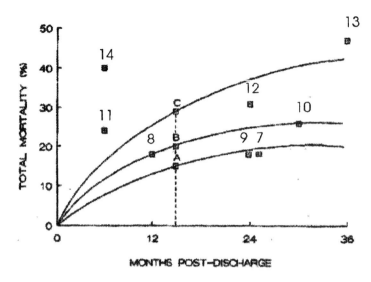

Figure 1   The projected "untreated" mortality of patients with clinical heart failure after myocardial infarction. (A) A "conservative" estimate of 15-month mortality (7,9); (B) A "realistic" estimate of 15-month mortality (8,10); (C) an "exaggerated" estimate of 15-month mortality (11–14). All curves are interpolated from the data of the Multicenter Postinfarction Research Group (15).

of between 25 and 30%, having allowed for the attenuating effect of cessation of randomized trial therapy in some patients.

PATIENT SELECTION

The inclusion and exclusion criteria utilized in AIRE have been previously published in detail, although the reasons for choosing them requires further explanation. In keeping with our desire to perform a clinically relevant trial, we sought to apply available scientific knowledge and prevailing clinical wisdom to the selection and exclusion of patients. Patients with overt severe heart failure after AMI, while never previously directly studied in a clinical survival study, were nevertheless expected to benefit from an ACE inhibitor based on the CONSENSUS-I findings. On ethical grounds such patients were excluded from randomization to permit prescription of an ACE inhibitor. The study protocol also required that any patients developing overt severe heart failure during the course of the study be treated with open-label ACE inhibition. This would have the predicted effect of attenuating the size of any difference between placebo and treatment group mortalities. Furthermore, the later publication of the SOLVD treatment data (17) redefined the level of severity based on a measurement of ejection fraction at which clinicians might wish to treat patients with open ACE-inhibitor therapy (17).

Standard contraindications to the use of ACE inhibitors were applied (e.g., a history of prior intolerance, angioedema, aortic or renal artery stenosis, excessive hypotension, and unstable angina). Furthermore, knowing that initiation of therapy would be expected to lower systolic blood pressure, we also considered it best to avoid the very early period after AMI (first 24 hours) during which time clinical stability can be difficult to predict.

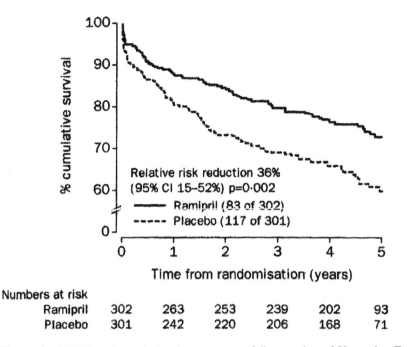

Figure 4 AIREX study survival estimates to mean follow-up time of 59 months. (From Ref. 35.)

AIRE IN CONTEXT

Countless reviews of the ACE-inhibitor trials have now been written. Most appear to accept subdivision into two groups evaluating *early nonselective* and *delayed selective* strategies (36,37). While there has been complete agreement regarding the appropriateness of treating patients with clinical signs of heart failure or impaired left ventricular systolic function, the value of very early treatment (less than 24 hours) of all patients with suspected AMI is still hotly disputed (38,39).

Physicians are currently being exhorted to practice "evidence-based medicine," in which individual patients are cared for on the basis of net statistical probabilities derived from meta-analyses and mega-trials. However, the utilitarian ethic that underpins such an approach (the greatest good of the greatest number at the lowest cost) is at odds with the Hippocratic ethic, which seeks to protect the rights of individual patients. According to the latter approach a physician undertakes to treat each patient as he or she would wish to be treated, i.e., as a unique and valued individual. Reflecting this long-established clinical ideal, the concept of "medicine-based evidence" has recently appeared in the medical literature (40).

When designing the AIRE study in 1987, we sought to benefit from all prevailing clinical wisdom and scientific knowledge. While acknowledging the important influence of other groups such as the CONSENSUS and ISIS investigators, we believe that the AIRE study itself now represents a milestone investigation. Conducted at a time when statistical power resulting from very large study size was frequently extolled as being a preeminent virtue, the AIRE Study has been successful because it achieved a good balance between clinical and scientific priorities. Specifically, the AIRE and AIREX investigations provide clinicians with persuasive medicine-based evidence.

REFERENCES

1. Hall AS, Winter C, Bogle SM, Mackintosh AF, Murray GD, Ball SG on behalf of the AIRE Study Investigators. J Cardiovasc Pharmacol 1991; 18(suppl 2):S105–S109.
2. CONSENSUS Trial Study Group. Effects of enalapril on mortality in severe congestive heart failure. N Engl J Med 1987; 316:1429–1435.
3. Yusuf S, Collins R, Peto RL. What do we need some large, simple randomized trials? Stats Med 1984; 3:409–420.
4. Pfeffer MA, Pfeffer JM, Fishbein MC, Fletcher PJ, Spadaro J, Kloner RA, Braunwald E. Myocardial infarct size and ventricular function in rats. Circ Res 1979; 44:503–512.
5. Pfeffer JM, Pfeffer MA, Steinberg C, Finn P. Survival after an experimental myocardial infarction: beneficial effects of long-term therapy with captopril. Circulation 1985; 72:406–412.
6. ISIS-2 Collaborative Group. Randomized trial of intravenous streptokinase, oral aspirin, both or neither among 17,187 cases of suspected acute myocardial infarction. Lancet 1988; 2:349–360.
7. Furberg CD, Hawkins CM, Lichstein E. Effect of propranolol in postinfarction patients with mechanical or electrical complications. Circulation 1984; 69:761–765.
8. Elmfeldt D, Wilhelmsen L. A study of representative post myocardial infarction patients aged 27–55. In: Tibblin G, Keyes A, Werko L, eds. Preventive Cardiology. Stockholm: Almquist and Wiksell, 1972:129.
9. Wilhelmsen C, Wilhelmsen L, Vedin JA, Tibblin G, Werko L. Reduction of sudden deaths after myocardial infarction by treatment with alprenolol. Preliminary results. Lancet 1974; 2:1157–1160.
10. Taylor GJ, Humphries JC, Mellits ED. Predictors of clinical course, coronary anatomy and left ventricular function after recovery from acute myocardial infarction. Circulation 1980; 62:960–970.
11. Bigger JT, Heller CA, Wenger TL, Weld FM. Risk stratification after acute myocardial infarction. Am J Cardiol 1978; 42:202–210.
12. Bigger JT, Coromilas J, Weld FM, Reiffel JA, Rolnitzkey LM. Prognosis after recovery from acute myocardial infarction. Annu Rev Med 1984; 35:127–147.
13. Norris RM, Cauchey DE, Deeming LW, Mercer CJ, Scott PJ. Coronary prognostic index for predicting survival after recovery from acute myocardial infarction. Lancet 1970; 2:485–487.
14. Murray DP, Salih M, Tan LB, Murray RG, Littler WA. Prognostic stratification of patients after myocardial infarction. Br Heart J 1987; 57:313–318.
15. The Multicenter Postinfarction Research Group. Risk stratification and survival after myocardial infarction. N Engl J Med 1983; 309:331–336.
16. Furberg CD, Yusuf S. Effects of vasodilators on survival in congestive heart failure. Am J Cardiol 1985; 55:1110–1112.
17. The SOLVD Investigators. Effect of enalapril on survival in patients with reduced ejection fractions and congestive heart failure. N Engl J Med 1991; 325:292–302.
18. Tardieu A, Virot P, Vancroux JC. Effects of captopril on myocardial perfusion in patients with coronary insufficiency: evaluation by exercise test and quantitative myocardial homoscintigraphy using thallium-201. Postgrad Med J 1986; 62 (suppl 1):38–41.
19. Hall AS, Ball SG. ACE inhibitors after AMI. Lancet 1989; 337:1527.
20. Todd PA, Benfield P. Ramipril: a review of its pharmacological properties and therapeutic efficacy in cardiovascular disorders. Drugs 1990; 39:110–135.
21. The Acute Infarction Ramipril Efficacy (AIRE) Study Investigators. Effect of ramipril on mortality and morbidity of survivors of acute myocardial infarction with clinical evidence of heart failure. Lancet 1993; 342:821–828.
22. Cleland JGF, Erhardt L, Hall AS, Winter C, Ball SG. Validation of primary and secondary outcomes and classification of mode of death among patients with clinical evidence of heart

failure after myocardial infarction. A report from the Acute Infarction Ramipril Efficacy (AIRE) Study Investigators. J Cardiovasc Pharmacol 1993; 22(suppl 9):S22–S27.

23. Cleland JGF, Erhardt L, Murray GD, Hall AS, Ball SG. Effect of ramipril on morbidity and mode of death among survivors of acute myocardial infarction with clinical evidence of heart failure. A report from the AIRE Study Investigators. Eur Heart J 1997; 18:41–51.

24. Pfeffer MA, Braunwald E, Moye LA, et al. on behalf of the SAVE investigators. Effect of captopril on mortality and morbidity in patients with left ventricular dysfunction after myocardial infarction. N Engl J Med 1992; 327:669–677.

25. Swedberg K, Held P, Kjekshus J, Rasmussen K, Ryden L, Wedel H, on the behalf of the CONSENSUS II study group. Effects of the early administration of enalapril on mortality in patients with acute myocardial infarction. N Engl J Med 1992; 327:678–684.

26. Hall AS, Tan LB, Ball SG. Inhibition of ACE/kininase-II, acute myocardial infarction and survival. Cardiovasc Res 1994; 28:190–198.

27. The TRACE Study Group. The TRAndolopril Cardiac Evaluation (TRACE) study: rationale, design and baseline characteristics of the screened population. Am J Cardiol 1994; 73:44–50C.

28. Kober L, Torp-Pedersen C, Carlsen JE, et al., for the TRACE study group. A clinical trial of the ACE inhibitor trandolapril in patients with left ventricular dysfunction after myocardial infarction. N Engl J Med 1995; 333:1670–1676.

29. Chinese cardiac study collaborative group. Oral captopril versus placebo among 13,634 patients with suspected acute myocardial infarction: interim report from the Chinese Cardiac Study (CCS-1). Lancet 1995; 345:686–687.

30. GISSI-3 Gruppo Italiano per lo Studio della Sopravvivenza nell'Infarto Miocardico. GISSI-3 study protocol on the effects of lisinopril, of nitrates, and of their association in patients with acute myocardial infarction. Am J Cardiol 1992; 70:62–69C.

31. Gruppo Italiano per lo Studio della Sopravvivenza nell' Infarto Miocardico. GISSI-3: effects of lisinopril and transdermal glyceryl trinitrate singly and together on 6-week mortality and ventricular function after acute myocardial infarction. Lancet 1994; 343:1115–1122.

32. ISIS-4 Collaborative Group. Fourth International Study of Infarct Survival: protocol for a large simple study of the effects of oral mononitrate, of oral captopril, and of intravenous magnesium. Am J Cardiol 1991; 68:87–100D.

33. ISIS-4 Collaborative Group. ISIS-4: a randomized factorial trial assessing oral captopril, oral mononitrate, and intravenous magnesium sulphate in 58,050 patients with suspected acute myocardial infarction. Lancet 1995; 345:669–685.

34. Kober L, C Torp-Pedersen, Cole D, Hampton JR, Camm AJ. Bayesian interim statistical analysis of randomised trials: the case against. Lancet 1997; 349:1168–1169.

35. Hall AS, Murray GD, Ball SG, on behalf of the AIREX study investigators. Follow-up study of patients randomly allocated ramipril or placebo for heart failure after acute myocardial infarction: AIRE Extension (AIREX) study. Lancet 1997; 349:1493–1497.

36. Pfeffer MA. ACE inhibition in acute myocardial infarction. N Engl J Med 1995; 332:118–120.

37. Latini R, Maggioni AP, Flather M, Sleight P, Tognoni G, for the meeting participants. ACE inhibitor use in patients with myocardial infarction. Summary of evidence from clinical trials. Circulation 1995; 92:3132–3137.

38. Latini R. ACE inhibitors post-MI: the case for early, nonselective treatment. Controversies Cardiol 1995; 6:9–12.

39. Hall AS. ACE inhibitors post-MI: the case for delayed, selective long-term treatment. Controversies Cardiol 1995; 6:5–8.

40. Knottnerus JA, Dinant GJ. Medicine based evidence, a prerequisite for evidence based medicine. Br Med J 1997; 7116:1109–1110.

25

TRACE

LARS KØBER and CHRISTIAN TORP-PEDERSEN

Køber L, Torp-Pedersen C, Carlsen JE, Bagger H, Eliasen P, Lyngborg K et al. for the Trandolapril Cardiac Evaluation (TRACE) Study Group. A clinical trial for the angiotensin-converting-enzyme inhibitor trandolapril in patients with left ventricular dysfunction after myocardial infarction. N Engl J Med 1995;333:1670–1676.

INTRODUCTION

In 1989, when the protocol for the Trandolapril Cardiac Evaluation (TRACE) study approached finalization, the use of left ventricular systolic function to identify high-risk patients after an acute myocardial infarction (AMI) was still a fresh concept, and we (and many others) thought it was superior to identifying high-risk patients on the basis of clinical findings of heart failure. The first CONSENSUS trial had been published, showing a remarkable reduction in mortality among patients with severe congestive heart failure (1). Small clinical studies indicated that angiotensin-converting enzyme (ACE) inhibition might be beneficial for AMI survivors with respect to left ventricular function. At this time there was also a belief that administration of an ACE inhibitor shortly after an AMI could be deleterious because of blood pressure reduction. A series of studies were therefore initiated to test whether ACE inhibition would be beneficial in patients with milder heart failure or left ventricular systolic dysfunction, either chronically or shortly following an AMI (2–9). We had no knowledge of the AIRE study, but the SAVE study had begun enrolling patients. The SAVE study was designed to test the benefit of ACE inhibition in patients with left ventricular dysfunction following AMI while excluding patients with overt heart failure or active ischemia. We thought that the uneasiness about giving patients an ACE inhibitor shortly after an infarction would still be present due to the exclusion of patients with ischemia. Specifically, we thought that there was a need for a trial testing whether routine determination of left ventricular function following myocardial infarction could be recommended in order to select patients for long-term ACE inhibition. Thus, like SAVE, TRACE was designed to test whether patients with severe left ventricular dysfunction shortly after an AMI would benefit from long-term ACE inhibition (10). In contrast to SAVE, only well-known contraindications to an ACE inhibitor excluded patients. To be able to extrapolate to a clinical recommendation of routine use of determination of left ventricular function, it was important for us to perform consecutive screening for entry and to document in detail which patients were enrolled and excluded from the study.

SCREENING

Consecutive male or female patients above 18 years of age who had myocardial infarction (MI) were screened for entry 2–6 days after the infarction. The diagnosis of an MI was established when chest pain or electrocardiographic signs of ischemia or infarction were present and accompanied by elevated cardiac enzymes to at least twice the upper limit of normal of the local laboratory. The participating 27 Danish departments agreed to screen consecutive patients admitted with an infarction as defined by these criteria. For patients screened, the following data were collected: a detailed medical history, circumstances around the infarction, a two-dimensional echocardiographic examination, and in-hospital complications for the entire hospital stay. Patients who had an MI confirmed by enzymes and who died prior to day 2 were screened by review of the medical history and in-hospital events. This was performed in order to obtain a complete registry of all MI patients for comparison with epidemiological data and to determine whether study patients were representative of all patients with MI. In Denmark, all hospitals have complete regional uptake, and the intention is that all patients with MI are admitted to the coronary care unit, irrespective of age.

The videotaped echocardiographic examination was transported by courier to the core lab, and wall motion index was determined by one of two examiners. Wall motion index was calculated using the nine-segment model of Heger et al. (11). When TRACE was planned, wall motion index was not routinely measured in Denmark, and most physicians were more used to ejection fraction. As radionuclide left ventriculography was not available in the majority of departments, and since an early examination was crucial, wall

Table 1 Baseline Characteristics of 7001 AMIs Screened for TRACE

Parameter	WMI ≤ 1.2	WMI > 1.2	WMI NA	Total	*p*
Number of infarctions	2606	3920	475	7001	
Age, years	70	67	73	69	<0.001
	(50–84)	(45–83)	(51–88)	(47–84)	
Wall motion index	1.0	1.7	—	1.4	
	(0.6–1.2)	(1.3–2.0)		(0.7–2.0)	
Male sex	69%	68%	57%	67%	<0.001
Smoker on admission	47%	55%	38%	51%	<0.001
History of hypertension	23%	23%	24%	23%	0.7
Diabetes mellitus	14%	8%	16%	11%	<0.001
Previous angina	46%	33%	40%	39%	<0.001
Previous AMI	37%	20%	26%	27%	<0.001
Anterior Q-wave AMI	43%	15%	21%	26%	<0.001
Thrombolysis given	39%	43%	28%	41%	<0.001
Congestive heart failure	74%	40%	73%	55%	<0.001

Age and wall motion index is shown as median (5–95 percentiles), other variables as percent present. The *p*-values show the probability of no difference between the three subgroups of WMI. AMI = Acute myocardial infarction, NA = not available, WMI = wall motion index.
Source: Reproduced with permission from Ref. 15.

motion index estimated from echocardiography was used. Segments in the wall motion index were scored as described by Berning et al. (12). This scoring system is the reverse of that used in the United States and includes grading segments for hyperkinesia. Grade −1 was used for dyskinesia, 0 for akinesia, 1 for hypokinesia, 2 for normokinesia, and 3 for hyperkinesia. Wall motion index was calculated by dividing the sum of the scores of each segment by 9. Thus, a normal left ventricle had a wall motion index of 2.0. A value of 1.2, which was used as the upper limit for entry into the main study, corresponds roughly to an ejection fraction of 0.35 (13). Doctors and technicians from the hospital centers performing the echocardiography participated in two 2-day sessions of intensive training with 4 weeks of self-training interposed. This ensured that they had all performed at least 50–100 examinations prior to the start of the study. The two-dimensional echocardiography included the following views: parasternal long axis, multiple parasternal short axis, and apical two- and four-chamber views. Subxiphoid projections were optional and only included if the examiner felt it added information.

DESIGN

TRACE was a double-blind placebo-controlled parallel group trial. Patients were randomly allocated to receive either the ACE inhibitor trandolapril or matching placebo 3–

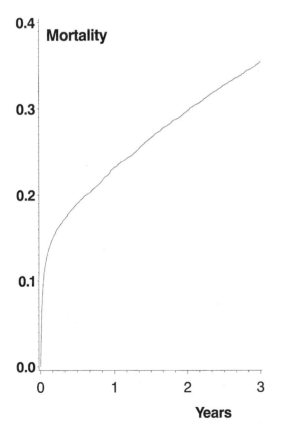

Figure 1 Mortality in 6676 patients with acute myocardial infarction screened for the TRACE study. (Reproduced with permission from Ref. 15.)

7 days following an MI, in addition to conventional therapy. Eligible patients were those with left ventricular systolic dysfunction (wall motion index ≤ 1.2) unless one of the following exclusion criteria was present: a definite need for or an absolute or relative contraindication to ACE inhibition; severe, uncontrolled diabetes mellitus; hyponatremia (sodium < 125 mmol/liter); an elevated serum creatinine (>2.3 mg/dl); pregnancy or lactation; acute pulmonary embolism; collagen vascular disease; severe aortic or mitral stenosis; unstable angina pectoris requiring immediate invasive therapy; severe liver disease; neutropenia; treatment with immunosuppressive or antineoplastic therapy; drug or alcohol abuse; treatment with another investigational drug; or lack of informed consent. Eligible patients were enrolled if they tolerated a test dose of 0.5 mg of trandolapril given on day 2–6. At randomization, patients received 1 mg of trandolapril or matching placebo, and after 2 days the dose was increased to 2 mg of trandolapril or matching placebo. After 4 weeks the dose was further increased to 4 mg once daily. If the increase in dose was not tolerated, the patients could continue with 1 or 2 mg once daily, but the drug was withdrawn if 1 mg was not tolerated. Treatment continued for at least 24 months. Follow-up was originally 12 months, but the Steering Committee, without having knowledge of the study results, extended the follow-up after SAVE reported that a beneficial treatment effect was not seen in the first year. Patients were seen after 1 and 3 months and every 3 months thereafter.

ENDPOINTS AND COMMITTEES

The primary endpoint was total mortality. Secondary endpoints were cardiovascular mortality, sudden death, recurrent MI, progression of heart failure, and change in left ventricular function at 12 months. All mortality endpoints were analyzed on an intention-to-treat basis, and the analysis of the primary endpoint was a comparison of survival in the two

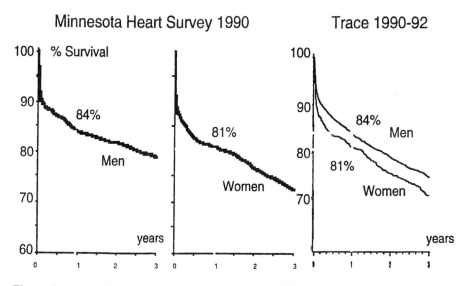

Figure 2   Survival in male and female patients less than 75 years of age screened for the TRACE study and from Minnesota Heart Study. (Reproduced with permission from Ref. 14.)

groups by a log rank test. Causes of death and the occurrence of recurrent MI were established by a Mortality Committee and a Reinfarction Committee, respectively. Progression
of heart failure was defined as hospitalization for heart failure or death due to heart failure.
Change in left ventricular function was measured as change in wall motion index at 3, 6,
and 12 months. Endpoints involving cardiovascular morbidity were analyzed on an on-
treatment basis. At the end of the study survival status was available for all patients and
all classifications were performed prior to unblinding.

A safety committee oversaw the conduct of the trial. Three preplanned interim analyses were performed and did not meet the criteria for stopping the study prematurely.

SAMPLE SIZE

Sample size was calculated using a one-tailed log rank test with an α risk of 0.025 and
a 25% relative reduction in mortality in the active group compared to placebo. One-year
mortality was expected to be 30% in the placebo group, and with a 10% risk of overlooking
an effect of treatment (β risk) 1500 patients were needed. This was increased to 1860 to
allow for a lower-than-expected placebo mortality. However, the Steering Committee decided that inclusion should end by July 1992 if more than 1500 patients had been included.

DATA ANALYSIS

Mortality data were available for all Danes screened by interrogation of the Danish Central
Person Register, where all deaths in the country are recorded within 2 weeks. The few
foreigners screened were censored at the time of discharge. Outcome data are presented
using rank sum tests and chi-square tests for the comparisons of continuous and discrete
variables. Monovariate comparisons of survival data were performed with the log rank
test, and risk reduction including confidence limits was performed using proportional hazard models. All p-values presented are two-sided.

Table 2 Mortality in Patients with Left Ventricular Systolic Dysfunction Divided
in Larger Subgroups According to Exclusion Criteria

Exclusion criteria	N	30-day mortality (%)	1-year mortality (%)
Test does not tolerated	39	54 ± 15	59 ± 15
ACE inhibitor indicated	150	22 ± 7	49 ± 8
Cardiogenic shock	101	81 ± 8	90 ± 6
Uremia	50	30 ± 13	54 ± 14
Dementia, abuse	142	34 ± 8	47 ± 8
No consent	218	15 ± 5	32 ± 6
Other	89	19 ± 8	44 ± 10
Early death	70		
Total	859	37 ± 2	54 ± 3

Mortality $\pm$ 95% confidence intervals is shown. ACE = Angiotensin-converting enzyme.
Source: Reproduced with permission from Ref. 15.

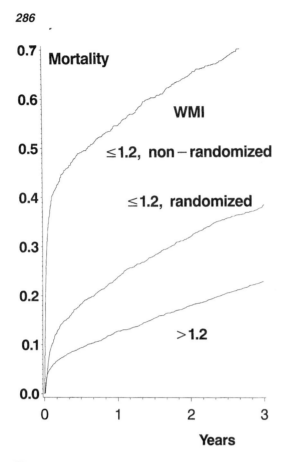

Figure 3   Mortality in patients with wall motion index > 1.2, wall motion index ≤ 1.2 for nonrandomized patients, and wall motion index ≤ 1.2 for randomized patients. (Reproduced with permission from Ref. 15.)

OUTCOME OF SCREENING

A total of 7001 infarctions occurring in 6676 patients were screened from May 1, 1990, until July 7, 1992, in the 27 participating Danish departments. Only patients not randomized at initial screening were rescreened in case of reinfarction. Baseline demographic data for the 6676 patients at their first screening are shown in Table 1, where patients are separated according to left ventricular function. The mortality of the screened patients is shown in Figure 1. In order to compare this mortality with a similar population from the same period, mortality of patients less than 75 years of age from the Minnesota Heart Survey are shown in Figure 2, separating men and women (14).

A total of 2606 patients had left ventricular dysfunction, and a total of 859 patients were excluded from TRACE for reasons listed in Table 2. Only 218 patients did not consent, but these patients had an increased mortality compared to patients included, which could not be explained by a treatment effect of trandolapril (Table 2) (15). Patients with left ventricular dysfunction but excluded from the study were a high-risk group, while patients with smaller infarctions (WMI [wall motion index] > 1.2) had a lower mortality (Fig. 3).

Table 3 Baseline Characteristics of 1749 Patients Assigned to Receive Trandolapril or Placebo

	Trandolapril ($n = 876$)	Placebo ($n = 873$)
Mean age (yr)	67.7	67.3
Male sex (% of patients)	72	71
Mean body-mass index	25.8	25.6
History of (% of patients)		
Hypertension	23	23
Diabetes mellitus	13	14
Angina pectoris	47	44
Previous myocardial infarction	37	34
Heart failure	21	23
Current or previous smoker	73	75
Anterior Q-wave	47	47
Mean time from infarction to randomization (days)	4.5	4.5
Events between infarction and randomization		
Killip class ≥ 2	59	59
Thrombolysis given	45	44
Mean wall motion index	1.0	1.0
Medications (% of patients)		
Aspirin	92	90
Beta-blocker	17	15
Diuretic	64	68
Calcium antagonist	28	28
Digoxin	26	29

Source: Reproduced with permission from Ref. 16.

OUTCOME OF THE STUDY

A total of 1749 patients (67% of those with wall motion index ≤ 1.2, plus 2 patients enrolled by error with a WMI > 1.2) were randomized: 876 in the trandolapril group and 873 in the placebo group. Baseline characteristics of the two groups are shown in Table 3. Randomization resulted in two well-matched groups without baseline differences. During the study period 369 patients (42.3%) in the placebo group died and 304 patients (34.7%) in the trandolapril group died, as shown in Figure 4 (16). The relative risk of death in the trandolapril group was 0.78 (CI 0.67–0.91%; $p < 0.001$) compared to the placebo group. This difference in mortality occurred early, and after 1 month there was an absolute difference in mortality of 2.4% (Fig. 5) corresponding to 24 lives saved per 1000 patients treated for one month. The effect of trandolapril on mortality in subgroups is shown in Table 4. The result was stable without any subgroup showing a tendency toward harm.

    Time-to-event curves for the secondary endpoints are shown in Figure 6. Cardiovascular death was reduced with trandolapril (226 vs. 288; relative risk 0.75; 95% CI 0.63–0.89%; $p = 0.001$). Sudden cardiovascular death defined as death within 1 hour of new symptoms was also significantly reduced with trandolapril (105 vs. 133; relative risk 0.76; 95% CI 0.59–0.98%; $p = 0.03$). The 14% risk reduction of reinfarction with trandolapril was not significant (95% CI 0.66–1.13%; $p = 0.29$). There was a significant reduction in progression to severe heart failure, and 82 patients receiving trandolapril compared to

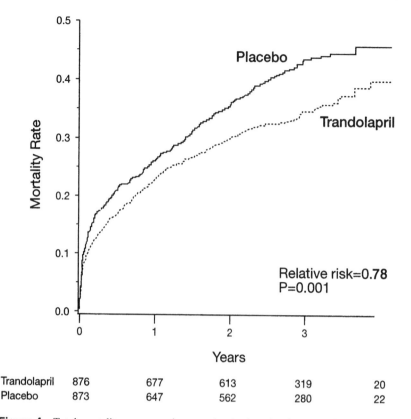

Figure 4 Total mortality among patients randomized to placebo or trandolapril. (Reproduced with permission from Ref. 16.)

103 receiving placebo died from heart failure. Change in wall motion index did not differ between the two groups after 6 and 12 months, while the mean change from baseline was significantly higher in the trandolapril group (0.09 vs. 0.06 WMI unit; $p = 0.03$) after 3 months.

The reduction in mortality with trandolapril was obtained using intention-to-treat analysis in spite of 328 patients (37.4%, excluding patients that died) being withdrawn from the trandolapril group and 310 (35.5%) from the placebo group. The most frequent reasons for withdrawal were need for open-label ACE inhibition (75 in the placebo group vs. 48 in the trandolapril group), cough (13 vs. 39, respectively), hypotension (7 vs. 18, respectively), and a reduction in kidney function (6 vs. 18, respectively).

PATIENT SELECTION IN PERSPECTIVE

When TRACE has been presented, the very high mortality of patients in this study has often caused surprise. Although unfounded, many cardiologists perceive the mortality of post-MI patients as being much lower than it actually is. We were therefore very pleased when McGovern et al. published their results from the Minnesota Heart Study. Only patients below 75 years of age were included in the study, and it is remarkable that the one-

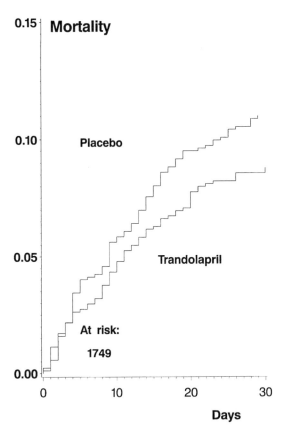

Figure 5   Total mortality in the initial 30 days among patients randomized to placebo or trandolapril. (Reproduced with permission from Am Heart J 1996; 132:235–243.)

year mortality of their patients is identical to that of patients below 75 years of age screened for inclusion into TRACE (Fig. 2). The average patient suffering an AMI has a high mortality, and from this background the high mortality observed in the final study population is not surprising. We believe that the high mortality observed is due to the influence of consecutive screening. Such screening required a continuous dialogue with the study office regarding every patient when the result of the WMI was communicated. It was our impression that this particular organization greatly strengthened the morale of the participants of the study. Epidemiological studies are often used as guidelines for selection of patients in trials, and often the mortality observed in trials is surprisingly low. TRACE is an exception, and the most likely explanation is that consecutive screening and enrollment ensured that representative patients were included in the study. An instrument to ensure recruiting representative patients could be an organization that carefully monitors all screened patients, irrespective of randomization. The registration of all those screened will enable other clinicians to judge for themselves the importance of the selection procedures used. As shown in Table 2, patients not randomized differ from those randomized, and patients not giving informed consent are a high-risk group for reasons not immediately explainable. In terms of our ambition of recommending determination of left ventricular function as a routine for selection of patients for ACE inhibition, the patient selection

Table 4 Relative Risk of Death from Any Cause in Subgroups of Patients Receiving Trandolapril or Placebo

| | No. of deaths/ No. of patients | | |
	Trandolapril ($n = 876$)	Placebo ($n = 873$)	Relative risk with trandolapril (95% CI)
Age ≥ 65 years	247/571	278/551	0.83 (0.70–0.98)
Age < 65 years	57/305	91/322	0.62 (0.45–0.86)
Male sex	203/627	256/621	0.74 (0.62–0.89)
Female sex	101/249	113/252	0.90 (0.69–1.18)
WMI < 0.8	53/89	62/90	0.87 (0.60–1.26)
WMI 0.8–1.0	136/308	173/322	0.76 (0.61–0.93)
WMI > 1.0	115/479	134/461	0.80 (0.62–1.03)
Anterior infarction	110/407	153/412	0.67 (0.53–0.86)
Nonanterior infarction	191/463	215/457	0.86 (0.71–1.05)
Killip class > 1	232/513	273/512	0.82 (0.69–0.98)
Killip class = 1	72/363	96/361	0.70 (0.52–0.96)
Diuretic treatment at randomization	247/558	307/591	0.82 (0.70–0.97)
No diuretic treatment	57/318	62/282	0.78 (0.54–1.12)
Aspirin given	271/803	318/788	0.81 (0.69–0.95)
Aspirin not given	33/73	51/85	0.64 (0.41–0.99)
Thrombolysis given	101/395	117/386	0.84 (0.64–1.09)
No thrombolysis	203/480	252/487	0.77 (0.64–0.92)
Residual angina	79/211	89/193	0.82 (0.66–1.00)
No residual angina	225/665	280/680	0.78 (0.66–0.93)

Source: Reproduced with permission from Ref. 16.

procedure was highly successful. Twenty-five percent of consecutive MI patients were enrolled in the trial as well as two-thirds of those with severe left ventricular dysfunction.

TRACE OUTCOME IN PERSPECTIVE

Studies of ACE inhibitor following myocardial infarction differ in several important aspects: different ACE inhibitors, day of initiating treatment, selection of patient population, and length of follow-up. Assuming that the effect of ACE inhibitors is a class effect, patient selection becomes an important issue when comparing the different trials. The studies aiming at treating all comers with acute myocardial infarction started ACE inhibitors early (within 24 hours) and applied short-term follow-up (approximately 1 month). Mortality reduction was modest (approximately 5 lives saved per 1000 treated). It is therefore debatable whether this effect is worthwhile compared to the effect of treating selected high-risk patients. The latter approach was used in SAVE, AIRE, and TRACE. While patients were selected on clinical grounds in the AIRE study, both SAVE and TRACE used an estimation of left ventricular systolic function for inclusion. Similar degrees of mortality reduction were observed in these three studies, and patients selected either on clinical grounds or by estimation of left ventricular systolic dysfunction will benefit from

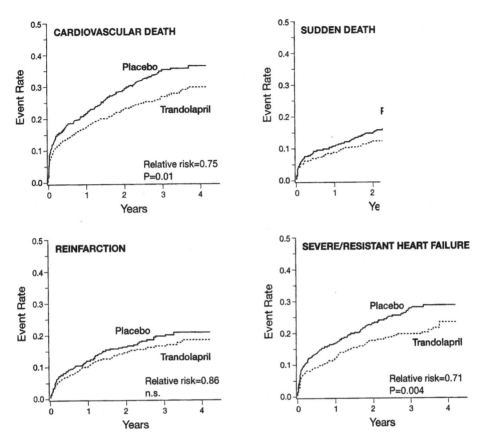

Figure 6   Time-to-event curves for the secondary endpoints among patients randomized to placebo or trandolapril. (Reproduced with permission from Ref. 16.)

ACE inhibition. Compared to our thoughts in 1987, this was a surprise, but clinical signs of heart failure are at least as important as measurement of left ventricular systolic function. Importantly, the mortality reduction found in TRACE was not exclusively found in patients with heart failure, but also in patients with asymptomatic left ventricular systolic dysfunction. TRACE differs from these other studies in more subtle, but yet critical aspects. Patients with residual angina were included in contrast to SAVE. There was a fear that lowering blood pressure in patients shortly after an infarction could aggravate ischemia and have a deleterious effect. This was not the case, as patients with ongoing ischemia had the same benefit as other patients (Table 4).

CONCLUSION

The results from TRACE indicate that at least two-thirds of patients with left ventricular systolic dysfunction determined by echocardiography are candidates for long-term treatment with trandolapril and that this treatment will result in lower mortality and morbidity. The result was obtained by screening consecutive patients with AMI in order to be able to translate the result into clinical practice. A main result of TRACE is then a clinical recommendation to perform a determination of left ventricular systolic function in all AMI survivors and to use this determination for selection of patients for long-term ACE inhibition. This recommendation is complementary to the AIRE study recommending ACE inhibition to all patients with clinical signs of congestive heart failure.

REFERENCES

1. The CONSENSUS Trial Study Group. Effects of enalapril on mortality in severe congestive heart failure. Results of the Cooperative North Scandinavian Enalapril Survival Study (CONSENSUS). N Engl J Med 1987; 316:1429–1435.
2. Pfeffer MA, Braunwald E, Moyé LA, Basta L, Brown EJ, Cuddy TE, et al. Effect of captopril on mortality and morbidity in patients with left ventricular dysfunction after myocardial infarction. Results of the Survival and Ventricular Enlargement trial. N Engl J Med 1992; 327: 669–677.
3. The Acute Infarction Ramipril Efficacy (AIRE) Study Investigators. The effect of ramipril on mortality and morbidity of survival of acute myocardial infarction with clinical evidence of heart failure. Lancet 1993; 342:821–828.
4. Swedberg K, Held P, Kjekshus J, Rasmussen K, Ryden L, Wedel H, et al. Effects of the early administration of enalapril on mortality in patients with acute myocardial infarction. Results of the Cooperative New Scandinavian Enalapril Survival Study II (CONSENSUS II). N Engl J Med 1992; 327:678–684.
5. ISIS-4 (Fourth international study of infarct survival) collaborative group. ISIS-4: a randomised factorial trial assessing early oral captopril, oral mononitrate, and intravenous magnesium sulphate in 58,050 patients with suspected acute myocardial infarction. Lancet 1995; 345:669–685.
6. Gruppo Italiano per lo Studio della Sopravvivenza nell'Infarto Miocardico. GISSI-3: effects of lisinopril and transdermal glyceryl trinitrate singly and together on 6-week mortality and ventricular function after acute myocardial infarction. Lancet 1994; 343:1115–1122.
7. The SOLVD Investigators. Effect of enalapril on survival in patients with reduced left ventricular ejection fractions and congestive heart failure. N Engl J Med 1991; 325:293–302.
8. The SOLVD Investigators. Effect of enalapril on mortality and the development of heart failure in asymptomatic patients with reduced left ventricular ejection fractions. N Engl J Med 1992; 327:685–691.
9. Ambrosioni E, Borghi C, Magnani B. The effect of the angiotensin-converting-enzyme inhibitor zofenopril on mortality and morbidity after anterior myocardial infarction. N Engl J Med 1995; 332:80–85.
10. TRACE Study Group. The TRAndolapril Cardiac Evaluation (TRACE) study: rationale, design and baseline characteristics of screened population. Am J Cardiol 1994; 73:44C–50C.
11. Heger JJ, Weyman AE, Wann IS, Rogers EW, Dillon JC, Feigenbaum H. Cross-sectional echocardiographic analysis of the extent of left ventricular asynergy in acute myocardial infarction. Circulation 1980; 61:1113–1118.
12. Berning J, Steensgaard-Hansen F. Early estimation of risk by echocardiographic determination of wall motion index in an unselected population with acute myocardial infarction. Am J Cardiol 1990; 65:567–576.
13. Berning J, Rokkedal Nielsen J, Launbjerg J, Fogh J, Mickley H, Andersen PE. Rapid estimation of left ventricular ejection fraction in acute myocardial infarction by echocardiographic wall motion analysis. Cardiology 1992; 80:257–266.
14. McGovern PG, Pankow JS, Shahar E, Doliszny KM, Folsom AR, Blackburn H, et al. Recent

trends in acute coronary heart disease. Mortality, morbidity, medical care, and risk factors. N Engl J Med 1996; 334:884–890.

15. Køber L, Torp-Pedersen C. Clinical characteristics and mortality of patients screened for entry into the trandolapril cardiac evaluation (TRACE) study. Am J Cardiol 1995; 76:1–5.

16. Køber L, Torp-Pedersen C, Carlsen J, Bagger H, Eliasen P, Lyngborg K, et al. A clinical trial of the angiotensin-converting-enzyme inhibitor trandolapril in patients with left ventricular dysfunction after myocardial infarction. N Engl J Med 1995; 333:1670–1676.

Section H
Cholesterol Reduction

Several important studies have recently established the efficacy of cholesterol reduction in decreasing adverse events and lowering mortality in patients who are either at risk for, or have evidence of, coronary artery disease. The CARE trial is unique in its focus on patients who had survived a myocardial infarction. The remarkable benefit of cholesterol reduction, even among patients with modest elevation of baseline lipids, should lead to the evaluation of lipids in all infarct patients and a low threshold for the institution of "statin" therapy. Evidence continues to accumulate that these potent agents are well tolerated and lead to better outcomes.

26

CARE

DAVID T. NASH

Sacks FM, Pfeffer MA, Moye LA, Rouleau JL, Rutherford JD, Cole TG, Brown L, Warnicka JW, Arnold JMO, Wun GC, Davis BR, Braunwald E, for the Cholesterol and Recurrent Events Trial Investigators. The effect of pravastatin on coronary events after myocardial infarction in patients with average cholesterol levels. N Engl J Med 1996;335:1001–1009.

The relationship between elevated serum cholesterol and increased risk of coronary heart disease is well established. The West of Scotland Coronary Prevention Study evaluated a reductase inhibitor, pravastatin, in preventing coronary events in men with high cholesterol levels and no history of myocardial infarction (1). Compared to placebo, pravastatin produced a significant reduction in the risk of the combined primary endpoint of definite nonfatal myocardial infarction and death from coronary heart disease of 31% ($p < 0.001$).

In 1994 the Scandinavian Simvastatin Survival Study (4S) was published (2). This study followed 4444 men and women with a history of angina pectoris or acute myocardial infarction (AMI) who had elevated levels of cholesterol and who were treated with simvastatin (20–40 mg) or matching placebo for 5 years. There was a significant reduction in total mortality from 12% to 8% in the simvastatin-treated group compared with placebo.

The relationship between plasma cholesterol and coronary events appears to be stronger in the elevated than in average ranges (3–6). Angiographic trials have demonstrated that cholesterol lowering slows progression and promotes regression of coronary atherosclerosis (7). These beneficial changes appear to relate to the pretreatment low-density lipoprotein (LDL) cholesterol level (6–8) with little benefit occurring in patients with average baseline LDL levels (9). Clinical trials in patients with rather elevated levels of cholesterol have shown that lowering LDL cholesterol from elevated levels prevents both first and recurrent coronary events (1,2,10–12). However, it had not been clear whether coronary events could be prevented by cholesterol-lowering therapy in patients who do not have hypercholesterolemia. This issue is important, because the large majority of patients with coronary disease have average, not elevated, cholesterol levels with a range (13–16) similar to that of the general population (17).

The Cholesterol and Recurrent Events (CARE) Trial was designed specifically to study the effectiveness of lowering average LDL cholesterol levels to prevent coronary events in a typical population after myocardial infarction. The entry criteria were plasma total cholesterol < 240 mg/dl (6.2 mmol/liter) and LDL cholesterol levels of 115–174 mg/dl (3.0–4.5 mmol/liter).

METHODS AND STUDY DESIGN

Men and postmenopausal women were eligible if they had experienced an acute myocardial infarction (AMI) between 3 and 20 months prior to randomization, were aged 21–75 years, and had fasting triglycerides < 350 mg/dl (4.0 mmol/liter), fasting glucose < 220 mg/dl (12 mmol/liter), left ventricular ejection fraction > 25%, and no symptomatic congestive heart failure. Criteria for a qualifying myocardial infarction included typical symptoms and an elevated serum creatine kinase (18). The lipid levels from two or three qualifying visits at least 8 weeks after hospital discharge for myocardial infarction and after 4 weeks of step 1 diet treatment (19) were averaged for eligibility. Patients continued on prescribed cardiac and other medications (Table 1). Plasma total cholesterol, high-density lipoprotein (HDL) cholesterol, and triglyceride levels were measured by the core laboratory at baseline, 6, and 12 weeks after randomization, quarterly for the first year, and semiannually thereafter. LDL cholesterol was calculated. For any patient with an LDL cholesterol > 175 mg/dl (4.5 mmol/liter), intensified (step 2) dietary counseling was initiated (19,20).

Pravastatin 40 mg or matching placebo was started in a random fashion once all the entry criteria had been met and the patient provided informed consent. Stratification by clinical center was achieved by a telephone call to the data center. After randomization the patients were followed every 3 months until the termination of the study. If the patient developed a persistently elevated LDL of >175 mg/dl, intensive diet counseling was provided (NCEP step 2), and if the LDL elevation persisted above 175 mg/dl, cholestyramine was added. To maintain the blinded design a patient in the other group matched for sex, age, and in the highest decile of LDL was provided with similar dietary and cholestyramine therapy.

The primary endpoint of the trial was death from coronary heart disease (fatal myocardial infarction definite or probable, sudden death, death during a coronary interventional procedure, other coronary death) or nonfatal myocardial infarction (symptomatic unless during noncardiac surgery), each confirmed centrally using serum creatine kinase measurements. The effect of therapy on the primary endpoint of the trial was assessed using log rank *p*-values (21). All other hypothesis tests and all risk reductions were assessed using the Cox proportional hazard model (22).

RESULTS

A total of 4159 patients were randomized: 2078 to the placebo group and 2081 to the pravastatin group. Characteristics of the patients before randomization were similar in both groups (Table 1). In the last year of follow-up, 86% of the placebo group and 94% of the treatment group were taking their study drug. This includes patients, comprising 6% of both treatment groups, who were taking cholestyramine according to the protocol. Eight percent of the patients in the placebo group and 2% in the treatment group discontinued study medication and started lipid treatment with open-label drug therapy, prescribed by their personal physicians.

The median duration of follow-up was 5.0 years (range 4.0–6.2 yr). Data were obtained to classify myocardial infarctions as confirmed or unconfirmed for all patients in

Table 1   Baseline Characteristics of Patients in the Placebo
and Pravastatin Groups

Characteristic	Placebo ($n = 2078$)	Pravastatin ($n = 2081$)
General		
Age (yr)	59 ± 9	59 ± 9
Sex (%)		
Female	14	14
Male	86	86
Race (%)		
White	92	93
Other	8	7
Country of residence (%)		
United States	66	66
Canada	34	34
Hypertension (%)	43	42
Current smoker (%)	21	21
Diabetes (%)	15	14
Body-mass index[a]	28 ± 4	28 ± 4
Blood pressure (mmHg)		
Systolic	129 ± 18	129 ± 18
Diastolic	79 ± 10	79 ± 10
Cardiovascular status		
Months from myocardial in-farction to randomization	10 ± 5	10 ± 5
Type of myocardial infarction (%)		
Q-wave	61	61
Other	38	38
Angina (%)	20	21
Congestive heart failure (%)	4	4
CABG (%)	28	26
PTCA (%)	32	34
CABG or PTCA (%)	54	54
Thrombolysis (%)	40	42
Ejection fraction (%)	53 ± 12	53 ± 12
Medication use		
Aspirin (%)	83	83
Beta-blocker (%)	39	41
Nitrate (%)	33	32
Calcium-channel blocker (%)	38	40
ACE inhibitor (%)	14	15
Diuretic agent (%)	11	11
Insulin (%)	2.6	2.4
Oral hypoglycemic agent (%)	7	5[b]
Estrogen (% of women)	10.3	8.4

Table 1   Continued

Characteristic	Placebo ($n = 2078$)	Pravastatin ($n = 2081$)
Plasma lipids[c]		
Cholesterol (mg/dl)		
Total	209 ± 17	209 ± 17
VLDL	27 ± 16	27 ± 16
LDL	139 ± 15	139 ± 15
HDL	39 ± 9	39 ± 9
Triglycerides (mg/dl)	155 ± 61	156 ± 61

Plus–minus values are means ± SD. Except for the use of oral hypoglycemic agents, differences between the groups were not significant. CABG denotes coronary-artery bypass grafting; PTCA, percutaneous transluminal coronary angioplasty; ACE, angiotensin-converting enzyme; VLDL, very-low-density lipoprotein; LDL, low-density lipoprotein; and HDL, high-density lipoprotein.

[a] The body-mass index is the weight in kilograms divided by the square of the height in meters.
[b] $p < 0.05$ for the comparison with the placebo group.
[c] To convert values for cholesterol to millimoles per liter, multiply by 0.02586. To convert values for triglycerides to millimoles per liter, multiply by 0.01129.

whom a myocardial infarction was reported. Vital status was ascertained for the first 4 years on all patients and at the end on all but one patient.

Pravastatin therapy lowered mean LDL cholesterol from 139 mg/dl (3.6 mmol/liter) by 32% maintaining mean levels of 97–98 mg/dl (2.5 mmol/liter) throughout the 5-year follow-up. The average differences in the lipid changes between the placebo and pravastatin groups during follow-up were: LDL cholesterol, 28%; total cholesterol, 20%; HDL cholesterol, 5%; and triglycerides, 14% (all $p < 0.001$).

Pravastatin treatment significantly lowered the rate of the primary endpoint, fatal coronary heart disease, and confirmed nonfatal myocardial infarction by 24% (95% CI 9–36, $p = 0.003$) (Table 2; Fig. 1). There were 274 (13.2%) patients who experienced a primary event in the placebo group compared to 212 (10.2%) in the pravastatin group. There were 173 patients who experienced nonfatal myocardial infarction in the placebo group compared with 135 in the pravastatin group, representing a 23% relative reduction ($p = 0.02$) (Table 2). In the placebo group, 119 patients died from coronary heart disease compared with 96 in the pravastatin group, constituting a 20% decrease ($p = 0.10$) (Table 2). Patients with a nonfatal myocardial infarction during the trial who subsequently died from a coronary event were counted only once in the primary endpoint. The rate of fatal myocardial infarction was reduced by 37% ($p = 0.07$) and total myocardial infarction, fatal or confirmed nonfatal, by 25% ($p = 0.006$) (Table 2). Pravastatin decreased the rate of coronary bypass surgery by 26% ($p = 0.005$), angioplasty by 23% ($p = 0.01$), and either procedure by 27% ($p < 0.001$) (Table 2; Fig. 1). Pravastatin treatment reduced the incidence of stroke by 31% ($p = 0.03$) (Table 2).

Pravastatin significantly lowered the rate of major coronary events in women (46%, $p = 0.001$) as well as in men (20%, $p = 0.001$) (Table 3). Pravastatin reduced major coronary events by comparable amounts in those with ages at baseline of 60–75 years or 24–59 years, in patients with or without hypertension, diabetes, or smoking, and in those with left ventricular ejection fraction 25–40% or >40% (Table 3). Pravastatin lowered major coronary events to a similar extent in patients who had pretreatment plasma lipid

Table 2 Cardiovascular Events According to Study Group

Event	Placebo (n = 2078)		Pravastatin (n = 2081)		Risk reduction with pravastatin (%) (95% CI)	p-value
	No. of patients	Incidence (%)	No. of patients	Incidence (%)		
Death from CHD or nonfatal MI[a]	274	13.2	212	10.2	24 (9–36)	0.003
Death from CHD	119	5.7	96	4.6	20 (−5 to 39)	0.10
Nonfatal MI	173	8.3	135	6.5	23 (4–39)	0.02
Fatal MI	38	1.8	24	1.2	37 (−5 to 62)	0.07
Fatal MI or confirmed nonfatal MI	207	10.0	157	7.5	25 (8–39)	0.006
Clinical nonfatal MI[b]	231	11.1	182	8.7	23 (6–36)	0.01
CABG	207	10.0	156	7.5	26 (8–40)	0.005
PTCA	219	10.5	172	8.3	23 (6–37)	0.01
CABG or PTCA	391	18.8	294	14.1	27 (15–37)	<0.001
Unstable angina	359	17.3	317	15.2	13 (−1 to 25)	0.07
Stroke	78	3.8	54	2.6	31 (3–52)	0.03

Risk reductions and p-values were based on Cox proportional-hazards analysis; p-values are identical to those derived by log-rank analysis. Patient-specific data were used to compute p-values and confidence intervals (CI). CHD denotes coronary heart disease; MI, myocardial infarction; CABG, coronary-artery bypass grafting; and PTCA, percutaneous transluminal coronary angioplasty.

[a] This combined variable was the specified primary endpoint. Nonfatal myocardial infarctions were confirmed by the core laboratory.

[b] This variable comprises all nonfatal myocardial infarctions reported by investigators.

levels that were above or below the median (Table 3). Qualitatively, similar subgroup results were obtained for the primary endpoint.

The pretreatment LDL level influenced the reduction in coronary events during treatment. Patients with baseline LDL > 150 mg/dl (3.9 mmol/liter) (n = 953), experienced a 35% reduction in major coronary events, compared to a 26% reduction in those with an LDL of 125–150 mg/dl (3.2–3.9 mmol/liter) (n = 2355), and a 3% increase for LDL < 125 mg/dl (3.2 mmol/liter) (n = 851) (p = 0.03 for interaction between baseline LDL and risk reduction) (Fig. 2; Table 3). Risk reduction was attenuated progressively in baseline LDL strata below the median.

In all, 196 patients in the control group died compared to 180 in the pravastatin group (9% reduction in risk, 95% CI −12 to 26%; p = 0.37). Deaths from noncoronary causes occurred in 75 and 84 patients in the placebo and pravastatin groups, respectively: 11 and 16 deaths due to cardiovascular but noncoronary causes, 45 and 49 due to cancer, 4 and 8 violent deaths, and 15 and 11 due to other causes, respectively, with no significant differences. The cause of death could not be determined for two patients in the placebo group.

Discontinuation of study medication due to an adverse event occurred in 74 (3.6%) and 45 (2.2%) patients in the placebo and pravastatin groups, respectively (p = 0.007). Elevated serum transaminase levels occurred in 73 and 66, elevated serum creatine kinase in 7 and 12, and myositis in 4 and 0 patients in the placebo and pravastatin groups, respectively, with no significant differences. There were 161 and 172 fatal and nonfatal primary

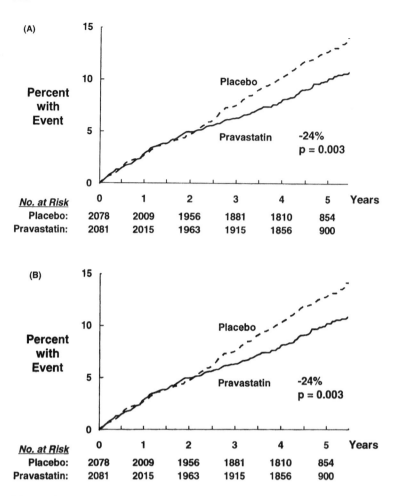

Figure 1 Kaplan-Meier curves and changes in relative risk in the pravastatin compared to the placebo group for fatal coronary heart disease (CHD) or nonfatal myocardial infarction (MI) (primary endpoint), and coronary bypass surgery or angioplasty. *p*-values based on Cox proportional hazards.

cancers in the placebo and pravastatin groups, respectively. The numbers of cancer cases at specific sites in the placebo and pravastatin groups were colorectal 21 and 12, other gastrointestinal 15 and 14, liver 1 and 0, lymphoma or leukemia 10 and 8, and melanoma 3 and 4, respectively. Breast cancer occurred in 1 patient in the placebo group and 12 in the pravastatin group ($p = 0.002$). Of the 12 cases in the pravastatin group, all were nonfatal; 3 occurred in patients with previous breast cancer, 1 was ductal carcinoma in situ, and 1 patient took pravastatin for only 6 weeks. The case in the placebo group was a death in a woman who had had previous breast cancer. There were no other significant differences between the groups in site-specific cancer incidence.

A prospective secondary analysis of CARE examined the efficacy in older (>65 yr) patients. There were 3028 younger patients and 1116 older patients. Baseline analysis revealed fewer smokers or diabetics but more hypertensives in the older population. Baseline lipids were similar in each group, but pravastatin effect was greater in the older group.

Table 3 Major Coronary Events in Subgroups Defined by Baseline Variables

Variable[a]	No. of patients		No. (%) of patients with event		Risk reduction (%) (95% CI)	p-value
	Placebo	Pravastatin	Placebo	Pravastatin		
Sex						
Female	290	286	80 (28)	46 (16)	46 (22–62)	0.001
Male	1788	1795	469 (26)	384 (21)	20 (8–30)	0.001
Age						
<60 yr	1003	1027	258 (26)	217 (21)	20 (4–33)	0.02
≥60 yr	1075	1054	291 (27)	213 (20)	27 (12–38)	<0.001
Hypertension						
Present	899	875	263 (29)	200 (23)	23 (8–36)	0.005
Absent	1179	1206	286 (24)	230 (19)	24 (9–36)	0.002
Diabetes						
Present	304	282	112 (37)	81 (29)	25 (0–43)	0.05
Absent	1774	1799	437 (25)	349 (19)	23 (11–33)	<0.001
Smoking						
Current	334	337	111 (33)	81 (24)	33 (11–50)	0.006
Other	1744	1744	437 (25)	349 (20)	22 (10–33)	<0.001
Left ventricular ejection fraction						
≤40%	353	353	112 (32)	84 (24)	28 (4–45)	0.02
>40%	1725	1728	436 (25)	346 (20)	23 (11–33)	<0.001
Previous CABG						
Yes	564	527	116 (21)	88 (17)	22 (−3 to 41)	0.08
No	1514	1554	433 (29)	342 (22)	25 (13–35)	<0.001
Previous PTCA						
Yes	668	701	188 (28)	153 (22)	25 (7–39)	0.009
No	1410	1380	361 (26)	277 (20)	23 (10–34)	<0.001
Previous CABG or PTCA						
Yes	1118	1127	269 (24)	218 (19)	22 (7–35)	0.006
No	960	954	280 (29)	212 (22)	25 (10–37)	0.002
Type of MI[b]						
Q wave	1277	1279	334 (26)	251 (20)	27 (14–38)	<0.001
Other	799	801	215 (27)	179 (22)	19 (1–34)	0.04
Total cholesterol						
≤209 mg/dl	1040	1032	260 (25)	211 (20)	19 (3–33)	0.02
>209 mg/dl	1038	1049	289 (28)	219 (21)	27 (13–39)	<0.001
LDL cholesterol						
≤137 mg/dl	1048	1042	269 (26)	210 (20)	23 (8–36)	0.004
>137 mg/dl	1030	1039	280 (27)	220 (21)	24 (10–36)	0.002
LDL cholesterol						
<125 mg/dl	441	410	93 (21)	89 (22)	−3 (−38 to 23)	0.85
125–150 mg/dl	1172	1183	311 (27)	239 (20)	26 (13–38)	<0.001
>150–175 mg/dl	465	488	145 (31)	102 (21)	35 (17–50)	0.008
HDL cholesterol						
≤37 mg/dl	1025	1033	290 (28)	236 (23)	21 (6–33)	0.008
>37 mg/dl	1053	1048	259 (25)	194 (19)	27 (12–39)	<0.001

Table 3   Continued

Variable[a]	No. of patients		No. (%) of patients with event		Risk reduction (%) (95% CI)	*p*-value
	Placebo	Pravastatin	Placebo	Pravastatin		
LDL:HDL ratio						
<3.7	1043	1036	251 (24)	190 (18)	26 (11–39)	0.002
≥3.7	1035	1045	298 (29)	240 (23)	21 (7–34)	0.006
Triglycerides						
<144 mg/dl	1049	1031	281 (27)	195 (19)	32 (18–43)	<0.001
≥144 mg/dl	1029	1050	268 (26)	235 (22)	15 (−1 to 29)	0.07

Major coronary events were the primary endpoint (death from coronary heart disease or nonfatal myocardial infarction [MI]), coronary artery bypass grafting (CABG), or percutaneous transluminal coronary angioplasty (PTCA), *p*-values for the interaction between subgroup and treatment were >0.10 except for sex ($p = 0.05$), LDL cholesterol level (<125, 125–150, and > 150 mg/dl; $p = 0.03$), and triglyceride level ($p = 0.08$). LDL denotes low-density lipoprotein and HDL high-density lipoprotein.

[a] The median values for all 4159 patients were as follows: total cholesterol, 209; LDL cholesterol, 137; HDL cholesterol, 37; LDL:HDL ratio, 3.7; and triglycerides, 144. To convert values for cholesterol to mmol/liter, multiply by 0.02586. To convert values for triglycerides to mmol/liter, multiply by 0.01129.

[b] The type of myocardial infarction could not be determined for three patients.

In comparison to placebo, reduction in CHD death or confirmed MI was 19% in younger patients and 32% in older patients.

A small subset of CARE patients was examined during the final 6 months of the study for brachial artery endothelium-dependent flow-mediated vasodilatation (FMD). The technique used high-resolution B-mode ultrasound following blood pressure cuff occlusion in 36 CARE participants. Pravastatin significantly improved FMD compared to the placebo group, and in the treated group FMD was similar to normal controls. Moreover, the percent diameter change was proportional to the percent LDL change. The increased FMD in the treated group supports the hypothesis that normalized endothelium-dependent vasoreactivity is a likely mechanism for the reduction in clinical events observed with lipid-lowering therapy.

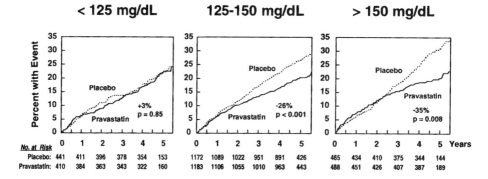

Figure 2   Major coronary events (coronary heart disease death, nonfatal myocardial infarction, CABG, or PTCA) according to baseline LDL cholesterol ranges: Kaplan-Meier curves and changes in relative risk in the pravastatin compared to the placebo group. *p*-value for interaction between baseline LDL level and treatment is 0.03 based on Cox proportional hazards.

Table 1 Entry to the Study and Reasons for Exclusion

	n
Admissions to coronary care units	7415
Randomized on admission	3498
Patients included in the study	1436
Treatment stopped	2062
Excluded on admission	3917
Reasons for exclusion[a]	
Arterial blood pressure < 90 mmHg	192
Cardiogenic shock	64
Pulmonary edema	217
Severe pulmonary congestion	704
Cardiac arrest on admission	249
PR > 0.3 sec	36
Second- and third-degree atrioventricular block	171
Sinoatrial block including heart rate < 45 beats/min	101
QRS ≥ 0.12 sec	264
Beta-blocker treatment	984
Calcium-antagonist treatment	452
Postoperative myocardial infarction	28
Valvular heart disease	68
Ventricular tachycardia	47
Other severe diseases	311
Living outside the catchment area	198
Previously included in the study	34
Did not want to participate	59
Administrative failure	103

[a] Two or more reasons for exclusion were present in 1040 admissions.

times daily or equivalent placebo for the following 6 months. Patients were randomized at each center. The study drug was discontinued permanently in case of (1) patients' unwillingness to continue participating; (2) second- or third-degree atrioventricular block; (3) severe congestive heart failure, including cardiogenic shock; (4) angina pectoris or arrhythmias necessitating treatment with beta-blockers or verapamil; (5) it being unreasonable or impossible to continue treatment (e.g., because of cerebral damages or other severe diseases); or (6) sinoatrial block with ventricular asystole > 3 sec.

Diagnosis

The diagnosis of acute myocardial infarction was based on a typical history of chest pain, changes in the electrocardiogram compatible with a Q-wave or non–Q-wave infarction or development of bundle branch block, and elevation of cardiac enzymes in serum to at least 50% above the upper normal limit. To be included in the final study group, patients had to meet all three diagnostic criteria.

Study Period

The study began in June 1979. Inclusion of patients was terminated on August 15, 1981, when 1436 patients with acute myocardial infarction had been included.

RESULTS

Description of Study Groups

During the study period 6631 patients were admitted a total of 7415 times to the participating coronary care units with a suspicion of acute myocardial infarction (Fig. 1). On admission 3917 were excluded (Table 1). Treatment was initially started on 3498 admissions. Treatment was stopped within 1 week in 2062 patients not fulfilling the diagnostic criteria for acute myocardial infarction.

The study group was comprised of 1436 patients who fulfilled all three criteria for acute myocardial infarction. Of these, 717 patients were randomized to treatment with

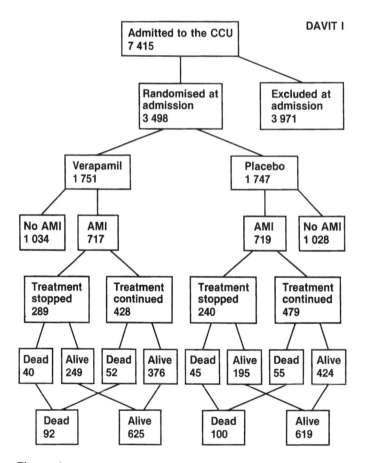

Figure 1 Number of patients evaluated for and randomized into DAVIT I, and total number of deaths at the end of the study period. CCU = Coronary care unit; AMI = acute myocardial infarction.

Table 2 Characteristics of 1436 Patients with Acute Myocardial Infarction Before Randomization and Mortality After 6 Months

	Verapamil			Placebo		
	Patient No.	Death		Patient No.	Death	
		No.	%		No.	%
Sex						
Male	565	63	11	585	79	14
Female	152	29	19	134	21	16
Age						
<65 years	425	49	12	426	36	8
≥65 years	292	43	15*	293	64	22
Previous history						
Previous AMI	106	21	20	98	25	26
Arterial hypertension	72	9	13	62	8	13
Angina pectoris	198	41	20	198	34	18
Heart failure	34	9	27	29	7	24
Diabetes	43	15	35	49	11	22
Smoker	423	43	10	439	48	11
Duration of symptoms						
<7 hours	422	57	14	406	51	13
≥7, ≤24 hours	180	17	9*	205	35	17
>24 hours	107	16	15	103	14	14
Not determined	8	2	—	5	0	—
Location and type of AMI						
Q-wave	534	71	13	548	84	15
anterior	255	44	17	262	52	20
inferior/posterior	279	27	10	286	32	11
Non–Q-wave	174	16	9	162	13	8
anterior	109	10	9	96	10	10
inferior/posterior	65	6	9	66	3	5
Not determined	9	5	—	9	3	—

* $p < 0.05$ compared to placebo.

verapamil and 719 to placebo treatment. No statistically significant differences were found between the two groups in relation to sex, age, previous history, duration of symptoms, or type and location of the index infarct (Table 2).

Endpoints

Death

After 6 months a total of 92 deaths were recorded in the 717 verapamil-treated patients and 100 deaths in the 719 placebo-treated patients. Six-month mortality rates were 12.8% and 13.9%, respectively (NS). Retrospective analyses demonstrated a significantly lower mortality rate in the verapamil group (3.7%) than in the placebo group (6.4%) ($p < 0.05$) in patients still alive on day 22 (Table 3).

Table 3 Time to, Number, and Percent of Deaths and Reinfarctions in Patients at Risk at Start of the Period

Period (day)	Patients at risk Verapamil No.	Placebo No.	Deaths Verapamil No.	%	Placebo No.	%	Reinfarctions Verapamil No.	%	Placebo No.	%
1–180	717	719	92	12.8	100	13.9	56	7.0	66	8.3
1–14	717	719	58	8.1	54	7.5	30	4.2	21	2.9
15–180	659	665	34	5.2	46	6.9	26	3.9**	45	6.8
22–180	649	661	24	3.7*	42	6.4	26	4.0	40	6.1

$*p < 0.05$; $**p < 0.03$ compared to placebo-treated patients.

Reinfarction

Fifty-six reinfarctions were recorded in 50 patients (7.0%) in the verapamil group, and 66 reinfarctions in 60 patients (8.3%) in the placebo group (NS). In both groups six patients had two reinfarctions. Retrospective analyses of patients alive on day 15 showed reinfarctions in 3.9% of verapamil- and 6.8% of placebo-treated patients ($p < 0.03$) (Table 3).

Subgroup Analyses

A retrospective subgroup analysis of mortality was performed in relation to age, gender, previous history, and duration of symptoms (Table 2). This demonstrated a significantly lower 6-month mortality with verapamil (9%) compared to placebo (17%) among patients who started treatment 7–24 hours after start of symptoms, but no difference in mortality among those treated within 6 hours.

A Cox analysis based on sex, age above or below 65 years of age, duration of symptoms as a continuous variable, and previous history demonstrated that the following variables were associated with an increased mortality: diabetes ($p < 0.001$), previous myocardial infarction ($p < 0.001$), age >65 years ($p < 0.001$), and heart failure ($p < 0.002$). Verapamil treatment was related to a decreasing mortality with increasing duration of symptoms ($p < 0.05$) and in patients above 65 years of age ($p < 0.01$). All other variables had no statistically significant influence (i.e., $p > 0.05$) when adjusting for the above-mentioned variables.

Adverse Events

The inpatient incidence of heart failure and atrioventricular block was significantly higher and the incidence of intermittent atrial fibrillation significantly lower in the verapamil compared to the placebo group (Table 4). Excluding death, treatment was withdrawn in 303 patients in the verapamil group and in 246 patients in the placebo group before the 6-month control (Table 5). The excess withdrawal in the verapamil group was limited to the first week and was due to second- and third-degree atrioventricular block. Trial medication was withdrawn in 103 of the verapamil-treated and in 47 of the placebo-treated patients during the first week because of atrioventricular block. In most cases, the block disappeared within 24 hours after termination of trial medication. No one was discharged with heart block. Eighteen of the 103 verapamil- and 14 of the 47 placebo-treated patients

Table 4 Adverse In-Hospital Events

	Verapamil No.	Placebo No.
Patients	717	719
No events	489	510
One event	183	177
Two or more events	45	32
Type of events		
Heart failure**	187	142
Cardiac arrest due to	57	52
Asystole	31	22
Ventricular fibrillation	20	26
Ventricular tachycardia	4	3
Unknown cause	2	1
Thromboembolic complications	13	22
Pulmonary embolism	6	8
Arterial embolism	4	3
Cerebral hemorrhage	3	7
Phlebothrombosis	0	4
Postmyocardial infarction syndrome	0	4
Pneumonia	9	15
Other major events	4	4
Electrocardiographic findings		
Ventricular fibrillation	23	36
Supraventricular tachycardia	45	61
Atrial fibrillation intermittent*	47	70
Sinoatrial block	67	52
Second- and third-degree atrioventricular block***	115	50
Asystole > 3 sec	33	22

$*p < 0.05$; $**p < 0.005$; $***p < 0.001$.

died in the following 6 months. Patients were withdrawn significantly more often from the placebo treatment because of angina pectoris and from the verapamil treatment because of sinoatrial block. Of patients alive after 6 months, 60.1% in the verapamil group and 68.7% in the placebo group were still under treatment ($p < 0.005$).

In patients initially treated but not included in the final study, no significant differences in adverse events were recorded between the two treatment groups.

DISCUSSION

The main purpose for very early intervention with verapamil in patients with acute myocardial infarction in the DAVIT-I was to reduce infarct size; treatment was continued for 6 months to prevent myocardial ischemia. By reducing infarct size and preventing myocardial ischemia, we hoped to improve survival and prevent reinfarction. There was, however, no significant reduction in mortality or first reinfarctions after 6 months in verapamil-compared to placebo-treated patients. It was supposed that very early intervention would improve survival, but the only a priori determined analysis of the results of DAVIT-I

Table 5 Reasons for Discontinuation of Study Medications

Reasons	Verapamil		Placebo	
	No.	%	No.	%
Death	38	5	49	7
Second- and third-degree atrioventricular block**	117	16	54	8
Heart failure	55	8	43	6
Sinoatrial block*	28	4	13	2
Angina pectoris*	18	3	35	5
Arrhythmias demanding treatment with beta-blocker or verapamil	17	2	29	4
Did not want to continue	54	8	59	8
Gastrointestinal complaints	10	1	6	1
Cancer	2	—	2	—
Arterial embolism	2	—	5	1
Six months treatment*	376	52	424	59
Number of patients	717	100	719	100

* $p < 0.05$; ** $p < 0.01$.

demonstrated that the 6-month mortality was not reduced in patients treated within 6 hours of start of symptoms; mortality rate was 13.5% in the verapamil group and 12.6% in the placebo group (NS). In contrast, the mortality in patients who started treatment 7–24 hours after start of symptoms was significantly reduced in the verapamil group (9.4% compared to 17.1% in the placebo group; $p < 0.05$) (Table 2). Also, the Cox analysis demonstrated that verapamil treatment was related to decreasing mortality with increasing duration of symptoms. These results may be evaluated in the light of coronary arteriographic findings published by de Wood et al. (48,49) and of animal experiments of treatment with verapamil after experimental coronary occlusion. In experimental coronary artery occlusion, vera-pamil has no or only limited effect on infarct size if administered after the occlusion in animals without collateral circulation (6,12), and the effect is most pronounced in small infarcts (7). De Wood et al. found significantly more often total or nearly total coronary artery occlusion at coronary arteriography in patients with Q-wave infarction (48) exam-ined within 6 hours of start of symptoms (86%) compared with patients who were exam-ined from 7 to 24 hours after start of symptoms (65%). In patients with non–Q-wave infarction (49) coronary arteriography demonstrated either nonoccluded coronary arteries or occluded coronary arteries with good collateral circulation when examined up to 7 days after start of symptoms. The results of DAVIT-I may be interpreted as demonstrating that verapamil only protects ischemic myocardium when the drug has access to the myocar-dium, as in patients without a totally occluded coronary artery or with good collaterals. Due to the special design of DAVIT-I, this point may be further evaluated by looking at the development of acute myocardial infarction in patients with and without a history of angina pectoris treated for at least 24 hours with trial medication. We know that patients with a history of angina pectoris more often have coronary collaterals (50) and are more likely to develop non–Q-wave rather than Q-wave infarctions (51), compared to patients without angina pectoris. In DAVIT-I we found a significant reduction in development of myocardial infarctions in patients with a history of angina pectoris treated with verapamil (163 of 414 patients, 39.4%) compared with patients treated with placebo (179 of 383 patients, 46.7%) ($p < 0.05$), but no difference in patients without a history of angina pectoris (46). As expected, verapamil prevented angina pectoris (Table 5). Thus verapamil seems to prevent development of myocardial infarction in patients with severe myocardial ischemia.

A number of clinical studies demonstrated that verapamil might prevent ventricular arrhythmias in patients with ischemic heart disease (21,23). DAVIT-I demonstrated a trend toward a lower incidence of ventricular fibrillation during stay in the coronary care unit in the verapamil group compared to the placebo group, though the difference was not statistically significant (Table 4), and a lower prevalence of ventricular ectopic beats after 6 months in patients still in treatment with verapamil (22 of 346 patients, 6.4%) compared with the placebo-treated (45 of 363, 11.7%) ($p < 0.03$) (47). These results are in accordance with animal experiments demonstrating reduction of ventricular fibrillation after coronary artery ligation (17,52) and prevention of the ischemia-induced conduction delay after treatment with verapamil (53).

The dosage of verapamil chosen was based on clinical and experimental findings. In chronic stable angina pectoris, optimal dosage has been repeatedly found to be 120 mg t.i.d. (28,30). Pharmacological studies in patients with rapid atrial fibrillation demonstrated that the peak effect after 5 mg verapamil intravenously occurred after 5–10 minutes and was maintained for 1–2 hours, and that the peak effect after 120 mg verapamil occurred after 1–2 hours and was maintained for 6–8 hours (54). Thus the IV administration of 0.1 mg/kg body weight and the simultaneous oral administration of 120 mg of verapamil on admission and the continued oral administration of 120 mg t.i.d. was assumed to give an immediate and permanent effect in the study period. Verapamil caused a significantly increased incidence of atrioventricular block compared to placebo during the first week. However, the number of deaths in patients with atrioventricular block was essentially the same in verapamil- and placebo-treated patients. Thus, the higher number of atrioventricular blocks in the verapamil group was not associated with an increased mortality rate. The significantly reduced prevalence of atrial fibrillation in the verapamil group is expected (19).

The more pronounced negative inotropic effects of verapamil in ischemic compared with normally perfused myocardium (55), the pronounced peripheral vasodilator effects (56,57), and the negative chronotropic effect during the acute episode of myocardial infarction (43,58) were thought to be potentially beneficial in acute myocardial infarction. Severe deterioration of left ventricular function after administration of verapamil is well described in patients with elevated left ventricular end-diastolic pressure (56). This may prevent the expected beneficial effect of verapamil and explain the higher incidence of congestive heart failure in the early part of the study period.

DAVIT-I demonstrated that (1) early intervention with verapamil in acute myocardial infarction did not significantly improve survival or prevent reinfarction, (2) verapamil prevented atrial fibrillation and angina pectoris, and (3) verapamil increased the incidence of atrioventricular block and of congestive heart failure during the acute event. Conclusions based on DAVIT-I include that verapamil is not indicated in early treatment of patients with acute myocardial infarction. Verapamil is a safe drug if indicated, e.g., for treatment of postinfarct angina pectoris or atrial fibrillation. Verapamil should not be administered to patients with acute myocardial infarction and congestive heart failure.

REFERENCES

1. Nayler WG, Ferrari R, Williams A. Protective effect of pretreatment with verapamil, nifedipine and propranolol on mitochondrial function in ischemic and reperfused myocardium. Am J Cardiol 1980; 45:242–248.
2. Wende W, Bleifeld W, Meyer J, Stühlen HW. Reduction of the size of acute experimental myocardial infarction by verapamil. Basic Res Cardiol 1975; 70:198–208.
3. Smith HJ, Sing BN, Nisbet HD, Norris RM. Effects of verapamil on infarct size following experimental coronary occlusion. Cardiovasc Res 1975; 9:569–578.
4. Reimer KA, Lowe JE, Jennings RB. Effects of the calcium antagonist verapamil on necrosis following temporary coronary artery occlusion in dogs. Circulation 1977; 55:581–587.
5. deBoer LWV, Strauss HW, Kloner RA, Rude RE, Davis RF, Maroko PR, Braunwald E. Autoradiographic method for measuring the ischemic myocardium at risk: effect of verapamil on infarct size after experimental coronary artery occlusion. Proc Natl Acad Sci 1980; 77:6119–6123.
6. Kloner RA, Braunwald E. Effects of calcium antagonists on infarcting myocardium. Am J Cardiol 1987; 59:84B–94B.
7. Yellon DM, Hearse DJ, Maxwell MP, Chambers DE, Downey JM. Sustained limitation of myocardial necrosis 24 hours after coronary artery occlusion: verapamil infusion in dogs with small myocardial infarcts. Am J Cardiol 1983; 51:1409–1413.
8. Reimer KA, Jennings RB. Temporary protection of severely ischemic myocardium without limitation of ultimate infarct size. Lab Invest 1984; 51:655–666.
9. Huey-Ming Lo, Kloner RA, Braunwald E. Effect of intracoronary verapamil on infarct size in the ischemic, reperfused canine heart: critical importance of the timing of treatment. Am J Cardiol 1985; 56:672–677.
10. Sullivan AT, Baker DJ, Drew GM. Effect of calcium channel blocking agents on infarct size after ischemia-reperfusion in anaesthetised pigs: relationship between cardioprotection and cardiodepression. J Cardiovasc Pharmacol 1991; 17:707–717.
11. Vanhoutte PM, Cohen R. Calcium entry blockers and cardiovascular diseases. Am J Cardiol 1983; 52:99A–103A.
12. Nayler WG. Calcium antagonists and the ischemic myocardium. Int J Cardiol 1987; 15:267–285.
13. Skolnick AE, Frishman WH. Calcium channel blockers in myocardial infarction. Arch Intern Med 1989; 149:1669–1677.
14. Rotevan S, Greve G, Øksendal N, Junge P. Tissue protection by verapamil in the calcium paradox. Scand J Lab Invest 1990; 50:595–604.
15. Tillmanns H, Neumann F-J, Parakh N, Waus W, Møller P, Zimmerman R, Steinhausen M, Købler W. Calcium antagonists and myocardial microperfusion. Drugs 1991; 42(suppl 1): 1–6.
16. Watson RM, Markle DR, McGuire DA, Vitale D, Epstein SE, Patterson RE. Effect of verapamil on pH of ischemic canine myocardium. J Am Coll Cardiol 1985; 5:1347–1354.
17. Kaumann JA, Aramendia P. Prevention of ventricular fibrillation induced by coronary ligation. J Pharmacol Exp Ther 1968; 164:326–340.
18. Bachour G, Bender F, Hochrein H. Antiarrhythmische Wirkungen und hämodynamische Reaktionen unter Verapamil bei akutem Herzinfarkt. Herz/Kreislauf 1977; 9:89–95.
19. Hagemeijer F. Verapamil in the management of supraventricular tachyarrhythmias occurring after a recent myocardial infarction. Circulation 1978; 57:751–755.
20. Krikler DM, Spurrell RAJ. Verapamil in the treatment of paroxysmal supraventricular tachycardia. Postgrad Med J 1974; 50:447–453.
21. Gülker H, Godejohann U, Dorsel T, Behrenbeck TH, Heuer H, Bender F. Prophylaxe belastungsinduzierter ventrikuläre Arrhythmien durch Verapamil. Zeitschr Kardiol 1987; 76:404–410.

22. Woelfel A, Foster JR, McAllister RG, Simpson RJ, Gettes LS. Efficacy of verapamil in exercise-induced ventricular tachycardia. Am J Cardiol 1985; 56:292–297.

23. Rolli A, Favaro L, Finadi A, Aurier E, Bonatti V, Botti G. Efficacité du vérapamil dans la prévention de la fibrillation ventriculaire à la phase aiguë de l'infarctus du myocarde. Arch Mal Coeur 1988; 81:907–911.

24. Peter T, Fujimoto T, Hamamoto H, Mandel WJ. Comparative study of the effect of slow channel-inhibiting agents on ischemia-induced conduction delay as relevant to the genesis of ventricular fibrillation. Am Heart J 1983; 106:1023–1028.

25. Opie LH. Calcium antagonists, ventricular arrhythmias, and sudden cardiac death: a major challenge for the future. J Cardiovasc Pharmacol 1991; 18(suppl 10):581–586.

26. Opie LH, Clusin WT. Cellular mechanism for ischemic ventricular arrhythmias. Annu Rev Med 1990; 41:231–238.

27. Andreasen F, Boye E, Christoffersen E, Dalsgaard P, Henneberg E, Kallenbach A, Ladefoged S, Lillquist K, Mikkelsen E, Norderø E, Olsen J, Pedersen JK, Pedersen V, Petersen GB, Schroll J, Schultz H, Seidelin J. Assessment of verapamil in the treatment of angina pectoris. Eur J Cardiol 1975; 2:443–452.

28. Livesley B, Catley PF, Campbell RC, Oram S. Double-blind evaluation of verapamil, propranolol, and isosorbide dinitrate against a placebo in the treatment of angina pectoris. Br Med J 1973; 1:375–378.

29. Subramanian VB, Bowles ML, Lahiri A, Davies AB, Raftery EB. Long-term antianginal action of verapamil assessed with quantitated serial treadmill stress testing. Am J Cardiol 1981; 48: 529–535.

30. Hansen JF, Grytter C, Thomsen S, Sigurd B. Verapamil and beta adrenoreceptor blockade in the treatment of stable angina pectoris. Clin Exp Pharmacol Physiol 1982; Suppl. 6:31–41.

31. Kholi RS, Rodrigues EA, Hughes LO, Lahiri A, Raftery EB. Sustained release verapamil, a once daily preparation: objective evaluation using exercise testing, ambulatory monitoring and blood levels in patients with stable angina. J Am Coll Cardiol 1987; 9:615–621.

32. Mauritson DR, Johnson SM, Winniford MD, Gary JR, Willerson JT, Hillis LD. Verapamil for unstable angina at rest. A short-termed randomized, double blind study. Am Heart J 1983; 106:652–658.

33. Mauri F, Mafrici A, Biraghi M, Cerri P, DeBiase AM. Effectiveness of calcium antagonist drugs in patients with unstable angina and proven coronary artery disease. Eur Heart J 1988; 9 (suppl N):158–163.

34. Hansen JF, Sandoe E. Treatment of Prinzmetal's angina due to coronary artery spasm using verapamil: a report of three cases. Eur J Cardiol 1978; 7:327–335.

35. Johnson SM, Mauritson DR, Willerson JT, Hillis LD. A controlled trial of verapamil for Prinzmetal's variant angina. N Engl J Med 1981; 304:862–868.

36. Parodi O, Simonetti I, Machelassi C, Carpeggiani C, Biagini A, L'Abbate A, Maseri A. Comparison of verapamil and propranolol therapy for angina at rest: a randomized crossover, controlled trial in the coronary care unit. Am J Cardiol 1986; 57:899–906.

37. Pallone MN. Effect of calcium antagonists in the treatment of silent ischemic heart disease. Curr Ther Res 1989; 45:339–346.

38. Walling A, Waters DD, Miller DD, Roy MD, Pelletier GB, Théroux P. Long-term prognosis of patients with variant angina. Circulation 1987; 76:990–997.

39. Lewis GRJ, Morley KD, Lewis BM. The treatment of hypertension with verapamil. NZ J Med 1978; 87:351–354.

40. Pedersen OL. Does verapamil have a clinically significant antihypertensive effect? Eur J Clin Pharmacol 1978; 13:21–24.

41. Holzgreve H, Distler A, Michaelis J, Philipp T, Wellek S, VERDI Trial Research Group. Verapamil versus hydrochlorothiazide in the treatment of hypertension: results of a long term double blind comparative trial. Br Med J 1989; 299:881–886.

42. Midtbø KA, Hals O, Lauve O, Van Der Meer J, Storstein L. Studies on verapamil in the treatment of essential hypertension, a review. Br J Clin Pharmacol 1986; 21:165S–171S.

43. Hansen JF, Sigurd B, Mellemgaard K, Lyngbye J. Verapamil in acute myocardial infarction. Dan Med Bull 1980; 27:105–109.

44. The Danish Study Group on Verapamil in Myocardial Infarction. Verapamil in acute myocardial infarction. Eur Heart J 1984; 5:516–528.

45. The Danish Study Group on Verapamil in Myocardial Infarction. Verapamil in acute myocardial infarction. Am J Cardiol 1984; 54:24E–28E.

46. The Danish Study Group on Verapamil in Myocardial Infarction. The Danish studies on verapamil in myocardial infarction. Br J Clin Pharmacol 1986; 21:197S–204S.

47. Hansen JF und Dänische Studien Gruppe. Verapamil bei akutem Myokardinfarkt: Sekundärprävention des Myokardinfarktes. In: Bender F, Fleckenstein A, eds. Therapie und Prävention mit Kalziumantagonisten. Darmstadt: Stenkopff Verlag 1988:61–71.

48. DeWood MA, Spores J, Notske R, Mouser LT, Burroughs R, Golden MS, Lang HT. Prevalence of total coronary occlusion during early hours of transmural myocardial infarction. N Engl J Med 1980; 303:897–902.

49. DeWood MA, Stifter W, Simpson CS, Spores J, Eugster GS, Judge TP, Hinnen ML. Coronary arteriographic findings soon after non-Q-wave myocardial infarction. N Engl J Med 1986; 315:417–423.

50. Hansen JF. Coronary collateral circulation: clinical significance and influence on survival in patients with coronary artery occlusion. Am Heart J 1989; 117:290–295.

51. Harper WH, Kennedy G, De Sanctis RW, Hutter AM. The incidence and pattern of angina prior to acute myocardial infarction: a study of 577 cases. Am Heart J 1979; 97:178–183.

52. Sugiyama S, Ozawa T, Suzuki S, Kato T. Effects of verapamil and propranolol on ventricular vulnerability after coronary reperfusion. J Electrocardiol 1980; 13:49–54.

53. Hamamoto H, Peter T, Fujimoto T, Mandel WJ. Effect of verapamil on conduction delay produced by myocardial ischemia and reperfusion. Am Heart J 1981; 102:350–358.

54. Follath F, Fromer M, Meier P, Vozeh S. Pharmacodynamic comparison of oral and intravenous verapamil in atrial fibrillation. Clin Invest Med 1980; 3:49–52.

55. Smith HJ, Goldstein RA, Griffith JM, Kent KM, Ebstein SE. Regional contractility: selective depression of ischemic myocardium by verapamil. Circulation 1976; 54:629–635.

56. Chew CYC, Hecht HS, Collett JT, McAllister RG, Singh BN. Influence of severity of ventricular dysfunction on hemodynamic responses to intravenously administered verapamil in ischemic heart disease. Am J Cardiol 1981; 47:917–922.

57. Vlietstra RE, Farias MAC, Frye RL, Smith HC, Ritman EL. Effect of verapamil on left ventricular function: a randomized placebo-controlled study. Am J Cardiol 1983; 51:1213–1217.

58. Berdeaux A, Coutte R, Guidicelli JF, Boissier JR. Effect of verapamil on regional myocardial blood flow and ST-segment: role of induced bradycardia. Eur J Pharmacol 1976; 39:287–294.

28

TRENT

ROBERT G. WILCOX

Wilcox RG, Hamptom JR, Banks DC, Birkhead JS, Brooksby IAB, Burns-Cox CJ, Hayes MJ, Joy MD, Malcolm AD, Mather HG, and Rowley JM. Trial of early nifedipine in acute myocardial infarction: The TRENT study. Br Med J 1986;293:1204–1208.

INTRODUCTION

The era of attempting to first anticipate and then to ameliorate the consequences of acute myocardial infarction began with the concept of the coronary care unit in the early 1960s. Alongside clinical initiatives were animal data detailing the morphological consequences of myocardial ischemia with the suggestion that damage could be either reduced or reversed by "metabolic protection" or reperfusion (1–4). Of the many strategies worthy of testing in acute myocardial infarction, immediate treatment with a calcium channel–blocking drug seemed persuasive.

Nifedipine is a substituted dihydropyridine with calcium channel–blocking properties (5). Compared with verapamil, it has very little cardiac electrophysiological effect (6). In experimental myocardial infarction in animals, pretreatment with nifedipine (in a dose carefully regulated to avoid a large fall in blood pressure and reflex tachycardia) causes an increase in coronary bloodflow in both normally perfused and ischemic areas of the heart, delays the release of cytoplasmic enzymes and the intracellular accumulation of calcium, preserves intracellular stores of adenosine triphosphate, and reduces infarct size (7–10). Nifedipine is active during periods of ischemia and also during subsequent reperfusion (7). This has led to speculation that the drug may have a cardioprotective action in humans.

In patients with angina, nifedipine has been shown to increase coronary perfusion and decrease afterload with minimal decrease in contractility (11,12) and is thereby thought to stabilize the imbalance between oxygen supply and oxygen demand. Roberts and coworkers have shown that nifedipine produces similar hemodynamic effects in patients with acute infarction, suggesting that in this condition the drug may be capable of improving a myocardial oxygen deficiency (13). Nifedipine also inhibits coronary artery spasm (14,15) and mildly inhibits platelet aggregation (16), both of which have been implicated in myocardial infarction (17).

The study by Roberts et al. also suggested that treatment with nifedipine within 12 hours of an infarct is safe provided that the dose is judiciously regulated to prevent hypotension (13). Of 17 patients examined, none developed increased chest pain or showed an increased incidence of ventricular arrhythmia. There was no sign of atrioventricular nodal blockade, which agrees with findings in dogs (18) and patients with angina (6). Preliminary results from open trials, including 164 patients with acute infarction in 11 different centers, also indicated that early treatment (i.e., within 24 hours) with nifedipine is safe (19). Evidently patients with myocardial infarction tolerate nifedipine quite well, even when they have been receiving long-term beta-blocker treatment (20).

In light of these encouraging theoretical, experimental, and limited clinical data, we considered that a large controlled trial of early treatment with nifedipine in patients with suspected acute myocardial infarction was both warranted and justified. The TRENT Trial records the results of this endeavor (21).

PATIENTS AND METHODS

Patients of either sex aged between 18 and 70 years and admitted within 24 hours of onset of symptoms of suspected acute myocardial infarction were considered. No ECG changes were mandatory. Patients were excluded from further consideration for the following reasons: pregnancy or ability to conceive within the next 4 weeks; systolic or diastolic blood pressure < 100 mmHg or < 50 mmHg, respectively, immediately prior to trial administration, or heart rate > 120/min similarly (reassessment was permissible at 2 and 4 hours provided the 24-hour inclusion period was not exceeded); severe heart failure requiring pharmacologic support; known serious renal or hepatic disease; current treatment with a calcium channel blocker; refusal to consent or inability to attend follow-up. All excluded patients had their index admission diagnosis and 1-month status recorded.

DRUG TREATMENT

Immediately after assessment in the coronary care unit (CCU), eligible patients were randomly assigned in a double-blind fashion to receive a capsule of 10 mg nifedipine or placebo sublingually. The second dose was given 4, 6, or 8 hours later if the systolic pressure exceeded 90 mmHg or heart rate was less than 120 beats/min. It at 8 hours from first dose these criteria were still not satisfied, the patient was withdrawn but follow-up continued. Otherwise double-blind treatment continued 6-hourly for 28 days (active dose nifedipine 10 mg) unless the hemodynamic criteria above were violated, severe heart failure supervened, the physician felt that treatment with a calcium channel blocker was essential, or the patient refused to continue because of side effects.

The only stratification of randomized treatment was for patients who had taken beta-blocking drugs within the 48 hours before admission. Beta-blockers could be continued or withdrawn at the discretion of the physician, but it was agreed the beta-blockers for secondary prophylaxis would not begin until the 28-day follow-up visit. No routine antiarrhythmic, anticoagulant, or antiplatelet drugs were permitted.

DEFINITIONS

The following definitions were used:

Definite myocardial infarction (MI)—Convincing history plus pathological Q waves in the ECG and peak enzyme levels exceeding twice the upper limit of normal.

Probable myocardial infarction—Convincing history plus either pathological Q waves or raised cardiac enzymes to twice the upper limit of normal.

Possible myocardial infarction—Convincing history plus ECG abnormalities not diagnostic of myocardial infarction and an increase of cardiac enzymes but to less than twice the upper limit of normal.

Ischemic heart disease (IHD)—Previous myocardial infarction or angina without new ECG or enzyme changes.

Chest pain of unknown cause (CP?C)—No history of previous myocardial infarction or angina and no ECG or enzyme evidence to suggest an event at this admission. No other cause for chest pain was found.

Bleeding complications were divided into major or minor categories, irrespective of the need for blood transfusion. Major bleeds comprised any hematemesis, melena, severe hemoptysis, or hematuria. Minor bleeds comprised slight hemoptysis or trace hematuria and skin or gum bleeding.

DATA HANDLING

Demographic and clinical data were recorded in the patient's study record file, checked by the local coordinator, and reviewed in the Department of Medicine, University Hospital, Nottingham, before forwarding for computer entry and subsequent statistical analysis in the Department of Mathematics, University of Nottingham. Only the independent ethical review committee received unblinded study progress reports, and they had prespecified rules for early termination of the trial.

STATISTICAL CONSIDERATIONS

The primary endpoint was all-cause mortality by 28 days from randomization. Based on our previous beta-blocker trials, we assumed a 10% mortality for control patients and a 30% reduction by nifedipine (assuming 2 $\alpha = 0.05$ and $\beta = 0.1$). After a few months it transpired that the overall death rate was lower than expected, and we were permitted to redefine our sample size based on a control mortality rate of 8%.

RESULTS

Recruitment

Recruitment began in November 1982 and ended in May 1985. During this time 9292 consecutive patients were considered for entry, but 4801 (52%) of these were excluded because of age or potential child-bearing (33%), symptoms > 24 hours (25%), already

Table 1 Comparability of Study Groups at Entry

	Placebo group (n = 2251)		Nifedipine group (n = 2240)	
	No.	%	No.	%
Men	1851	82.2	1178	79.4
Women	400	17.8	462	20.6
Age (yr)				
>40	148	6.6	116	5.2
41–50	393	17.5	427	19.1
51–60	889	39.5	871	38.9
61–70	816	36.3	815	36.4
Unknown	5	0.2	11	0.5
Previous History				
Myocardial infarction				
Definite	350	15.5	372	16.6
Suggestive	225	10.0	219	9.8
Angina	767	34.0	783	34.9
Hypertension	453	20.1	444	19.8
Diabetes	100	4.4	117	5.2
Smoking				
Never	475	21.1	503	22.4
Stopped >6 months	533	23.6	538	24.0
1–10/day	178	7.9	184	8.2
10–20/day	482	21.4	449	20.0
>20/day	368	16.3	375	16.7
Pipe or cigars	191	8.5	173	7.7
Unknown	24	1.1	18	0.8
Drugs				
Diuretics	320	14.2	356	15.9
Digoxin	47	2.1	63	2.8
Beta-blockers	421	18.7	406	18.1
Other hypotensives	89	3.9	85	3.8
Antiarrhythmics	14	0.6	13	0.6
Others	684	30.3	679	30.3

taking a calcium blocker (21%), severe heart failure (7%), or miscellaneous (14%). Thus, 4491 patients were randomized to either placebo (2251) or to nifedipine (2240).

Included Patients

Clinical Course

The two randomized groups were well matched for baseline demographic features (Table 1) and the distribution of time from symptom onset to the first sublingual capsule (32% within 4 hours, 68% by 8 hours, 81% by 12 hours, and most of the remainder within the next 4 hours). The index diagnostic classification and in-hospital clinical events were comparable (Tables 2 and 3): 1442 (64%) control and 1429 (64%) nifedipine-treated patients had acute myocardial infarction.

Table 2 Diagnostic Categorization of Patients in Study Groups

	No. of patients (%)	
	Placebo group (n = 2251)	Nifedipine group (n = 2240)
Myocardial infarction	1442 (64.2)	1429 (63.8)
Definite	1080 (48.0)	1087 (48.5)
Probable	205 (9.1)	180 (8.0)
Possible	157 (7.0)	162 (7.2)
Anterior	669	662
Inferior	628	603
Unsited	138	156
Not recorded	7	8
Ischemic heart disease	389 (17.3)	370 (16.5)
Chest pain of unknown cause	326 (14.5)	342 (15.3)
Other diagnosis	94 (4.2)	99 (4.4)

Withdrawals

Of the patients allocated to nifedipine, 608 (27%) were withdrawn from assigned treatment before day 28, as were 572 (25%) of patients randomized to placebo for reasons listed in Table 4. Most withdrawals occurred in the first few days of treatment. More control patients were withdrawn in order to receive elective treatment with a calcium channel blocker, usually for persistent angina (113 vs. 76), whereas more patients were withdrawn from nifedipine because of headache (49 vs. 20), indigestion (49 vs. 30), and dizziness (24 vs. 17).

Table 3 Treatment and Complications In Hospital and Treatment on Discharge from Hospital

	Placebo group				Nifedipine group			
	In hospital (n = 2251)		On discharge (n = 2148)		In hospital (n = 2240)		On discharge (n = 2135)	
	No.	%	No.	%	No.	%	No.	%
Treatment								
Diuretics	738	34.7	565	26.3	817	36.4	566	26.5
Beta-blockers	475	21.1	385	17.9	439	19.5	350	16.4
Antiarrhythmics	242	10.7	73	3.4	220	9.8	60	2.8
Digoxin	121	5.4	82	3.8	136	6.1	100	4.7
DC shock	144	6.4	—	—	120	5.3	—	—
Pacemaker	49	2.2	17	0.8	54	2.4	10	0.5
Complications								
Recurrent MI	33	1.5	—	—	49	2.2	—	—
Ventricular fibrillation	133	5.9	—	—	114	5.1	—	—
Asystole	28	1.2	—	—	36	1.6	—	—
Pulmonary embolism	10	0.4	—	—	16	0.7	—	—
Other[a]	377	16.7	—	—	384	17.1	—	—

[a] Heart failure, other embolism, other serious arrhythmia, ventricular septal rupture, mitral regurgitation, etc.

Table 4 Reasons for Withdrawal from Assigned Treatment Before Day 28

| | No. of patients (%) | | | | | |
	Hypotension	Tachycardia	Heart failure	Treatment with calcium channel blockers	Side effects	Others[a]
Placebo group (n = 572)	127 (22.2)	46 (8.0)	34 (5.9)	113 (19.7)	96 (16.7)	176 (30.8)
Nifedipine group (n = 608)	151 (24.8)	53 (8.7)	45 (7.4)	76 (12.5)	148 (24.3)	171 (28.1)

Note: Some patients had more than one reason for withdrawal.
[a] Errors, protocol noncompliance, etc.

Mortality by 28 Days

By 28 days 150 (6.7%) of those allocated nifedipine and 141 (6.3%) of those allocated placebo had died, a relative increase of 7% (95% CI +30% to −16%). Of the total 291 study deaths, 280 (96%) occurred in patients who had an index diagnosis of acute myocardial infarction. Their 28-day infarct mortality rate was 10.2% (146/1429) for the nifedipine group and 9.3% (134/1442) for the placebo group.

There were more deaths in both groups among patients withdrawn from assigned study medication, usually for persistent hypotension, tachycardia, or severe heart failure (Fig. 1).

Subgroup Analysis

Patients who had taken beta-blockers within 48 hours of randomization comprised the only predetermined subgroup for treatment stratification and analysis. There were 406 (18.2%) such patients given nifedipine and 421 (18.7%) allocated to placebo. They dif-

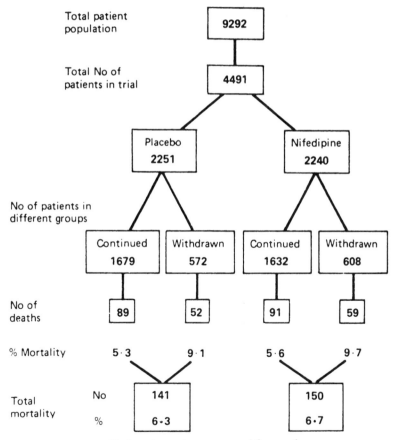

Outcome at 28 days in patients entered for study.

Figure 1   Outcome at 28 days according to allocated treatment and whether withdrawn prematurely.

Table 5   Total and Infarct Mortality at 28 Days Among Patients Taking and Not Taking Beta-Blockers on Admission

	Placebo group ($n = 2251$)	Nifedipine group ($n = 2240$)
Not taking beta-blockers on admission		
Number of patients	1830	1834
Number (%) dead	103 (5.6)	112 (6.1)
Number (%) with MI	1198 (65.4)	1178 (64.2)
Number (%) death	98 (8.2)	109 (9.2)
Taking beta-blockers on admission		
Number of patients	421	406
Number (%) dead	38 (9.0)	38 (9.3)
Number (%) with MI	244 (57.9)	251 (61.8)
Number (%) death	36 (14.7)	37 (14.7)

fered from patients not taking prior beta-blockers with regards to the prevalence of proven previous myocardial infarction (31% vs. 13%), suspected previous infarction (16% vs. 8%), angina pectoris (63% vs. 28%), and hypertension (55% vs. 12%).

Although the proportion of patients diagnosed as having an index acute myocardial infarction was lower in the prior beta-blocker group irrespective of trial assignment, the overall infarct fatality rate was higher (overall 14.7% vs. 8.7%; Table 5). There was also no evidence of an interaction between prior beta-blocker treatment and assignment to nifedipine.

Excluded Patients

The excluded patients comprised 52% of all registered patients. The in-hospital diagnosis was available for 4798 of 4801 excluded patients, of whom 2926 (61%) had an index acute myocardial infarction. The 28-day outcome was known for 97.4% of the excluded group: among these 4674 patients the overall fatality rate was 18.2% (as compared with 6.3–6.7% of the trial population). This difference was largely due to a much higher mortality in patients with diagnosed infarcts (26.8% vs. 10.2% in the nifedipine group vs. 9.3% in the placebo group), perhaps a reflection of their older age and poorer cardiovascular state on admission to the coronary care units.

DISCUSSION

The TRENT trial provided no evidence to suggest that in patients with suspected acute myocardial infarction, the use of nifedipine capsules 10 mg 6-hourly would confer an early (28-day) survival benefit. There was also no evidence to suggest a beneficial or deleterious interaction with prior beta-blocker treatment, nor was any subgroup identified that appeared to benefit and was thus worthy of a further specific trial. At the inception of the study we were concerned about a potentially deleterious interaction between nifedipine and beta-blockers (22,23). We saw no such interaction; neither did we observe an acute withdrawal syndrome as described for verapamil and diltiazem (24).

The optimal dose of nifedipine is uncertain. We used a dose schedule and rate of administration that had been shown to result in "therapeutic" plasma concentrations of nifedipine and to be clinically safe, avoiding any large falls in blood pressure. We were perhaps unduly worried by the possibility of an unfavorable fall in systolic blood pressure or increase in heart rate that a larger dose might have caused. Gottlieb et al. gave placebo or oral nifedipine 120 mg daily for 10 days to 30 patients with acute myocardial infarction (25). Using two-dimensional echocardiography they found a significant reduction in what they termed early infarct expansion. They attributed this ostensibly advantageous effect of nifedipine to the modest reduction in systolic blood pressure (mean 9 mmHg). In our study, using a much smaller daily dose, we found a mean fall in systolic blood pressure of 5 mmHg.

Because the participating coronary care units keep a register of admitted patients, we were able to assess not only the proportion of patients who *might* have been eligible for nifedipine treatment (48%), but also the characteristics of ineligible patients and their early outcome. The ineligible group did not differ significantly from the eligible patients, but their mortality was substantially higher (18.2% vs. 6.3–6.7% overall). This emphasizes the importance of keeping a register during the assessment of new strategies or therapies, not only to appreciate differences between eligible and ineligible patients, but also to determine the overall likely benefit of introducing a new intervention.

During this trial several other clinical studies were reported suggesting that the optimism engendered by animal studies for using calcium channel–blocking drugs in myocardial ischemia was not supported by clinical experience. In a large Danish multicenter study of acute infarction, verapamil was given first intravenously, then by mouth in a daily dose of 120 mg for 6 months. Of 3498 patients randomized to verapamil or placebo, there was no difference either in the number who progressed to proved myocardial infarction or in the fatality rates at 6 months (26).

Sirnes et al. entered 227 patients with suspected acute myocardial infarction within 12 hours from onset of symptoms to treatment with nifedipine or placebo in a manner comparable to our study (27). They found no evidence that nifedipine reduced infarct size as determined by enzyme kinetics. They considered nifedipine to be safe in this setting, however, and its use was associated with a reduction in furosemide requirements during the first 4 days. This may reflect a beneficial effect of nifedipine on left ventricular function and is in keeping with invasive studies showing that nifedipine reduced myocardial oxygen requirements and enhanced cardiac and peripheral hemodynamics with subsequent improvement in cardiac output (28,29). In our study, however, we saw no difference in the incidence of or treatment for heart failure between the nifedipine- and placebo-treated patients.

Muller et al. screened almost 10,000 patients admitted to four coronary care units and ultimately randomized 243 patients with symptoms suggestive of myocardial ischemia of less than 6 hours' duration to either placebo or nifedipine 20 mg every 4 hours for 14 days (30). They found no evidence of a reduced progression from "threatened" to acute myocardial infarction, no difference in cardiac enzyme kinetics in those with proved myocardial infarction, and no difference in mortality at 6 months. They attributed this neutral effect of nifedipine to the delay between the onset of symptoms and the beginning of treatment (mean 4.6 hr). We did not randomize patients separately according to time from symptoms, but in our much larger study retrospective stratification by time did not disclose a potential advantage in those patients treated early. As with other "cardioprotective" strategies, however, the time interval between symptoms and treatment may be crucial (32,33).

In the few years following the publication of the TRENT trial, several other outcome studies of longer duration appeared using nifedipine (33,34), diltiazem (35), or verapamil (36,37) in similar clinical settings. Those with nifedipine confirmed the findings of the TRENT trial. The diltiazem trial gave an identical mortality rate after a mean follow-up of 25 months, and the verapamil trials (one early, one late administration) at least showed no harm.

The TRENT trial was an example of the interdependence of the clinical trialists, the study statistician, the independent safety-monitoring board, and the study sponsor. While no single study should be cited to recommend changes in or reservations about clinical practice, the conclusion of the TRENT trial was clear and unambiguous in its limited objective—acute short-term use of nifedipine capsules 40 mg/day confers no short-term benefit to patients with suspected acute myocardial infarction. No subsequent trial challenged this stance or provided the clinician with alternative circumstances in which acute treatment with any calcium channel–blocking drug would unequivocally benefit the patient admitted with suspected acute myocardial infarction.

ACKNOWLEDGMENTS

In this invited historical review of the TRENT study, the author wishes to thank his co-investigators, all of whom are noted in the original paper, and the *British Medical Journal* for permission to reproduce and quote liberally from the publication as referenced. The study was supported by an educational grant from Bayer Clinical Research.

REFERENCES

1. Jennings RB, Sommers HM, Smyth GA, Flack HA, Linn H. Myocardial necrosis induced by temporary occlusion of a coronary artery in the dog. Arch Pathol 1960; 70:68–78.
2. Neely JR, Rovetto MJ, Whitmer JT, Morgan HE. Effects of ischaemia on function and metabolism of the isolated working rat heart. Am J Physiol 1973; 225:651–658.
3. Reimer KA, Lowe JE, Rasmussen MM, Jennings RB. The wave-front phenomenon of ischaemic cell death. I. Myocardial infarct size vs. duration of coronary occlusion in dogs. Circulation 1977; 56:786–794.
4. Nayler WG, Fassold E, Yepez C. The pharmacological protection of mitochondrial function in hypoxic heart muscle: effect of verapamil, propranolol and methylprednisolone. Cardiovasc Res 1978; 12:151–161.
5. Bossert F, Vater W. Dihydropyridine, eine Gruppe stark wirksamer Koronartherapeutika. Naturwissenschaften 1971; 58(suppl II):578–579.
6. Rowland E, Evans T, Krikler D. Effect of nifedipine on atrioventricular conduction as compared with verapamil: intracardiac electrophysiological study. Br Heart J 1979; 42:124–127.
7. Henry PD, Schuchleib R, Davis J, Weiss ES, Sobel BE. Myocardial contracture and accumulation of mitochondrial calcium in ischemic rabbit heart. Am J Physiol 1977; 233:H677–684.
8. Henry PD, Schuchleib R, Borda LJ, Robers R, Williamson JR, Sobel BE. Effects of nifedipine on myocardial perfusion and ischemic injury in dogs. Circ Res 1978; 43:372–380.
9. Welman E, Carrol BJ, Scott Lawson J, Selwyn AP, Fox KM. Effects of nifedipine on creatinine kinase release during myocardial ischaemia in dogs. Eur J Cardiol 1978; 7:379–389.
10. Nayler WG, Ferrari R, Williams A. Protective effect of pretreatment with verapamil, nifedi-

pine, and propranolol on mitochondrial function in the ischemic and reperfused myocardium. Am J Cardiol 1980; 46:242–248.

11. Lichtlen P, Engel HJ, Amende I, Rafflenbeul W, Simon R. Mechanisms of various antianginal drugs. Relationships between regional flow behaviour and contractility. In: Jatene AD, Lichtlen PR, eds. Third International Adalat Symposium. Oxford: Excerpta Medica, 1976:14–29.

12. Serruys PW, Brower RW, Ten Katen HJ, Bom AH, Hugenholtz PG. Regional wall motion from radiopaque markers after intravenous and intracoronary injections of nifedipine. Circulation 1981; 63:584–589.

13. Roberts R, Jaffe AS, Henry PD, Sobel BE. Nifedipine and acute myocardial infarction. Herz 1981; 60:90–97.

14. Heupler FA, Proudfit WL. Nifedipine therapy for refractory coronary arterial spasm. Am J Cardiol 1979; 44:798–803.

15. Antmann E, Muller J, Goldberg S, MacAlpin R, Rubenfire M, Tabatznik B, Lian C-S, Heupler F, Achuff S, Reichek N, Geltman E, Kerin NZ, Neff RK, Braunwald E. Nifedipine therapy for coronary artery spasm. N Engl J Med 1980; 302:1269–1273.

16. Johnsson H. Effect of nifedipine (Adalat) on platelet function in vitro and in vivo. Thromb Res 1981; 21:523–528.

17. Oliva PB. Pathophysiology of acute myocardial infarction. Ann Intern Med 1981; 94:236–250.

18. Fujimoto T, Thomas P, Hamamoto H, McCullen AE, Mandel WJ. Effects of nifedipine on conduction delay during ventricular myocardial ischemia and reperfusion. Am Heart J 1981; 102:45–52.

19. Bayer Ltd. Planning meeting on acute myocardial infarction. Ressort medizin, Elberfeld, West Germany, 17 December 1981 (Available from datafile at Bayer).

20. Emanuelsson H, Hjalmarson A. Acute haemodynamic effects of nifedipine after myocardial infarction. In: Puech P, Krebs R, eds. Fourth International Adalat Symposium. Oxford: Excerpta Medica, 1980:212–219.

21. Wilcox RG, Hampton JR, Banks DC, Birkhead JS, Brooksby IAB, Burns-Cox CJ, Hayes MJ, Joy MD, Malcolm AD, Mather HG, Rowley JM. Trial of early nifedipine in acute myocardial infarction: the TRENT Study. Br Med J 1986; 293:1204–1208.

22. Robson RH, Vishwanath MC. Nifedipine and beta-blockade as a cause of cardiac failure. Br Med J 1982;284:104.

23. Opie LH. Calcium antagonists. Mechanisms, therapeutic indications and reservations: a review. Q J Med 1984; 209:1–16.

24. Subramanian VB, Bowles MJ, Khurmi NS, Davies AB, O'Hara MJ, Raftery EB. Calcium antagonist withdrawal syndrome: objective demonstration with frequency-modulated ambulatory monitoring. Br Med J 1983; 286:520–521.

25. Gottlieb SO, Gerstenblith G, Shapiro EP, Chandra N, Healy B, Weisfeldt ML, Weiss JL. Nifedipine reduced early infarct expansion: results of a double-blind randomised trial. Circulation 1985; 72(suppl III):274.

26. Danish Study Group on Verapamil in Myocardial Infarction. Verapamil in acute myocardial infarction. Eur Heart J 1984; 5:516–528.

27. Sirnes PA, Overskeid K, Pedersen TR, Bathen J, Drivenes A, Froland GS, Kjekshus JK, Landmark K, Rokseth R, Sirnes KE, Sunday A, Torjussen BR, Westland KM, Wik BA. Evolution of infarct size during the early use of nifedipine in patients with acute myocardial infarction: the Norwegian nifedipine multicenter trial. Circulation 1984; 70:638–644.

28. Ludbrook PA, Tiefenbrunn AJ, Reed FR, Sobel BE. Acute hemodynamic responses to sublingual nifedipine: dependence on left ventricular function. Circulation 1982; 65:489–498.

29. Hanrath P, Kremer P, Bleifeld W. Influence of nifedipine on left ventricular dysfunction at rest and during exercise. Eur Heart J 1982; 3:325–330.

30. Muller JE, Morrison J, Stone PH, Rude RE, Rosner B, Roberts R, Pearle DL, Turi ZG, Schneider JF, Serfas DH, Tate C, Scheiner E, Sobel BE, Hennekens CH, Braunwald E. Nifedipine

therapy for patients with threatened and acute myocardial infarction: a randomised, double-blind, placebo-controlled comparison. Circulation 1984; 69:740–747.

31. Miura M, Thomas R, Ganz W, Sokol T, Shell WE, Toshimitsu T, Kwan AC, Singh BN. The effect of delay in propranolol administration on reduction of myocardial infarct size after experimental coronary artery occlusion in dogs. Circulation 1979; 59:1148–1157.

32. Hillis LD, Fishbein MC, Braunwald E, Maroko PR. The influence of the time interval between occlusion and the administration of hyaluronidase on salvage of ischemic myocardium in dogs. Circ Res 1977; 41:26–31.

33. The SPRINT Study Group. Secondary prevention reinfarction Israeli nifedipine trial (SPRINT). A randomised intervention trial of nifedipine in patients with acute myocardial infarction. Eur Heart J 1988; 9:354–364.

34. The SPRINT Study Group. The secondary prevention reinfarction Israeli nifedipine trial (SPRINT) II: design, methods, results. Eur Heart J 1988; 9(suppl I):350.

35. The Multicenter Diltiazem Postinfarction Trial Research Group. The effect of diltiazem on mortality and reinfarction after myocardial infarction. N Engl J Med 1988; 319:385–392.

36. The Danish Group on Verapamil in Myocardial Infarction. Verapamil in acute myocardial infarction. Eur Heart J 1984; 5:516–528.

37. The Danish Group on Verapamil in Myocardial Infarction. Effect of verapamil on mortality and major events after myocardial infarction (the Danish Verapamil Infarction Trial-DAVIT II). Am J Cardiol 1990; 66:779–785.

Section J
Calcium Channel Blockers: Delayed Use

There are no data to support the routine use of diltiazem or nifedipine following myocardial infarction. The studies discussed in this section represent the most thorough and careful examination of this issue. As is highlighted in each chapter, it is extremely unlikely that a beneficial effect was missed as a matter of chance. Rather, it appears as though these drugs may pose a hazard to patients with impaired ventricles. Such patients are already at higher risk for adverse outcomes and benefit from beta-blockers, ACE inhibitors, and coronary revascularization. While MDPIT found that patients who had suffered minimal left ventricular impairment may derive some benefit from diltiazem, the effect was small and statistically uncertain, and these patients have an excellent prognosis without calcium channel blockers. Similarly, the favorable results with the use of verapamil in DAVIT-II were concentrated in patients without heart failure. As the author concludes, verapamil should be considered only as a second-line agent in select patients. In general, none of these drugs should be considered as part of the routine management of patients with myocardial infarction, and they should be avoided in patients with left ventricular dysfunction or heart failure.

29

MDPIT

ROBERT E. GOLDSTEIN

Multicenter Diltiazem Postinfarction Trial Research Group. The effect of diltiazem on mortality and reinfarction after myocardial infarction. N Engl J Med 1988;319:385–392.

CALCIUM CHANNEL BLOCKERS AFTER MYOCARDIAL INFARCTION

L-type calcium channel blockers have multiple effects on myocardium and blood vessels, some of which may be beneficial for patients after myocardial infarction. Blockers acting directly on the myocardium, such as diltiazem or verapamil, reduce the intensity and spontaneous frequency of contractile activation. In susceptible tissues, e.g., the atrioventricular and sinoatrial nodes, these calcium channel blockers also diminish the speed and reliability of electrical wavefront propagation. All L-type calcium channel blockers lower the intensity of calcium-calmodulin interaction, resulting in smooth muscle relaxation, dilation of many vascular beds, and consequent reduction in arterial blood pressures and impedance to ventricular emptying. Attenuation of heart rate, systemic arterial pressure, and myocardial contractility each tend to decrease myocardial metabolic activity and oxygen consumption. For a given level of external bodily work, the myocardial oxygen demands and, hence, requirements for coronary blood flow are less. This effect would render perfusion-limited myocardium less vulnerable to ischemia.

These actions likely explain the established beneficial effects of calcium channel blockers on symptoms of stable effort angina, when coronary perfusion increment is limited by proximal stenosis and ischemia is precipitated by rising myocardial oxygen demands. Calcium channel blockers might also provide some measure of protection for myocardium rendered ischemic by reduction in baseline coronary blood flow due to progression in arterial occlusion, although the experimental basis for such speculation is less certain. The adverse effects of excess calcium accumulation in ischemic myocytes are well known. These include faulty diastolic relaxation, abnormal electrical activation and recovery, and damage or even lethal destruction of metabolic machinery. If calcium channel blockers effectively attenuate excessive calcium levels within ischemic myocytes, calcium-related adverse effects may be averted in patients predisposed to myocardial ischemia. In addition, vasodilatory and possibly platelet inhibitory actions of calcium channel blockers may prevent the coronary spastic or thrombotic events underlying ischemic episodes in patients with atherosclerotic coronary disease.

Although the basis for postinfarction benefit from calcium channel blockers is well established, there are also theoretical reasons for concern about detrimental effects. Vasodilation could lead to reflex-mediated neuroendocrine activation, with important negative long-term consequences. A rise in catecholamines brought about through this mechanism could augment the frequency and lethal potential of arrhythmias in postinfarction patients. Increased catecholamine stimulation might also hasten the deterioration of surviving myocardium by enhancing myocardial metabolic requirements or by other adverse effects on myocyte survival known to occur with catecholamine-induced cardiomyopathy. Similar concerns are also introduced by other neuroendocrine agonists that might be increased with vasodilators, particularly angiotensin II, which may potentiate ischemia and unfavorable left ventricular remodeling. The negative inotropic and chronotropic influence of verapamil and diltiazem could be further sources of problems for vulnerable postinfarction hearts. The action of these drugs on injured tissues could precipitate significant bradycardia or congestive heart failure, especially in patients with extensive left ventricular damage. The capacity of other drug actions—vasodilator-related reduction in afterload or reflex-mediated adrenergic increase—to buffer the primary myocardial action of calcium channel blockers over long periods is open to question. Although a favorable balance of effects is likely in the majority of postinfarction patients, in whom global left ventricular performance is preserved, buffering of cardiodepressant influence may not occur in the minority with deteriorated cardiovascular function due to inadequate adrenergic responses or depleted myocardial reserve.

POSTINFARCTION CLINICAL TRIALS OF CALCIUM CHANNEL BLOCKERS

Despite the previously cited theoretical reasons for postinfarction benefit from calcium channel blockers, demonstration of such benefit in patient populations has been elusive. Thirteen published trials of nifedipine, a dihydropyridine calcium channel blocker, showed no improvement in postinfarction mortality or reinfarction rates or the incidence of recurrent ischemic symptoms. These data clearly show that consistent mortality benefit after myocardial infarction is not a generic property of calcium channel blockers. If the benefit suggested by theory is to be realized, potent adverse actions need to be reversed or neutralized.

Verapamil, a calcium channel–blocking phenylalkamine, has special features of potential value. Its attenuation of adrenergic influence on myocardium opposes an enhancement of adrenergic activity favored by its vasodilator action. There is evidence (1) that verapamil can reduce recurrent coronary events, but the overall benefit appears modest. Mortality reduction, if present, is only apparent in patients without overt left ventricular dysfunction.

Diltiazem, a benzothiazapine calcium channel blocker, shares verapamil's capacity to inhibit adrenergic responses and other receptor-mediated influences on sarcolemmal calcium flux. Like verapamil, diltiazem's specific properties might yield net benefit after infarction even though dihydropyridine calcium channel blockers failed to do so. This hypothesis was tested in the 576-patient Diltiazem Reinfarction Study, a randomized comparison of diltiazem, 90 mg every 6 hours, versus placebo beginning 1–3 days after non–Q-wave infarction (2). The primary endpoint was reinfarction (defined as MB-CK rising 50% above baseline) during a 14-day observation period. Postinfarction angina, revascularization, and death within 14 days were secondary endpoints. At 14 days, reinfarction rate was 12.9% in the placebo group and 6.3% in the diltiazem group, a difference that was statistically significant ($p = 0.029$) by the prespecified one-sided t-test but was not significant by conventional two-sided t-testing. Postinfarction angina was also reduced in patients taking diltiazem, but there was no difference in mortality (9 in the placebo group and 11 in the diltiazem group). The meaning of this short-term investigation is limited by the small number of study subjects and primary endpoints as well as the study's exclusive focus on the first 14 days after non–Q-wave infarction. Use of aspirin and heparin, which might well affect reinfarction rates, was not specified for the two treatment groups. Nevertheless, the Diltiazem Reinfarction Study attracted much interest: it was a first look at diltiazem's effect on recurrent coronary events after acute myocardial infarction, and it presented positive findings that aligned with theoretically grounded hopes for a beneficial effect. Questions regarding the long-term effects of diltiazem in a larger, more broadly defined postinfarction population remained unaddressed.

THE MULTICENTER DILTIAZEM POSTINFARCTION TRIAL

Overview

MDPIT was conducted to assess long-term treatment with diltiazem in the broad spectrum of postinfarction patients with no recognized contraindication to this drug. Treatment was begun as soon as practical to evaluate diltiazem's impact on recurrent coronary events, which often appear soon after infarction, and also to examine potential adverse actions during this critical early period. Treatment was maintained throughout the many months when risk of recurrent events remains elevated in the wake of antecedent infarction. The principal aim of MDPIT was to identify or exclude a significant overall beneficial effect of diltiazem on recurrent myocardial infarction or death. Nonfatal reinfarction and death were combined as a single MDPIT endpoint, termed "coronary events," to increase the study's statistical power but also to accommodate the reciprocity between the two outcomes: death excludes the possibility of coincident nonfatal reinfarction and the converse. Important secondary aims included identification of major patient subsets likely to have beneficial or detrimental consequences of diltiazem therapy. To implement these aims, 12 patient characteristics were identified based upon prior published experience. Each of these was analyzed as a covariate to ascertain whether the presence or absence of these characteristics conditioned patient response to diltiazem. This analytic plan was developed and finalized before opening the data base.

Study Procedures

MDPIT was a randomized, double-blind, placebo-controlled trial of diltiazem in 2466 postinfarction patients with follow-up for 12–52 (mean 25) months to a common termination date, June 30, 1987. A complete description of MDPIT policies and procedures has been published (3). In brief, patients from 38 collaborating hospitals were enrolled and assigned to start diltiazem, 240 mg/day, or placebo 3–15 days after a documented acute myocardial infarction. Enrolling hospitals were organized into 23 centers, each with a principal investigator and one or more specially trained study coordinators, who were responsible for recruitment and follow-up of patients.

Enrollment Criteria

Patients aged 25–75 admitted to the coronary care unit of an enrolling hospital were judged eligible for enrollment if acute myocardial infarction was suggested by clinical features and electrocardiograms and confirmed by one of the following enzymatic findings: MB isoenzyme more than 4% of total creatine kinase level; a qualitatively positive MB band; elevation of total lactic dehydrogenase with abnormal reversal of the ratio isoenzyme 1 : isoenzyme 2; or an otherwise-unexplained elevation of two or more serum enzyme levels—creatine kinase, aspartate transaminase, or lactic dehydrogenase—to at least twice the upper limit of normal while in the coronary care unit. A total of 13,618 patients met these criteria during the enrollment period.

Exclusion Criteria

Patients who exhibited any of the following were excluded from MDPIT enrollment: ongoing cardiogenic shock or symptomatic hypotension; pulmonary hypertension with right ventricular failure; second- or third-degree atrioventricular block; a resting heart rate below 50 beats/min or a history suggesting sinus node dysfunction; history of adverse reaction to diltiazem; no use of medically prescribed contraceptive measures (in women of childbearing potential); Wolff-Parkinson-White syndrome; other conditions likely to be treated with calcium channel blockers before the planned end of the trial; any comorbid condition associated with a diminished probability of survival during the trial period, e.g., cancer, uremia, or advanced liver disease; nonatherosclerotic precipitation of the qualifying myocardial infarction, e.g., surgery, shock, or trauma; strong likelihood of cardiac surgery in the near future; or various administrative problems, e.g., residence outside the study area or unwillingness to provide written informed consent. Of the 13,618 satisfying enrollment criteria, 11,152 were excluded for one or more of these reasons. The most common reasons for exclusion were need for open-label treatment with a calcium channel blocker, as determined by the managing physician (3506 or 31%) and patient or physician unwillingness to participate (3115 or 28%). Only 518 patients (4.6%) were excluded due to bradycardia, atrioventricular block, or cardiogenic shock. A total of 2466 patients (18% of the potentially eligible population) were enrolled in MDPIT.

Treatment Assignment and Follow-Up

After providing written consent for MDPIT and while still in the hospital, patients were randomly selected to receive either diltiazem or placebo in a double-blind manner, 3–15 days following the onset of the index myocardial infarction. To assure balance between treatment categories within each enrolling hospital, MDPIT employed a permuted block randomization procedure. Within each hospital the randomization also included dichotomous blocking on number of days from myocardial infarction to treatment assignment (≥ 5 days vs. <5 days), New York Heart Association functional category 1 month prior to admission (Class I vs. Class II–IV), and current use of beta-blockers (yes or no). The standard diltiazem dose was 60 mg four times daily, but the center physician could reduce the dose to as little as twice daily if this was judged necessary. Patients were followed with periodic clinic visits throughout the trial. At each visit, study medication was counted to monitor compliance. A final clinic evaluation was performed soon after the study's completion. In the course of the study, patients were followed for 12–52 months, and mean duration of follow-up was 25 months.

Information Acquisition and Management

MDPIT participation did not require any specific testing except enzyme measurements to satisfy entry criteria. However, several commonly acquired test results of particular interest were collected to satisfy secondary study objectives. At pretreatment baseline, radionuclide ejection fraction was determined in 42%, 24-hour Holter-monitor recording obtained in 68%, and at least one chest roentgenogram taken in the coronary care unit prior to starting trial medication in 97%. Holter recordings and qualifying electrocardiograms were analyzed at MDPIT centers, the latter employing then-new Manhattan criteria (4) for acute infarction type (Q-wave or non–Q-wave) and acute and old infarct location (anterior-lateral or inferior-posterior). Based upon official hospital reports, study coordinators identified a roentgenogram for each patient showing the most severe pulmonary congestion and coded this on a four-level scale. These data were later dichotomized (no congestion vs. any congestion) for analytic purposes. Study coordinators recorded all data on study forms in accordance with a written MDPIT manual of operations. These forms were transmitted to the Coordination and Data Center and entered into a unified data bank. Accuracy of data entry was monitored by Center personnel, who also performed frequent site visits to enrolling hospitals. Fatal outcomes were reviewed by a four-member mortality subcommittee, who collected detailed information on the causes and circumstances of each death, along with appropriate documentation. The subcommittee categorized each death as due to either cardiac or noncardiac causes and classified the mechanism of cardiac deaths according to Hinkle-Thaler criteria (5). Nonfatal reinfarctions were examined by a three-member subcommittee, which evaluated pertinent information obtained by study coordinators from patients hospitalized again with a suspected acute coronary event on or before June 30, 1987. The criteria for diagnosis of recurrent nonfatal infarction were the same as those used for the index infarction. Both committees applied written criteria in the absence of any information regarding patient treatment assignment.

Statistical Methods

MDPIT was originally planned to have sufficient power to discriminate a 15% coronary event rate in diltiazem-treated patients from a 20% event rate in placebo-treated patients (i.e., identify a 25% diltiazem-associated reduction) with 80% probability. The putative statistical test would accept as significant a one-sided $p \leq 0.05$. The initial design was based on the rationale that adverse outcome was unlikely and would be sought by the independent safety-monitoring subcommittee. This plan implied that 2000 patients would be needed, allowing for noncompliance, patient cross-overs, and beta-blocker effects. When blinded early MDPIT data revealed an unexpectedly low total mortality, targeted recruitment was increased to 2500 patients. Concomitantly, the primary endpoint was shifted from total mortality to coronary event rate (cardiac death or nonfatal reinfarction, whichever came first) and the plans for test of significance based on two-sided $p \leq 0.05$.

In all statistical analyses, differences in duration of follow-up were accommodated by special life-table methods (6). The primary data analysis employed a Cox proportional-hazards regression model (computer program BMDP-2L), with enrolling hospitals entered as stratification factors and treatment and the three blocking variables (beta-blocker use, functional category, and time to enrollment) included in the model as main effects. Findings are expressed as hazard ratios, i.e., risk of endpoint event per unit time among diltia-zem-assigned patients relative to the risk among those randomly assigned to placebo. In all cases, analyses were based upon treatment groups defined at study enrollment (intention-to-treat principle).

One-year event rates in each treatment group were determined for each patient subset defined by 12 prespecified, clinically meaningful, dichotomized covariates using the method of Kaplan and Meier (6). Interactions between these covariates and treatment assignment were assessed by the Cox model. Interaction was deemed to occur if the hazard ratio for diltiazem versus placebo among patients in one category of a dichotomized covariate was significantly different from the same hazard ratio for patients in the other category of this covariate.

Study results were originally reported based upon an analytic data base released November 1, 1987. However, none of the reported results was significantly altered by the minor corrections introduced into later analytic data bases for MDPIT.

MDPIT: THE PRIMARY ANALYSIS

MDPIT Population Characteristics

Patients in MDPIT were fairly young (mean age 58) with about 12% aged 70–75 and none older. They were largely males (80%) presenting with a first infarction (79%) and no prior symptoms (82%). Many smoked cigarettes (50%) and received treatment for hypertension (38%), but few had diabetes mellitus (9%). A small group had earlier bypass surgery (6%). About 9% (118 patients assigned to diltiazem and 99 patients assigned to placebo) received streptokinase, then the only available thrombolytic agent, at the time of the index infarction; none were treated with immediate coronary angioplasty. Approximately 70% of patients had Q-wave index infarctions, and 25% had non–Q-wave infarctions. The index infarction was significant in some, producing clinically assessed creatine kinase values above 1000 units in 49%, radiographic evidence of pulmonary congestion in 20%, and in-hospital radionuclide ejection fraction (when assessed) below 0.40 in 30%. About 7% (87 patients assigned to diltiazem and 86 patients assigned to placebo) had new-onset atrial fibrillation or atrial flutter. Frequency of beta-blocker use remained the same (about 54%) at study enrollment and during follow-up. When assessed after 12 months of follow-up, aspirin use was only 34% and other anticoagulant therapy rare (4%). Use of digoxin (14%) or antiarrhythmic agents (10%), evaluated at this same time, was uncommon. Less than 8% took angiotensin-converting enzyme (ACE) inhibitors. Throughout the course of MDPIT, few patients had coronary bypass surgery (13%) and virtually none (37 patients or 1.5%) had coronary angioplasty. As might be expected in this large, randomized trial, each of the features just cited was represented equally in the group assigned to diltiazem treatment ($n = 1232$ patients) and the group assigned to placebo ($n = 1234$ patients).

Despite the fact that MDPIT enrollees represent a modest fraction of eligible patients, the demographic features of the study population were characteristic of most coronary care unit patients. Important subgroups—women and minorities—were not fully represented in MDPIT, reflecting the features of eligible patients at the 38 enrolling hospitals. There were no patients in MDPIT over age 75. The applicability of MDPIT conclusions to these subgroups is limited and somewhat uncertain. The use of beta-blockers in half the MDPIT population was helpful in that it allowed a meaningful analysis of interaction between beta-blockers and diltiazem, a possibility further strengthened by a randomization procedure that stratified on receipt of beta-blocker therapy. Infrequent use of other drugs now commonly employed in postinfarction patients—aspirin and ACE inhibitors, in particular—and the rarity of coronary angioplasty make MDPIT patients appear undertreated by contemporary standards. Paucity of anti-ischemic interventions and incompleteness of anti-ischemic drug therapy might accentuate anti-ischemic benefits of diltiazem and thereby improve MDPIT outcomes relative to what might be observed with current background therapy. At the same time, sparse use of ACE inhibitors might cause MDPIT to exaggerate adverse actions of diltiazem in patients with impaired left ventricular function. In fact, ACE inhibitors have not been shown to enhance the margin of safety for diltiazem in postinfarction patients. A suggestion that this may be the case must be regarded as speculative.

Use of Trial Medication

By 6 months after study enrollment, approximately 74% of MDPIT patients in either treatment group were still taking blinded trial medication. This figure fell to 63% for either group at 2 years. It should be noted that these are complete figures: only 3.2% of the study population was lost to follow-up. Unless patients had clear contraindications, study medication was restarted as quickly as possible after discontinuation. At least half of the prescribed dose of study medication was taken by more than 95% of patients receiving trial medication at 6 months and 2 years. These figures indicate a high level of acceptability for diltiazem in postinfarction patients and a willingness of participating patients and physicians to follow the study protocol. While not ideal, these adherence data indicate that MDPIT represented a solid, if not perfect, test of the study's primary hypothesis regarding the impact of diltiazem on recurrent coronary events in postinfarction patients.

The most frequent cause for discontinuation of study drug was occurrence of an adverse experience, which appeared in 357 patients taking placebo and 406 patients taking diltiazem. Most adverse experiences, including new congestive heart failure, were noted with equal frequency in patients taking diltiazem and patients taking placebo. Unstable angina, reported as an adverse event, also appeared with equal frequency in the two treatment groups, suggesting no prophylaxis against unstable angina with diltiazem. There was a modest excess of atrioventricular block, atrial bradycardia, and hypotension in the diltiazem group, as might be expected from the known pharmacodynamic actions of this calcium channel blocker. However, the effects were not inordinate or suggestive of a particular problem in postinfarction patients. There was no indication that adverse experiences limited drug utilization in the entire group taking diltiazem. If present, such limitation would have compromised the drug's potential value for prevention of undesired outcomes in unselected postinfarction populations.

Primary Trial Endpoints

As its primary hypothesis, MDPIT postulated that patients assigned to diltiazem treatment would have fewer recurrent cardiac events (defined as cardiac death or nonfatal reinfarction, whichever came first) when compared with patients assigned to placebo. The data showed that event rates during the course of the trial were similar in the two groups

Table 1 Endpoint Events in the MDPIT Trial

	Diltiazem group (*n* = 1232)	Placebo group (*n* = 1234)	Hazard ratio (D/P)[b]	95% Confidence limits
First recurrent cardiac event[a]				
Cardiac death	103	110		
Nonfatal reinfarction	99	116		
Total events	202	226	0.90	0.74, 1.08
Mortality during trial				
Cardiac death	127	124		
Noncardiac death	38	43		
Unclassified death	1	0		
Total mortality	166	167	1.02	0.82, 1.27

[a] Either cardiac death or nonfatal reinfarction, whichever occurred first after enrollment (subsequent events not included).

[b] Hazard ratio is the risk of events in the diltiazem-treated group relative to the risk in the placebo-treated group. A ratio of less than 1.0 indicates diltiazem-associated benefit and a ratio of more than 1.0 indicates diltiazem-associated detriment.

(Table 1; Fig. 1). The hazard ratio, 0.90 (risk for diltiazem group/risk for placebo group), was bracketed by 95% confidence intervals (CI) that included 1.0, the number expected if diltiazem treatment had no net effect on rate of recurrent cardiac events. Thus, MDPIT showed either a mild and equivocal overall benefit associated with diltiazem treatment or no overall benefit. MDPIT was designed to detect a 25% decrease in event rates, a benefit deemed biologically and clinically significant. The trial satisfied the expectations of its designers regarding total event rates, patient characteristics, drug utilization, data collection, and other aspects of trial design and conduct. MDPIT should have shown an overall diltiazem-associated benefit of importance to patient management, if such existed. The fact that MDPIT did not demonstrate such a benefit represents a significant and enduring negative statement regarding the value of diltiazem as a treatment for all patients with no contraindication in an effort to suppress recurrent cardiac events.

This conclusion is reinforced by MDPIT mortality data. Cardiac and noncardiac death rates, considered separately, as well as total mortality in the diltiazem-treated group and the placebo-treated group were each virtually identical throughout the study period (Table 1; Fig. 1). The Cox proportional-hazards ratio was close to unity (Table 1). Whatever benefit is suggested by the data on first recurrent events did not translate into a long-term diltiazem-associated decrement in mortality for all persons assigned to take diltiazem.

MDPIT Interaction Analysis

MDPIT was designed to evaluate the influence of diltiazem treatment on postinfarction prognosis, regardless of specific patient attributes. It was assumed that the potentially beneficial pharmacodynamic actions described above would reduce recurrent cardiac events in a broad variety of postinfarction patients. Nevertheless, even before trial results became available, MDPIT planners recognized that diltiazem might have unique and important effects in different patient subsets. In statistical terms, this would be evident as an interaction between hazard ratio—the prime measure of benefit—and the presence or

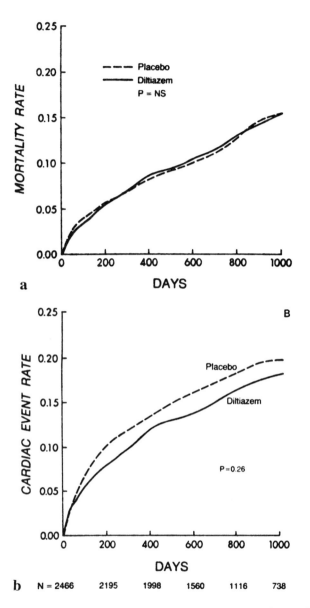

Figure 1   Kaplan-Meier plots show cumulative rate of total (all-cause) mortality (a) and first recurrent cardiac events (cardiac death or nonfatal reinfarction) (b) for patients assigned to placebo (dashed) or diltiazem (solid). Numbers below each panel indicate patients at risk for any given length of follow-up. NS implies no statistical significance between the two treatment groups. (From Ref. 3.)

absence of a critical clinical variable. Twelve clinical and laboratory variables were selected for inclusion in an interaction analysis of the hazard ratio for recurrent cardiac events based upon the ability of each variable to alter the pathophysiologic environment that shaped the risk of recurrent cardiac events (Table 2). For example, a drug affecting propensity to lethal arrhythmia might have measurable influence on cardiac events in the

Table 2 Baseline Variables Evaluated in the
MDPIT Interaction Analysis

Functional class (New York Heart Association)
Use of beta-blockers
Days after index infarction at randomization
Age
Gender
Pulmonary congestion
Radionuclide ejection fraction
Acute anterior-lateral Q-wave
Acute inferior-posterior Q-wave
Acute non–Q-wave infarction
Frequent ventricular ectopics on Holter
  monitoring
Blood urea nitrogen > 35 mg/dl

subgroup with pretreatment evidence of arrhythmia yet exert no such influence either in the subgroup lacking that evidence or in the study population taken as a whole.

Among the 12 preselected clinical variables, only one had significant interaction ($p < 0.01$) with treatment assignment: the presence or absence of pulmonary congestion on chest roentgenogram. The two-sided p-value for this interaction, 0.0042, indicated persistent high-level significance for the association between diltiazem and pulmonary congestion even after correction for the number of covariates tested using the method of Bonferroni. Kaplan-Meier plots demonstrated a ''bidirectional'' interaction: hazard ratio was greater, 1.41 (95% CI 1.01–1.96%), showing *more recurrent cardiac events on diltiazem* in the 490 patients (20% of the total MDPIT population) *with pulmonary congestion*; and this hazard ratio was reduced, 0.77 (95% CI 0.61–0.98%), showing *fewer recurrent cardiac events on diltiazem* in the 1909 patients *without pulmonary congestion* (Fig. 2). A similar bidirectional interaction was observed between diltiazem and pulmonary congestion when cardiac mortality was used as the endpoint (two-sided p-value = 0.0013). These data suggested that the presence of left ventricular dysfunction, which was the preponderant cause of pulmonary congestion soon after acute myocardial infarction, led to detrimental responses to diltiazem and a consequent increase in cardiac events. These detrimental responses appeared to overwhelm and reverse favorable actions of diltiazem suggested by the reduced hazard ratio in patients without pulmonary congestion.

This interpretation was supported by data derived from radionuclide ejection fraction, an independently assessed variable reflecting impairment of left ventricular function. Although the interaction was of only borderline significance (two-sided p-value = 0.05), the hazard ratio for recurrent cardiac events was 1.31 (95% CI 0.87–1.98%) in 321 patients with ejection fraction below 0.40 and 0.73 (95% CI 0.48–1.11%) in 726 patients with ejection fraction at or above 0.40. These results favor the concept that patients with impaired global left ventricular performance are likely to have more cardiac events when given diltiazem, while this is not true for the majority of patients, who do not have such impairment. Qualitatively similar results were obtained from the borderline-significant (two-sided p-value = 0.04) interaction with acute anterior-lateral Q-wave infarction, which is commonly associated with more extensive left ventricular damage. In addition, a more detailed analysis of findings disclosed an ordinal relationship between hazard ratio

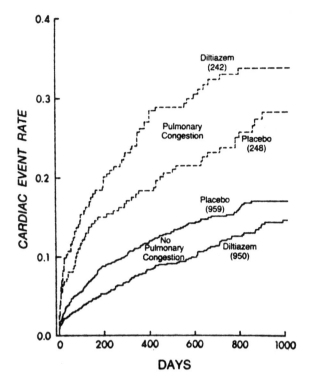

Figure 2 Kaplan-Meier plots show cumulative rates of first recurrent cardiac events (cardiac death or nonfatal reinfarction) according to treatment assignment and the presence or absence of radiographic pulmonary congestion soon after index infarction. Upper two plots demonstrate worsened outcomes for congested patients given diltiazem (higher of pair) compared with congested patients given placebo (lower of pair). Lower two plots demonstrate improved outcomes for noncongested patients given diltiazem (lower of pair) compared with noncongested patients given placebo (higher of pair). The values in parentheses are numbers of patients in each subset. Two-sided *p*-value = 0.0042 for this "bidirectional interaction" between pulmonary congestion at outset and assigned treatment group. (From Ref. 3.)

for recurrent cardiac events and either severity of pulmonary congestion or decrement of radionuclide ejection fraction—the more impressive the evidence of depressed left ventricular function, the higher the risk of recurrent cardiac events in patients receiving diltiazem treatment. Hazard ratio was as high as 2.5 in the small subgroup with ejection fraction below 0.20.

Further review failed to reveal another covariate equivalent to pulmonary congestion in its interaction with diltiazem, showing the absence of a surrogate for pulmonary congestion among the remaining 11 covariates. In addition, use of beta-blockers did not have a measurable influence on the interaction between pulmonary congestion and diltiazem.

The absence of interaction with diltiazem was, itself, notable for several variables, particularly in light of the suggestion of substantial, directionally opposite actions of diltiazem in postinfarction patient subsets, as shown by the data just reviewed. Beta-blockers appeared neither to potentiate a diltiazem-related detriment nor conceal a diltiazem-related benefit on recurrent cardiac event rate. Similarly, age and gender (within limits imposed by MDPIT demography), functional status, and the presence of frequent ventricular ectopy all had neither positive nor negative influence on recurrent cardiac event rates.

MDPIT: SECONDARY ANALYSES

Numerous secondary analyses have been conducted employing some portion of the MDPIT data base. The most salient of the analyses focusing on use of diltiazem in post-infarction patients will be summarized and discussed in the ensuing sections.

Diltiazem and Increased Cardiac Mortality

The primary analysis of MDPIT showed that long-term diltiazem treatment after acute myocardial infarction had no overall effect on either recurrent cardiac events or total mortality. A significant ($p < 0.01$) bidirectional interaction was noted with a single covariate, pulmonary congestion on chest roentgenogram: those with pulmonary congestion had increased recurrent cardiac events, while those without this abnormality had fewer such events. A secondary analysis, examining covariate interactions with cardiac death as the endpoint, found that three variables reflecting left ventricular dysfunction, singly and in combination, predicted greater cardiac mortality in patients assigned to diltiazem treatment (7). Conversely, those without these indicators of left ventricular dysfunction had reduced cardiac mortality when assigned to diltiazem. Hazard ratios (risk of cardiac death per unit time for those assigned to diltiazem/risk per unit time for those assigned to placebo) were 1.85 (95% CI 1.24–2.75%) in patients with pulmonary congestion ($p = 0.0013$) and 1.52 (95% CI 1.03–2.23%) in patients with acute anterior-lateral Q-wave infarction ($p = 0.0092$). A similar trend was observed when radionuclide ejection fraction was <0.40; these patients had a hazard ratio of 1.67 (95% CI 1.04–2.71%; $p = 0.096$). Patients with two of the three indicators of left ventricular dysfunction had markedly increased cardiac mortality when assigned to diltiazem (hazard ratios 1.70–3.80). Patients without these indicators had consistently reduced cardiac mortality when assigned to diltiazem (hazard ratios 0.55–0.98). The finding that each of three different indicators of left ventricular dysfunction was independently and collectively associated with greater mortality in diltiazem-treated patients provided important support for the concept that diltiazem has preponderant adverse actions in patients with impaired global left ventricular function after acute myocardial infarction, leading to an increase in lethal outcomes. The results of this secondary analysis strengthen the recommendation that diltiazem not be prescribed to patients with advanced left ventricular dysfunction.

Diltiazem and Increased Late-Onset Congestive Heart Failure

As noted previously, new or worsened congestive heart failure (CHF) developing during long-term follow-up (subsequently termed late CHF) was observed with equal frequency in diltiazem-treated and placebo-treated patients. The bidirectional interaction of either recurrent cardiac events or cardiac mortality with indicators of left ventricular impairment suggested that more detailed analysis might be fruitful. The same pattern observed for cardiac events and cardiac mortality was also noted for late CHF: assignment to diltiazem treatment appeared to increase the occurrence of late CHF in patient groups with pulmonary congestion, acute anterior-lateral Q-wave infarction ($p = 0.041$), or radionuclide ejection fraction < 0.40 ($p = 0.004$) (8). By contrast, diltiazem treatment had no effect on occurrence of late CHF in any of the corresponding groups with normal baseline variables. Examination of the interaction of pulmonary congestion, ejection fraction, and late CHF revealed that diltiazem-associated enhancement of late CHF was only seen in patients with ejection fraction < 0.40. Patients who had pulmonary congestion but also an ejection fraction of at least 0.40 had more late CHF than those without pulmonary congestion but there was no further increase in late CHF when assigned to diltiazem therapy. These findings and the preeminent statistical association between reduced ejection fraction and late CHF suggested that left ventricular systolic dysfunction played a particularly important role in diltiazem-related increment of late CHF.

The relation between baseline ejection fraction and late CHF was further examined by comparing placebo- and diltiazem-assigned subgroups within each of four ejection fraction categories (Fig. 3). Late CHF occurred infrequently when baseline ejection fraction was normal (at least 0.45), and its occurrence was not influenced by diltiazem therapy. Progressively more severe impairment of baseline ejection fraction was associated with progressively greater occurrence of late CHF. Although this rise was observed for both placebo- and diltiazem-assigned subgroups, patients receiving diltiazem had a more rapid increase. Hence, the more severe the reduction in baseline ejection fraction, the greater the increment in diltiazem-related occurrence of late CHF relative to placebo.

The association between diltiazem treatment and increased occurrence of late CHF in patients with reduced ejection fraction was also apparent on life-table analysis of the 623 individuals with ejection fraction < 0.40. Throughout the period of observation, the curve for the 297 patients receiving diltiazem showed consistently greater occurrence of late CHF than the curve for the 326 patients receiving placebo ($p = 0.0017$ by Tarone-Ware test). Similar results were obtained when the endpoint was either cardiac death or late CHF ($p = 0.028$ by Tarone-Ware test). An analysis of covariates among patients with ejection fraction < 0.40 demonstrated a balance of nonpharmacologic risk factors for poor left ventricular performance in groups assigned to diltiazem and placebo.

To explore possible influences of beta-blockers, the occurrence of late CHF was compared in placebo- and diltiazem-treated patients grouped by beta-blocker use and ejection fraction. Diltiazem treatment was associated with increased late CHF in both patient groups having ejection fraction < 0.40—those not using beta-blockers as well as those using beta-blockers; the link to diltiazem assignment was strongest in patients with ejection fraction < 0.40 and *not* using beta-blockers. Although outcomes may be influenced by the nonrandom use of beta-blockers, this analysis found no tendency for treatment with beta-blockers to enhance diltiazem-associated rise in late CHF, even among those with reduced ejection fraction.

This secondary analysis demonstrated that patients with impaired left ventricular function following an acute myocardial infarction are more likely to develop new or worsened congestive heart failure when treated with diltiazem. Risk enhancement appeared particularly evident for those with reduced ejection fraction. Taken together, the MDPIT findings indicate that diltiazem use in the presence of postinfarction left ventricular impairment poses several important long-term risks, including increased recurrent cardiac events, cardiac death, and overt congestive heart failure. The actions of diltiazem that enhance problems in the subgroup with left ventricular dysfunction are unclear. The fact that heart failure is most closely linked to reduced ejection fraction while recurrent cardiac events are more firmly tied to pulmonary congestion may reflect a diversity of diltiazem-

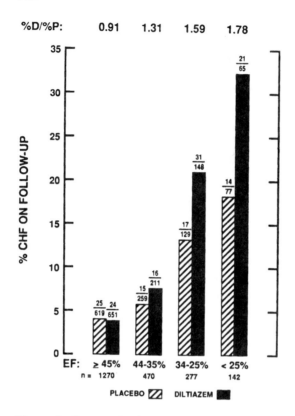

Figure 3 Percent of patients with new or worsened congestive heart failure (CHF) during long-term follow-up is shown for four groups defined solely by baseline ejection fraction (EF): ≥0.45, 0.44–0.35, 0.34–0.25, and <0.25. Paired bars show occurrence of late CHF in placebo- and diltiazem-treated subsets. Number of patients with CHF (numerator) and total number in each subset (denominator) are displayed above each bar. At top of figure, value for each group shows percentage of patients with late CHF among those given diltiazem (D) divided by percent of patients with last CHF among those given placebo (P). Data are shown for 2159 patients with baseline measurement of EF, including all measurements made before (1066) or 1–6 days after (1093) initiation of study drug [the primary MDPIT analysis (3) did not include EF measurements made after drug was started]. Diltiazem-associated increase in late CHF is progressively larger as baseline EF is reduced. (From Ref. 8.)

associated detrimental actions in these patients. Nevertheless, the most certain implication is a reinforcement of concern regarding prescription of diltiazem to postinfarction patients with impaired left ventricular function: the adverse consequences now seem multiple and demonstrable utilizing a variety of independent measures.

Diltiazem and Reduced Nonfatal Reinfarction After Non–Q-Infarction

Both primary and secondary MDPIT analyses identified postinfarction subgroups that appeared to have an improved prognosis when treated with diltiazem. Patients lacking pulmonary congestion, anterior-lateral Q-wave infarction, or reduced radionuclide ejection fraction seemed to experience fewer recurrent cardiac events or cardiac deaths (there was no diltiazem-associated change in their already-low occurrence of late CHF). This effect was generally modest and of borderline statistical significance or without significance. Particular attention has focused on use of diltiazem in non–Q-wave infarction, a commonly occurring event whose clinical management remains an enduring source of debate. The Diltiazem Reinfarction Study, conducted exclusively in patients with antecedent non–Q-wave infarction, suggested short-term decrease in recurrent nonfatal infarction with diltiazem treatment. A secondary analysis of MDPIT patients with non–Q-wave index infarction revealed that, within the first 6 months of observation, 17 of 279 patients assigned to placebo had recurrent nonfatal infarction while only 2 of 235 patients assigned to diltiazem had such an event ($p < 0.001$) (9). The recurrent infarcts tended to occur in the same myocardial region as the index infarct, suggesting that diltiazem retarded recurrence or progression of the coronary lesion responsible for the index infarct. After the first 6 months an equal number of nonfatal infarctions (13–14) occurred in both placebo and diltiazem treatment groups. Mortality rates were modest and not different between groups. Although their data were suggestive, the authors indicated that the character of the analysis implied a need for a prospective trial before therapeutic recommendations could be made. Another subgroup analysis examined recurrent cardiac events and cardiac mortality in several subgroups defined by electrocardiographic classification of the index infarction (10). Hazard ratios suggested that diltiazem treatment led to equally favorable outcomes in patients entering with a first non–Q-wave or with a first inferior Q-wave infarction. These two infarct categories were also very likely to have patients with preserved left ventricular function, leading the authors to propose that postinfarction left ventricular function rather than electrocardiographic features of the index infarction was the key feature in determining the impact of diltiazem on long-term prognosis. This latter study was severely limited by the small size of its subgroups and the consequent lack of statistical significance in the numerical assessments underpinning its assertions.

APPLICATIONS OF MDPIT TO CURRENT THERAPEUTIC PRACTICE

Study Strengths

Because of the effort and expense involved, it is unlikely that a trial similar to MDPIT will be conducted in the foreseeable future, even though certain questions persist regarding the use of diltiazem in postinfarction patients. Fortunately, MDPIT strengths are sufficient to assure that its data provide a solid basis for most, if not all, contemporary therapeutic decisions regarding diltiazem after acute myocardial infarction. MDPIT was a moderately large, very carefully conducted, randomized, blinded, placebo-controlled trial in a representative population. Drug dosage, patient compliance, data management, and statistical analysis were each more than adequate to provide a reliable, enduring assessment of the key issues for clinical therapeutics. The principal question MDPIT asked was: Does diltiazem treatment improve prognosis with respect to recurrent cardiac events (i.e., cardiac death or nonfatal myocardial infarction, whichever comes first) when given generally to patients with acute myocardial infarction? This was (and is) a particularly important issue, because the answer to this same question for a closely related drug group, the beta-blockers, is yes, especially for patients with mild or moderate pulmonary congestion or other evidence of left ventricular impairment. MDPIT showed that the answer for diltiazem is no. Despite its favorable side-effect profile, diltiazem should not be substituted for beta-blockers (or any other drug) as a means of improving postinfarction prophylaxis.

What about diltiazem use in patient subgroups? MDPIT is particularly strong in that it evaluated a *prespecified* group of key covariates using state-of-the-art (even a decade later) statistical methods to define the context in which diltiazem is likely to be beneficial or detrimental. MDPIT results are clearest for the "downside" of diltiazem: this drug is likely to increase recurrent cardiac events, cardiac death, and the late development or worsening of congestive heart failure in patients with early postinfarction left ventricular dysfunction. Such patients should not receive long-term treatment with diltiazem except in very unusual extenuating circumstances, e.g., no acceptable alternative for controlling ischemic problems. These conclusions, similar to those derived for verapamil in secondary analysis of the second Danish Verapamil Trial, suggest a common pattern of postinfarction response for calcium channel blockers that have strong influence on myocardial as well as vascular function.

The "upside" of diltiazem was suggested by MDPIT data but not clearly proven. Long-term diltiazem administration may reduce recurrent cardiac events, particularly recurrent nonfatal myocardial infarction, in postinfarction patients with unimpaired left ventricular function, as defined by absence of pulmonary congestion in the coronary care unit, normal radionuclide ejection fraction, or the absence of an anterior-lateral Q-wave index infarction. This reduction in recurrent infarction seems particularly evident in the first few months after the index infarction. Because the magnitude of the apparent beneficial effect on recurrent cardiac events was modest, MDPIT lacked power to define a precise context for benefit. Importantly, a claim of benefit should be substantiated by a prospective trial and not rely exclusively on subset analysis from a single trial.

Study Limitations

Although MDPIT offered an impressive array of facts pointing to an adverse effect of diltiazem on the impaired left ventricle, there is no clear explanation of the mechanism(s) involved or a possible remedy for this problem. Of course, MDPIT was not designed to provide such information. Nevertheless, lack of pathophysiologic grounding weakens the credibility of MDPIT interpretations and introduces uncertainty as to exactly how MDPIT should be applied in patient management. One potential explanation—the possibility that left ventricular impairment led to slowed metabolism of diltiazem and accumulation of toxic plasma levels of diltiazem—has been examined and discarded (11). Other possible explanations involve the impact of diltiazem's negative inotropic influence on the impaired left ventricle. Such explanations are difficult and convoluted, in part because negatively inotropic beta-blockers improve prognosis in postinfarction patients with left ventricular dysfunction and many positively inotropic drugs such as the phosphodiesterase inhibitors worsen prognosis in this patient group. Diltiazem may enhance some as-yet poorly understood aspect of progressive left ventricular deterioration after myocardial infarction, such as sustained or accelerating rise in myocyte apoptosis. If this is the case, there is no known way to antagonize such an effect in the clinical setting. One cannot assume that drugs, e.g., ACE inhibitors, that might superficially undo an adverse component of diltiazem will, in fact, mitigate diltiazem's tendency to worsen prognosis in postinfarction patients with left ventricular impairment.

With the passage of time, MDPIT results lose some of their clinical relevance because of changes in the therapeutic milieu. It is true that widespread use of mechanical intervention with angioplasty and stent placement plus the frequent administration of thrombolytic agents, ACE inhibitors, and an array of anticoagulant drugs have brought about major shifts in the pathophysiologic and pharmacologic environment in which diltiazem is used. In addition, more subtle changes such as quicker transportation of patients, more rapid progression from coronary care unit to step-down unit to home, and less frequent use of previously common postinfarction treatments such as antiarrhythmic agents and digoxin may change conditions appreciably. It is hard to assess such imponderables. However, there may also be more frequent appearance of circumstances relating directly to MDPIT conclusions. With the survival of older and sicker hearts, the problem of medically managing the patient with an impaired left ventricle after acute myocardial infarction may become increasingly commonplace. In addition, with increasing efforts to salvage jeopardized myocardium and recurrent problems with coronary restenosis after mechanical intervention, the need for an array of relatively nontoxic anti-ischemic agents may increase. MDPIT implies that diltiazem should be avoided in postinfarction patients with left ventricular impairment yet may play a benign and even beneficial role in postinfarction patients without such impairment. The clinical trial data substantiating this information may well remain highly relevant even if viewed across an increasing span of years and through an increasingly complex array of change in treatment algorithms.

ACKNOWLEDGMENT

The author is grateful to Mary Brown, R.N., M.S., for her assistance in reviewing and newly analyzing elements of the MDPIT data base.

REFERENCES

1. Danish Study Group on Verapamil in Myocardial Infarction. Effect of verapamil on mortality and major events after acute myocardial infarction. The Danish Verapamil Infarction Trial II (DAVIT-II). Am J Cardiol 1990; 66:779–785.
2. Gibson RS, Boden WE, Theroux P, Strauss HD, Pratt CM, Gheorghiade M, Capone RJ, Crawford MH, Schlant RC, Kleiger RE, Young PM, Schechtman K, Perryman MB, Roberts R, Diltiazem Reinfarction Study Group. Diltiazem and reinfarction in patients with non-Q-wave myocardial infarction. Results of a double-blind, randomized, multicenter trial. N Engl J Med 1986; 315:423–429.
3. Multicenter Diltiazem Postinfarction Trial Research Group. The effect of diltiazem on mortality and reinfarction after myocardial infarction. N Engl J Med 1988; 319:385–392.
4. Greenberg H, Gillespie J, Dwyer EM Jr, Multicenter Post-Infarction Research Group. A new electrocardiographic classification for post-myocardial infarction clinical trials. Am J Cardiol 1987; 59:1057–1063.
5. Hinkle LE Jr, Thaler HT. Clinical classification of cardiac deaths. Circulation 1982; 65:457–464.
6. Kaplan EL, Meier P. Nonparametric estimation for incomplete observations. J Am Stat Assoc 1958; 53:457–481.
7. Moss AJ, Oakes D, Benhorin J, Carleen E, Multicenter Diltiazem Post-Infarction Research Group. The interaction between diltiazem and left ventricular function after myocardial infarction. Circulation 1989; 80(suppl IV):IV-102–106.
8. Goldstein RE, Boccuzzi SJ, Cruess D, Nattel S, Adverse Experience Committee, Multicenter

Diltiazem Postinfarction Research Group. Diltiazem increases late-onset congestive heart failure in postinfarction patients with early reduction in ejection fraction. Circulation 1991; 83: 52–60.

9. Wong SC, Greenberg H, Hagar WD, Dwyer EM Jr. Effects of diltiazem on recurrent myocardial infarction in patients with non-Q wave myocardial infarction. J Am Coll Cardiol 1992; 19:1421–1425.

10. Boden WE, Krone RJ, Kleiger RE, Oakes D, Greenberg H, Dwyer EJ Jr, Miller P, Abrams J, Coromilas J, Goldstein R, Moss AJ, Multicenter Diltiazem Post-Infarction Trial Research Group. Electrocardiographic subset analysis of diltiazem administration on long-term outcome after acute myocardial infarction. Am J Cardiol 1991; 67:335–342.

11. Nattel S, Talajic M, Goldstein RE, McCans J, Multicenter Diltiazem Postinfarction Trial Research Group. Determinants and significance of diltiazem plasma concentrations after acute myocardial infarction. Am J Cardiol 1990; 66:1422–1428.

30

SPRINT

SOLOMON BEHAR

The Israeli SPRINT Study Group. Secondary prevention of reinfarction in Israeli nifedipine trial (SPRINT). A randomized intervention trial of nifedipine in patients with acute myocardial infarction. Eur Heart J 1988; 9:354–364.

The management and prognosis of patients with acute myocardial infarction (AMI) changed dramatically with the advent of reperfusion therapy in the late 1980s (1–3). In a recent national survey performed in 1996 in all operating coronary care units (CCUs) in Israel, the 30-day mortality of patients after AMI was 9% compared to 19% in a similar study carried out in 1981–83. Mortality after discharge also declined, but less significantly during the same period (3,4). Thus, mortality after AMI remains substantial. Risk stratification and secondary prevention after AMI continue to be of great importance and concern.

INTRODUCTION

The development of calcium channel blockers (CCBs) in the 1970s and their rapidly increasing clinical use opened up new vistas in the management of patients with acute and chronic coronary syndromes. This group of drugs (in particular nifedipine) was aimed at the prevention and alleviation of coronary spasm, as well as improving coronary blood flow and reducing left ventricular workload (5–7). In animal experiments, nifedipine was shown to protect the myocardium from ischemia and reperfusion injury (8,9). During the same period several publications emphasized the role of coronary spasm in the pathogenesis of myocardial infarction and its major complications, including extension of the infarction area, impairment of left ventricular function, and possibly provocation of life-threatening arrhythmias (10–12).

By virtue of their properties on coronary spasm and smooth arterial muscle, CCBs seemed the ideal "cardioprotective" drugs for treatment and prevention for patients with coronary artery disease. This was the background of the Secondary Prevention Reinfarction Israeli Nifedipine Trial (SPRINT) conducted in 14 cardiac departments throughout Israel in 1981–83. A detailed description of the rationale, methods, and results of the SPRINT study was published in 1988 (13). In this chapter the findings and results of the SPRINT study, the clinical implications of CCB use after AMI, and the long-term prognosis of SPRINT patients will be reviewed.

PATIENT POPULATION AND METHODS

From July 1981 to August 1983, 5839 consecutive MI patients were hospitalized in 14 out of 21 operating CCUs in Israel (SPRINT Registry). Clinical characteristics and data on hospital course were recorded for all of them. Of the total 4808 hospital survivors, 2276 patients (47%) who fulfilled the inclusion criteria and signed informed consent were randomized to short-acting nifedipine or placebo (SPRINT study). The aim of this randomized double-blind, placebo-controlled study was to assess whether routine use of short-acting nifedipine, on top of conventional therapy, reduces cardiac events following AMI.

The study was supervised by a Steering Committee including the directors of all participating CCUs and members of the Coordinating Center. An independent International Review Committee was responsible for the ethical and safety issues of the study. Regular reports from all participating centers and the Coordinating Center were submitted for assessment and analysis to a Data Monitoring and Quality Control Committee. Critical events including all deaths were reviewed and ascertained by an independent Critical Events Committee. The operational aspects of the study were organized and supervised by the Coordinating Center of the study located at the Heart Institute of the Sheba Medical Center, Tel Hashomer.

Eligibility and Exclusion Criteria

Patients of both genders, aged 30–74, were eligible for the study and recruited 7–21 days after a recent myocardial infarction. The diagnostic criteria of the infarction included (1) typical symptoms lasting for at least 1 hour, (2) unequivocal ECG changes based on Minnesota Code interpretation, and (3) elevated serum enzyme levels (at least 1.5 times the upper normal limit of CK-MB or two of the enzymes CK, SGOT, and LDH).

Patients with a typical history and high enzyme levels were included with Q- and non–Q-wave infarction on the ECG. For those lacking a typical history or high enzyme levels, major new and sequential Q/QS changes on the ECGs were required for inclusion. Patients were asked to sign informed consent prior to randomization, and the study was approved by the Helsinki Committees of each participating hospital.

The main reasons for excluding patients from the study were (1) lack of diagnostic or age-eligible criteria for inclusion; (2) need for treatment with a calcium channel blocker; and (3) inability of the patients to cooperate or refusal to sign informed consent.

Stratification and Follow-Up

Short-acting nifedipine (10 mg 3 times/day) or placebo was randomly assigned in a double-blind manner in each of the 14 participating centers within the following three strata:

(1) males with a first infarction; (2) males with a prior history of infarction; and (3) females admitted with an AMI.

Study medication was initiated between days 7 and 21 from hospital admission, when the patient's status was stabilized. Prior to randomization, 24-hour Holter monitoring was performed on 80% of patients. (This procedure was not an obligatory condition for inclusion in the study.) Follow-up visits were scheduled 1, 2, 4, 6, and 12 months after randomization. Medication was distributed monthly. Laboratory study data were collected at the first and last follow-up visit. Exercise tests were done 3 months after hospital discharge in patients able to exercise.

The study was ended in December 1983 upon recommendation of the International Review Committee. Therefore, 1-year follow-up was completed by 83% of the study group. The mean follow-up period for all patients of the study was 10 months. Patients were assessed 1 month from study medication discontinuation for possible withdrawal effects.

Endpoints, Adverse Events, and Compliance

The primary endpoints of the study (critical events) were total mortality and nonfatal recurrent AMI. The secondary endpoints included stroke, angina, heart failure, and need for cardiac surgery. Adverse events (side effects) were reported periodically to the Coordinating Center.

Compliance was assessed by two methods: capsule count at each medication visit and urine fluorescence test. All study capsules contained 5 mg of rifboflavin, which is excreted in the urine and easily detected under ultraviolet light. Urine tests were performed in three patient samples during the study. By the pill count method, 83% of patients demonstrated a high degree of adherence (over 90% of presented medication), and 95% of urine tests performed produced positive results for compliance.

Statistical Analysis

The sample size of 2000 patients was calculated based on the following assumptions: (1) a 10% mortality rate in the year following AMI was anticipated; (2) 25% mortality reduction (subject to a type I error of $\alpha = 0.05$ and a power of 80%) was hypothesized in the active treatment group in comparison to the group assigned to placebo. Eventually 2276 patients were enrolled.

Analyses were done on an intent-to-treat basis. Comparison of rates and means between the two groups was performed using the χ^2 and two-sided t tests. The relative odds of mortality were estimated for clinical variables associated with prognosis. Life-table rates were calculated using the Kaplan-Meier method, log-rank analysis, and the Cox proportional hazard analysis.

RESULTS

The two treatment groups were well matched. Characteristics, clinical data, hospital course, and therapy on discharge were virtually identical in both the nifedipine and placebo groups (Table 1). The rate of study medication withdrawal not due to primary endpoints was similar in both the nifedipine (14.9%) and placebo (14.5%) groups. The major causes

Table 1 Comparison of Medication Groups: Baseline Characteristics

	Placebo	Nifedipine
No. of patients	1078	1068
Age (mean ± SD), years	58 ± 9	58 ± 9
Men (%)	75	75
History (%)		
Previous myocardial infarction	18	17
Angina	46	44
Hypertension	43	43
Diabetes	21	22
Smoking	48	45
Admission data		
Systolic blood pressure (mmHg)	137	137
Diastolic blood pressure (mmHg)	86	86
Heart rate (beats/min)	77	77
Congestive heart failure (%)	21	21
Concomitant therapy on discharge (%)		
Beta blockers	19	18
Digitalis	10	9
Diuretics	24	26
Antiarrhythmic drugs	30	27
Vasodilators	40	41
Anticoagulants	1	1
Antiplatelets	19	17

Table 2 Mortality and Nonfatal Myocardial Infarction by Medication

	Placebo ($n = 1146$)		Nifedipine ($n = 1130$)	
	No.	%	No.	%
Total mortality	65	5.7	65	5.8
All cardiac deaths	53	4.6	53	4.7
Noncardiac death	12	1.0	12	1.1
Nonfatal recurrent infarction	55	4.8	50	1.1
Primary endpoints	120	10.5	115	10.2

Table 3 Mortality: Distribution by Cause and Study Medication

Cause	Total	Placebo	Nifedipine
All definite or presumed coronary mortality	106	53	53
Acute MI	41	19	22
Sudden death without evidence of acute MI	43	23	20
Pump failure—no MI	22	11	11
Cerebrovascular accident	2	1	1
Malignancy, trauma, or other causes	22	11	11
Total	130	65	65

MI = Myocardial infarction.

Table 4 Primary Endpoints by Strata and Medication

	Stratum I: Men with a first MI		Stratum II: Men with recurrent MI		Stratum III: Women	
	Placebo ($n = 817$)	Nifedipine ($n = 807$)	Placebo ($n = 158$)	Nifedipine ($n = 153$)	Placebo ($n = 171$)	Nifedipine ($n = 170$)
Cardiac death	28	35	15	8	10	10
	3.4%	4.3%	9.5%	5.2%	5.9%	5.9%
Noncardiac death	3	9	4	2	5	1
	0.4%	1.1%	2.5%	1.3%	2.9%	0.8%
Total mortality	31	44	19	10	15	11
	3.8%	5.5%	12.0%	6.5%	8.8%	6.5%
Nonfatal recurrent MI	42	32	8	8	5	10
	5.1%	4.0%	5.1%	5.2%	2.9%	5.2%
All critical events	73	76	21	18	20	21
	8.9%	9.4%	13.8%	11.8%	11.7%	12.4%

of trial deviation included need for calcium antagonist therapy (5.3% in the placebo group vs. 4.9% in those randomized to nifedipine) and side effects (3.9% in the nifedipine and 1.9% among the placebo group of patients). The most frequent side effects were gastrointestinal disturbances (1.7% in the nifedipine group and 0.7% in the placebo group) and dizziness or fatigue (1.8 and 1.1%, respectively). Ankle edema was experienced by 19 patients in the nifedipine group and by a single patient in the placebo group.

Primary Endpoints

Primary endpoints (death and nonfatal AMI) occurred in 115 and 120 patients in the nifedipine and the placebo groups, respectively. The crude mortality rate was 5.8% in the nifedipine group versus 5.7% among placebo counterparts. Rates of nonfatal recurrent AMI were 4.4 and 4.8%, respectively. Eighty-two percent of deaths were from cardiac origin in both treatment groups (Table 2). The causes of death are presented in Table 3. Death from coronary causes, cerebrovascular accident, malignancy, trauma, and others were identical in both treatment groups.

Table 4 presents the primary endpoint rates by strata of randomization. The event rates were higher among men with recurrent MI (stratum II) and women (stratum III), without a significant difference between the study medication groups in each stratum.

Figure 1 depicts the incidence of primary endpoints as a function of time elapsed since hospital discharge. Events were most frequent in the first 3 months after discharge.

Secondary Endpoints (Additional Monitored Events)

The rate of rehospitalization and the frequency of angina, congestive heart failure, stroke, and need for coronary artery bypass grafting (CABG) according to treatment are presented in Table 5. Rehospitalizations for any reason, as well as the occurrence of stroke or the

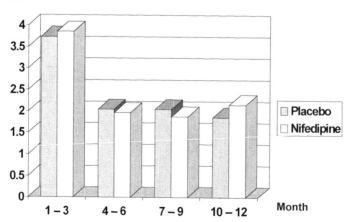

Figure 1   Time trend of primary endpoints in the first year after hospital discharge in the SPRINT study.

Table 5 Additional Monitored Events by Medication

	Placebo		Nifedipine	
	No.	%	No.	%
Reason for hospitalization:				
Cardiac	264	24	265	25
Noncardiac	62	6	43	4
Anginal syndrome[a]	392	36	394	37
Congestive heart failure[a]	61	6	58	5
Stroke	6	<1	6	<1
Coronary artery bypass grafting	10	1	9	<1

[a] At the last follow-up visit.

need for CABG, were similar in both nifedipine and placebo groups. Only 1% of patients underwent CABG in the year following the AMI.

Table 6 presents the mortality rates and odds ratios of independent risk predictors in the SPRINT study population. Increased age, history of MI, previous angina, hypertension, anterior MI site, and treatment with digitalis or diuretics were independent predictors of high mortality risk in the SPRINT study.

Long-Term Follow-Up

Patients of the SPRINT study were followed for mortality 13–15 years (mean 14 years) from inclusion. Five-year mortality rates were quite similar in both the nifedipine (18.5%)

Table 6 Mortality Rates and Odds of Risk Indicators

	Present		Absent			
Risk indicator	n	Rate (%)	n	Rate (%)	Relative odds	95% CI
Elevated serum (LDH ≥4 times upper normal limit)	303	10.6	1973	5.0	2.3	(1.5–3.4)
Age (≥60 yr)	1032	8.1	1244	3.7	2.3	(1.6–3.3)
Treated hypertension	545	7.9	1731	5.0	1.6	(1.1–2.4)
Previous MI	373	10.5	1903	4.8	2.3	(1.6–3.4)
Anterior MI	1216	7.4	1060	3.8	2.0	(1.4–3.0)
Digitalis	245	16.3	2031	4.4	4.2	(2.9–6.1)
Diuretics	566	11.3	1710	3.9	3.2	(2.3–4.5)
	None		Mild		Moderate or severe	
Anginal syndrome in month preceding MI	1406	4.3	557	7.4	164	13.4

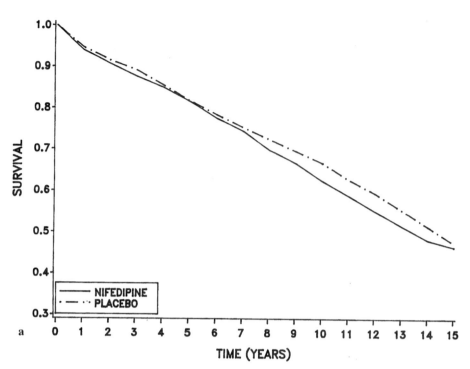

Figure 2 Long-term survival curves of the SPRINT study population according to the study medication.

and placebo groups (18.6%, respectively). Figure 2 presents the long-term survival curves according to treatment at randomization. However, no information is available on the treatment of these patients after the end of the study.

COMMENTS

Several clinical trials using CCBs for a variety of coronary syndromes, including AMI, were performed during the 1980s. Most of these studies did not show any beneficial effect of routine CCB treatment in patients with unstable angina or after AMI (14–18). One of the first secondary prevention trials with CCBs in the postacute myocardial infarction phase was the SPRINT study using short-acting nifedipine. The study, conducted among 2276 post-MI patients during 1981–1983 showed no differences between the study and control groups regarding primary and secondary endpoints. Since the completion of the SPRINT study several clinical or experimental studies have also reported no beneficial effects of nifedipine on infarct size, clinical course, or mortality (19–21) between the active and placebo treatment groups.

Two reasons have been suggested to explain the results of the SPRINT study: the nifedipine dosage used (30 mg/daily) was too low, and the time of initiation of therapy (7–21 days after the MI) was too late. In addition, patients in strata II (men with recurrent infarction) on placebo exhibited a twofold increased death rate compared to patients on nifedipine. We therefore conducted a second modified study (SPRINT-2) during 1985–86 in which a higher dosage of short-acting nifedipine was administered to 1358 high-risk patients with suspected AMI as soon as possible upon hospital admission but in no case later than 48 hours from pain onset (22). The dosage of nifedipine was titrated up to 60 mg/daily. This study was prematurely stopped by the advisory board because the 6-day mortality was higher among the nifedipine-treated group (7.8%) than the controls (5.5%). We therefore concluded from both SPRINT-1 and SPRINT-2 studies that nifedipine as a prophylactic treatment in patients after AMI was ineffective. Moreover, early routine administration of short-acting nifedipine after acute AMI may be hazardous and seems to be contraindicated (SPRINT-2).

The negative effect of short-acting nifedipine in patients after AMI was likely due to its vasodilatory properties, which can cause reduction of coronary perfusion, thereby compromising blood flow to the jeopardized myocardium. Furthermore, by elevating heart rate, nifedipine increases the myocardial oxygen demand, thus contributing to the possibility of damage to the compromised infarcted myocardium. At present, other formulations of nifedipine are in use for treatment of hypertension and angina. Prospective studies are also being conducted with long-acting nifedipine for efficacy and safety purposes (23,24).

The low rate of cardiac intervention (1%) after AMI was an acceptable policy in our country in the early 1980s. Thus the data of the present study reflect the natural history of patients after AMI unexposed to interventional procedures. The low rate of cardiac events and heart failure that developed during the study period denotes a low-risk group of patients recruited to SPRINT. Moreover, despite the relatively low rate of aspirin (<10%) and β-blocker use (20%) in the year following the acute event, the 1-year mortality and reinfarction rates were relatively low, significantly less than the anticipated critical events rates in both the nifedipine and the placebo group. Nevertheless, the low cardiac event rate did not alter the study conclusions as the difference in primary endpoints between the two treatment groups was insignificant.

The probability of missing a positive effect of nifedipine because the calculated power was based on a different assumption from the findings achieved seems very low. Assuming no difference at all between the two groups, i.e., assuming that the true rate in the nifedipine group is also 5.7%, the probability of achieving a rate of 5.8% or less (the *p*-value) is 0.56, which is quite high. Thus, it is very likely that there really is no difference between the two groups.

In summary, on the basis of the two SPRINT (and other) studies, short-acting nifedipine should not be recommended for prophylactic use in patients during or after AMI.

REFERENCES

1. GISSI Study Group. Effectiveness of intravenous thrombolytic treatment in acute myocardial infarction. Gruppo Italiano per lo Studio della Streptochinasi nell'Infarto Miocardico (GISSI). Lancet 1986; 1:397–402.
2. ISIS-2 (Second International Study of Infarct Survival) Collaborative Group. Randomized trial of intravenous streptokinase, oral aspirin, both, or neither, among 17,187 cases of suspected acute myocardial infarction. ISIS-2. Lancet 1988; 2:349–360.
3. Behar S, Barbash GI, Copel L, Gottlieb S, Goldbourt U, for the SPRINT Study Group and

the Israeli Thrombolytic Survey Group. Improved survival of hospitalized patients with acute myocardial infarction from 1981–1983 to 1992 in Israel.

4. de Vreede JJM, Gorgels APM, Verstraaten GMP, Vermeer F, Dassen WRM, Wellens HJJ. Did prognosis after acute myocardial infarction change during the past 30 years? A meta-analysis. J Am Coll Cardiol 1991; 18:698–706.

5. Theroux P, Waters DD, Lateur JG. Clinical manifestations and pathophysiology of myocardial ischaemia with special reference to coronary artery spasm and the role of slow channel calcium blockers. Prog Cardiovasc Dis 1982; 25:157–168.

6. Stone PH, Antman EM, Muller JE, Braunwald E. Calcium channel blocking agents in the treatment of cardiovascular disorders. II. Haemodynamic effects and clinical applications. Ann Intern Med 1980; 93:886–904.

7. Moskovitz RM, Piccini PA, Nacarelli GV, Zelis R. Nifedipine therapy for stable angina pectoris: preliminary results of effects on angina frequency and treadmill exercise response. Am J Cardiol 1979; 44:811–816.

8. Nayler WG. The role of calcium in the ischaemic myocardium. Am J Pathol 1981; 102:262–270.

9. Henry PD, Shuchleib R, Burda LJ, Roberts R, Williamson JR, Sobel BE. Effects of nifedipine on myocardial perfusion and ischemic injury in dogs. Circ Res 1978; 43:372–380.

10. Conti CRM, Pepine CJ, Curry JC. Coronary artery spasm: an important mechanism in the pathophysiology of ischaemic heart disease. Curr Prob Cardiol 1979; 4:9–70.

11. Olivia PB, Breckenridge JC. Arteriographic evidence of coronary arterial spasm in acute myocardial infarction. Circulation 1977; 56:366–374.

12. Cipriano PR, Koch FH, Rosenthal SJ, Baim DS, Ginsburg R, Schroeder JS. Myocardial infarction in patients with coronary artery spasm demonstrated by angiography. Am Heart J 1983; 105:542–547.

13. The Israeli SPRINT Study Group. Secondary prevention reinfarction Israeli nifedipine trial (SPRINT). A randomized intervention trial of nifedipine in patients with acute myocardial infarction. Eur Heart J 1988; 9:354–364.

14. The Danish Study Group on Verapamil in Myocardial Infarction. Effect of verapamil on mortality and major events after acute myocardial infarction (The Danish Verapamil Infarction Trial II—DAVIT II). Am J Cardiol 1990; 66:779–785.

15. Gibson RS, Boden WE, Theroux P, Strauss HD, Pratt CM, Gheorghiade M, Capone RJ, Crawford MH, Schlant RC, Kleiger RE, Young PM, Schechtman K, Perryman MB, Roberts R. Diltiazem and reinfarction in patients with non-Q-wave myocardial infarction. N Engl J Med 1986; 315:423–429.

16. The Multicenter Diltiazem Postinfarction Trial Research Group. The effect of diltiazem on mortality and reinfarction after myocardial infarction. N Engl J Med 1988; 319:385–392.

17. Yusuf S, Furberg CD. Effects of calcium channel blockers on survival after myocardial infarction. Cardiovasc Drugs Ther 1987; 1:343–344.

18. Yusuf S, Held P, Furberg C. Update of effects of calcium antagonists in myocardial infarction or angina in light of the second Danish Verapamil Infarction Trial (DAVIT-II) and other recent studies (editorial). Am J Cardiol 1990; 66:779–785.

19. Sirnes PA, Overskeid K, Pedersen TR, Bathen J, Drivenes A, Froland GS, Kjekshus JK, Landmark K, Rokseth R, Sirnes KE, Sundoy A, Torjussen BR, Westlund KM, Wik BA. Evolution of infarct size during the early use of nifedipine in patients with acute myocardial infarction: The Norwegian Nifedipine Multicenter Trial. Circulation 1984; 70:638–644.

20. Muller JE, Morrison J, Stone PH, Rude RE, Rosner B, Roberts R, Pearle DL, Turi ZG, Schneider JF, Serfas DH, Tate C, Scheiner E, Sobel BE, Hennekens CH, Braunwald E. Nifedipine therapy for patients with threatened and acute myocardial infarction: a randomized, double-blind, placebo-controlled comparison. Circulation 1984; 69:740–747.

21. Wilcox RG, Hampton JR, Banks DC, Birkhead JS, Brooksby IAB, Burns-Cox CJ, Hayes MJ,

Joy MD, Malcolm AD, Mather HG, Rowley JM. Trial of early nifedipine in acute myocardial infarction. The TRENT Study. Br Med J 1986; 293:1204–1208.

22. Goldbourt U, Behar S, Reicher-Reiss H, Zion M, Mandelzweig L, Kaplinsky E, for the SPRINT Study Group. Early administration of nifedipine in suspected acute myocardial infarction. The Secondary Prevention Reinfarction Israel Nifedipine Trial 2 Study. Arch Intern Med 1993; 153:345–353.

23. Hansson L, Zanchetti A. The Hypertensive Optimal Treatment (HOT) Study—patient characteristics: randomization, risk profiles, and early blood pressure results. Blood Press 1994; 3: 322–327.

24. Lubsen J, Poole-Wilson PA. ACTION: a 30,000 patient-years double-blind, placebo-controlled trial of nifedipine GITS in stable angina. ACTION research group. Br J Clin Prac Suppl 1997; 88:23–26.

31

DAVIT-II

JØRGEN FISCHER HANSEN

The Danish Study Group on Verapamil in Myocardial Infarction. The effect of verapamil on mortality and major events after acute myocardial infarction (the Danish verapamil infarction trial II–DAVIT-II). Am J Cardiol 1990;66:779–785.

INTRODUCTION

Verapamil is used in the treatment of ischemic heart disease due to its antihypertensive (1,2), antiarrhythmic (3–5), and anti-ischemic (6–8) effects. Verapamil inhibits liberation of norepinephrine from the myocardium during ischemia (9) and reduces plasma norepinephrine at rest in patients with ischemic heart disease. It also inhibits platelet aggregation (10). Apart from these effects, three observations related to verapamil might be of importance in long-term therapy to prevent cardiovascular events. First, verapamil has no adverse effect on blood lipids and may even increase high-density lipoprotein (HDL) cholesterol (11). Second, left ventricular hypertrophy and ventricular ectopic activity are reduced by verapamil (12); left ventricular mass is an independent and important risk factor for ischemic heart disease (13) and is associated by increased prevalence of ventricular ectopic activity (14,15). Third, verapamil has a pronounced antiatherosclerotic effect in animal models (16).

In the Danish Verapamil Infarction Trial (DAVIT)-I, a post hoc analysis found that the late mortality and reinfarction rate was significantly reduced in patients treated with verapamil (17). This was the main reason for the decision to perform DAVIT-II. The purpose of DAVIT-II was to examine if treatment with verapamil from the second week after an acute myocardial infarction and the following 12–18 months might prevent death and first reinfarction (18–21).

METHODS

Design

The study was a multicenter, double-blind, randomized, placebo-controlled trial of verapamil. All patients below 76 years of age with diagnosis of acute myocardial infarction were eligible. Consecutive patients were recruited from 20 coronary care units from day 7 to day 15 after admission. Treatment was planned for 18 months with the last included patients treated for at least 12 months. When a patient was included in the study, the following information was recorded: history before admission, treatment and complications in the hospital, type and location of the infarction, and status at the initiation of study treatment (heart rate, systemic blood pressure, chest x-ray, electrocardiogram, and ongoing therapy). The clinical status was evaluated again at discharge from the hospital and after 1 and 3 months, and then every third month up to 18 months after randomization. Patients who stopped treatment prematurely were seen after 18 months or at the end of the study period. If a reinfarction was diagnosed in the observation period, trial medication was continued unless contraindications developed.

Exclusion Criteria

These included uncontrolled congestive heart failure, defined as signs of heart failure despite treatment with digoxin and diuretics corresponding to 160 mg of furosemide per day; sinoatrial block within the last 3 days before randomization; heart rate below 45 beats per minute; second or third degree atrioventricular block present after day 3 or PR > 0.28 seconds; systolic blood pressure < 90 mmHg at repeated measurements the last 3 days before randomization; indication for treatment with beta-blocking agents or calcium antagonists (e.g., due to angina pectoris, arterial hypertension, or arrhythmias); valvular or congenital heart disease; peri- or postoperative myocardial infarction; other serious diseases such as pulmonary diseases, cancer, uremia, or psychiatric diseases; living outside the catchment area of the hospital; refusal to participate; earlier inclusion in the study; and other reasons at the discretion of the responsible physician.

Endpoints

Endpoints were death and major event (first reinfarction or death) in the study period. Results were evaluated on an intention-to-treat basis.

Study Medication

Verapamil 120 mg 3 times daily or matching placebo were given. Medication was reduced to 1 or 2 tablets per day in case of supposed adverse drug reactions. Patients were block randomized at each center. Study medication was terminated for the following reasons: patient unwillingness to continue participation, second and third degree atrioventricular block, severe intractable congestive heart failure, angina pectoris or arrhythmias necessitating treatment with beta-blockers or calcium antagonists, or inability to continue treatment because of other severe disease.

Diagnosis of Acute Myocardial Infarction

Patients were considered for inclusion if they had chest discomfort and electrocardiographic changes compatible with Q-wave or non–Q-wave infarction or developed bundle branch block and an increase of at least 25% above the upper normal limit in the serum enzymes routinely used in the coronary care units, such as creatine phosphokinase MB, lactate dehydrogenase 1, or aspartate aminotransferase.

Study Period

Enrollment of patients began in February 1985. Inclusion of patients terminated January 1988, and the last included patients stopped treatment in January 1989.

RESULTS

Description of Study Groups

During the study period 11,447 patients were admitted to hospitals a total of 13,771 times; 6966 patients did not have acute myocardial infarction. Of 4481 patients with infarction, 490 died before randomization; 2216 patients were excluded. Major reasons for exclusion were heart failure (13%), sinoatrial or second or third atrioventricular block (11%), treatment with beta-blockers (18%) or calcium antagonists (19%), other severe disabling diseases (12%), patients not wishing to participate (16%), and patients living outside the catchment area (8%).

Of 1775 patients randomized, 878 patients received treatment with verapamil and 897 placebo treatment. The two groups showed no statistically significant differences in any of the recorded baseline parameters (Table 1). Patients were randomized 9 ± 2.7 days (mean $\pm$ 1 SD) after admission. For men the mean age was 59 ± 9 years, and for women it was 62 ± 9 years ($p < 0.01$). At randomization mean heart rate was 75 ± 11 beats/min, systolic blood pressure 120 ± 16 mmHg, and diastolic blood pressure 76 ± 10 mmHg for both groups.

Duration of Follow-Up

The mean observation time from start of treatment to follow-up via the Danish Central Person Register, which includes information about all deaths, was 492 days in the placebo group and 504 days in the verapamil group. This corresponds to the follow-up time for death. The mean observation time from start of treatment to death or until the patient was last seen alive in the study was 467 days in the placebo group and 478 days in the verapamil group. This corresponds to the follow-up time for reinfarction. The mean time from start of treatment to permanent treatment stop was 383 days in the placebo group and 361 days in the verapamil group.

Endpoints

Death

One hundred and nineteen deaths were recorded in the placebo group and 95 in the verapamil group. This corresponds to 18-month event rates of 13.8% in patients randomized to placebo and 11.1% in patients randomized to verapamil ($p = 0.11$, hazard ratio (HR) 0.80, 95% CI 0.61–1.05%). Of the total number of deaths, 72 in the placebo group and 48 in the verapamil group took place with the patients still on trial medication ($p = 0.07$, HR 0.72, CI 0.50–1.04%). Of the remaining deaths in the placebo and verapamil groups, 8 and 7 occurred in the first week, respectively, and 39 and 40 more than 1 week after premature permanent treatment stop.

Table 1 Baseline Characteristics of 1775 Randomized Patients

	Placebo (%) (n = 897)	Verapamil (%) (n = 878)
Sex		
Male	79.6	80.0
Female	20.4	20.0
Age		
<65 years	64.3	67.1
≥65 years	35.7	32.9
History		
Previous myocardial infarction	17.9	15.7
Hypertension	13.9	14.2
Angina pectoris	26.1	27.0
Diabetes	5.6	5.5
Cigarette smoking	61.5	63.4
Complications in coronary care unit		
Shock	3.9	3.6
Heart failure	36.0	33.1
Cardiac arrest	4.5	4.0
Status at randomization		
CT index < 50	53.8	52.3
CT index ≥ 50	30.4	32.3
CT index not measurable	15.7	15.4
Congestion, chest x-ray	6.5	5.7
Atrial fibrillation	3.0	2.6
Bundle branch block	7.2	6.7
Diuretics	41.8	39.7
Digoxin	12.4	11.2
Antiarrhythmics	2.3	2.5
Nitrates other than sublingual	8.4	7.9
AMI type and location		
Anterolateral Q-wave	36.7	36.2
Inferoposterior Q-wave	35.1	37.0
Non–Q-wave	17.9	16.1
Other	10.3	10.7

AMI = Acute myocardial infarction; CT = cardiothoracic.

Major Event

A first reinfarction or death from any cause was recorded in 180 patients in the placebo group and 146 patients in the verapamil group. Eighteen-month event rates were 21.6% and 18.0%, respectively (p = 0.03, HR 0.80, CI 0.64–0.99%) (Fig. 1). A major event was recorded in 139 (18.6%) placebo and 96 (14.6%) verapamil-treated patients still on trial medication (p = 0.01, HR 0.73, CI 0.57–0.95%).

The diagnosis of reinfarction was based on clinical findings and autopsy (19). A total of 129 reinfarctions were recorded in patients allocated to placebo and in 91 patients allocated to verapamil corresponding to 29% fewer reinfarctions in verapamil-treated patients. Of the reinfarctions, 102 in the placebo and 66 in the verapamil group were recorded

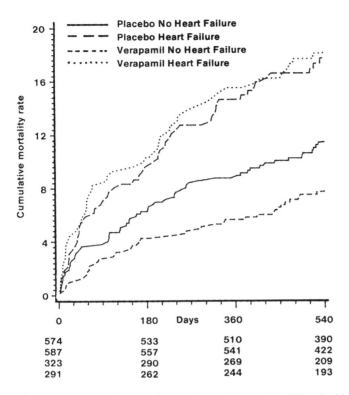

Figure 1 Cumulative mortality rates in patients with (NS) and without ($p = 0.02$, HR 0.64, CI 0.44–0.94%) congestive heart failure. The number of patients at risk are shown at the bottom (no heart failure—placebo 574, verapamil 587; heart failure—placebo 323, verapamil 291). (From Ref. 18.)

in patients still on trial medication, 3 and 4 infarcts were diagnosed in the first week post infarction, and 24 and 21, respectively, more than 1 week after premature permanent treatment stop. If a first nonfatal reinfarction is defined as an infarct not followed by death within 21 days, the 18-month first nonfatal reinfarction rate was 9.4% ($n = 76$) and 7.2% ($n = 54$) in patients allocated to placebo and verapamil, respectively ($p = 0.03$, HR 0.70, CI 0.50–0.99%); this is a post hoc analysis.

Sudden death was a predetermined secondary endpoint. Sixty-three deaths in the placebo group and 46 in the verapamil group were classified as sudden, corresponding to 18-month event rates of 7.4% and 5.6% ($p = 0.10$, HR 0.74, CI 0.50–1.08%). During treatment with trial medication sudden death was recorded in 50 placebo and 29 verapamil-treated patients, corresponding to 18-month event rates of 6.8% and 4.4% ($p = 0.04$, HR 0.63, CI 0.40–0.99%).

Sudden event means first reinfarction or sudden death. It was decided to examine this after the study was first published. Sudden events were recorded in 153 placebo and 121 verapamil-treated patients. After 18 months, event rates were 18.3% in placebo and 15.3% in verapamil-treated patients ($p = 0.02$, HR 0.78, CI 0.62–0.99%).

Congestive heart failure was defined as observation of pulmonary rales over the lower third of the lungs with the patient sitting, or a third heart sound, or congestion on any chest x-ray followed by diuretic treatment. According to the protocol, subgroup analy-

Table 2 Number of Endpoint Events (*n*) and 18-Month Event Rates (%) According
to Treatment Group and Heart Failure

| | Placebo | | Verapamil | | | Hazard | |
	n	%	*n*	%	*p*-value	ratio	95% CI
No heart failure	574		587				
Death	64	11.8	43	7.7	0.02	0.64	0.44–0.94
first major event	104	19.7	78	14.6	0.01	0.70	0.52–0.93
first sudden event	89	16.8	71	13.5	0.03	0.78	0.62–0.99
Heart failure	323		291				
Death	55	17.5	52	17.9	0.77	1.05	0.72–1.54
first major event	76	24.9	68	24.9	0.96	1.00	0.72–1.39
first sudden event	64	21.1	50	19.2	0.44	0.87	0.60–1.27

First major event = first reinfarction or death; first sudden event = first reinfarction or sudden death.

ses were planned in patients with and without heart failure. A statistically significant reduction in event rates was seen in patients without heart failure allocated to verapamil compared with patients allocated to placebo with respect to death, major events, and sudden events (Table 2). No significant differences between treatment groups were found in patients treated for congestive heart failure in the coronary care unit.

Follow-Up

Patients were followed in the outpatient clinics. Results at the follow-up closest to 12 months showed (Table 3) significantly lower resting heart rate and systolic and diastolic blood pressures in the verapamil compared to the placebo group. Fewer verapamil-treated patients reported angina pectoris or used diuretics, antiarrhythmics, sublingual nitroglycerine, or other nitrates compared to the placebo group.

Adverse events that caused permanent premature treatment stop occurred significantly more often due to atrioventricular block, gastrointestinal complaints, and sinoatrial block (Table 4) in the verapamil group.

DISCUSSION

The results of DAVIT-II are in agreement with the retrospective analysis of DAVIT-I (18), which was the basis for starting DAVIT-II.

Study Performance

As we anticipated when planning the study, 40% of the patients with acute myocardial infarction had no exclusion criteria and were randomized. Mortality rates in the placebo group after 12 and 18 months were 10.8% and 13.8%, respectively, well in accordance with the expected values based on the placebo groups of DAVIT-I and the Norwegian Timolol Trial (22) of 10% and 13%. The study included 1775 patients; we initially planned to include 2100. The enrollment was lower because two departments stopped inclusion of patients for administrative reasons and one department was closed. Because of the

Table 3 Clinical Findings and Concomitant Medicine at 12 Months Outpatient Clinic Visit

		Placebo		Verapamil	
		N	%	N	%
No. of patients		600	100	558	100
No. of tablets/day	3**	583	97.2	516	92.5
	2	9		29	
	1	4		7	
	0	4		6	
Treatment					
Digoxin		62	10.3	45	8.1
Diuretics**		215	35.8	154	27.6
Antiarrhythmics***		14	2.3	4	0.7
NSAIDS		33	5.5	25	4.5
Antihypertensives		15	2.5	6	1.1
Psychoactive drugs		43	7.2	58	10.4
Nitroglycerin***		180	30.0	138	24.7
Other nitrates***		118	19.7	84	15.1
Any nitrate***		225	37.5	174	31.1
Clinical findings					
Angina pectoris***		210	35.0	163	29.2
Dyspnea		91	15.2	87	15.6
Peripheral edemas		20	3.3	24	4.3
Pulmonary congestion		9	1.5	3	0.5
Smoker***		215	35.8	232	41.6
NYHA group					
I		437	72.8	422	75.6
II		151	25.2	129	23.1
III–IV		12	2.0	7	1.3
Treatment and clinical findings					
Dyspnea and diuretics		58	9.7	44	7.9
Angina pectoris and nitroglycerin		154	25.7	119	21.3
Angina pectoris and other nitrates		85	14.2	58	10.4
		Mean ± SD		Mean ± SD	
Heart rate* (beats/min)		76 ± 11		71 ± 11	
Systolic blood pressure* (mmHg)		141 ± 20		137 ± 18	
Diastolic blood pressure* (mmHg)		86 ± 11		82 ± 10	
Mean follow-up (days)		363 ± 25		363 ± 26	

$*p < 0.001$; $**p < 0.01$; $***p < 0.05$.

lower number of patients, the statistical power of the study was slightly reduced compared with the study plan. There was a 100% confirmation of mortality. Nonfatal reinfarctions were likewise recorded with great certainty, because patients were normally readmitted to the same department, and only 110 patients in the placebo and 111 patients in the verapamil group were not seen in the outpatient clinic at the end of the study period.

The aim of DAVIT-II was to examine if treatment with verapamil reduced total death and major events. The intention-to-treat analyses demonstrated a 20% reduction of deaths (NS) and of major event ($p = 0.03$). The nonfatal first reinfarction rate was reduced

Table 4 Events Causing Permanent Withdrawal of Trial Medication

	Placebo		Verapamil	
Event	N	%	N	%
Death**	72	8.0	48	5.5
Second or third degree AV block*	7	0.8	23	2.6
Did not want to continue	61	6.8	68	7.7
Heart failure	43	4.8	50	5.7
Angina pectoris	95	10.6	74	8.4
Antiarrhythmic treatment	14	1.6	13	1.5
Antihypertensive treatment*	10	1.1	0	—
Constipation; abdominal pain*	11	1.2	27	3.1
Sinus bradycardia; SA block**	2	0.2	9	1.0
Cannot take oral medication	11	1.2	7	0.8
Hypotension; dizziness	14	1.6	17	1.9
Administrative reasons	25	2.8	37	4.2
Other reasons	16	1.8	19	2.2
According to protocol	516	57.5	486	55.4
Total	897	100.0	878	100.0

$* p < 0.01$; $** p < 0.05$.
AV = Atrioventricular; SA = sinoatrial.

by 30% ($p = 0.03$). A reduction of nonfatal reinfarctions was also seen in the verapamil group in the Calcium Antagonist Reinfarction Italian Study (CRIS) (23). CRIS included in a secondary postinfarct trial of low-risk patients 531 patients to treatment with verapamil 360 mg/day and 542 patients to placebo treatment. Overall mortality was 5.5% after 2 years with no difference between the groups; reinfarction rates were 7.3% ($n = 39$) in verapamil and 9.0% ($n = 49$) in placebo-treated patients (NS, risk ratio 0.81, CI 0.53–1.34%); fewer verapamil-treated patients developed angina pectoris (18.8% vs. 24.3%, $p < 0.005$, risk ratio 0.8, CI 0.5–0.9%).

Efficacy Analyses

The results of the as-treated analyses demonstrate that verapamil prevents reinfarctions and sudden death during treatment. As soon as treatment stops, the protection of verapamil disappears. The reduction of sudden death combined with the pronounced effect on prevention of reinfarction are in accordance with the theory of Nayler (24) and Opie (25) that the beneficial effects of verapamil are related primarily to a reduction of sudden death and reinfarction. To evaluate this point further, a retrospective analysis of 18 months' sudden event rates was calculated, and the total effect of verapamil might be explained by prevention of sudden events with a reduction of 22% compared with placebo-treated patients. Sudden events were observed in 153 placebo and 121 verapamil-treated patients and nonsudden events in 27 and 25 patients, respectively.

Heart Failure

The question of interaction between calcium antagonists and postmyocardial infarction heart failure has been of great concern since the demonstration of a significantly increased cardiac event rate in postinfarct patients with congestion on chest x-ray treated with diltiazem compared to placebo-treated patients (26). Treatment for congestive heart failure during the acute event was preselected for subgroup analysis in the DAVIT-II. The analysis demonstrated that in patients without heart failure, verapamil significantly reduced event rates by about one third compared with placebo, while no significant difference was found in patients treated for heart failure (Table 2).

The risk of developing heart failure during verapamil treatment was also evaluated in light of the information that diltiazem increased the incidence of heart failure of postinfarct patients with depressed left ventricular function (27). The following retrospective analyses were performed: (1) congestive heart failure as reason for premature permanent treatment stop was recorded in 5.7% of verapamil compared to 4.8% of placebo-treated patients (NS) (Table 4); (2) in patients with congestive heart failure prior to randomization, congestive heart failure was the cause of premature permanent treatment stop in 10.6% in the verapamil group and 8.7% in the placebo group (NS); (3) the number of patients in need of diuretic treatment decreased over time from 41.8% at randomization to 33.4% ($p < 0.005$) after 18 months in the placebo group and from 39.7% to 28.1% ($p < 0.0001$), respectively, in the verapamil group. After 12 months (Table 3) 35.8% of placebo and 27.6% of verapamil-treated patients were in diuretic treatment ($p < 0.005$). Of the patients in diuretic treatment at randomization seen at follow-up after 12 months, 43.5% in the verapamil and 30.9% in the placebo group had stopped diuretic treatment ($p < 0.01$). Of the patients not in diuretic treatment at randomization, 13.2% in the verapamil group and 14.7% in the placebo group (NS) were in diuretic treatment.

Based on these analyses, it is concluded that no deleterious effect in patients treated for heart failure prior to randomization and no increase in incidence of heart failure was found during verapamil treatment in DAVIT-II. On the contrary, verapamil seems to prevent congestive heart failure. This is in accordance with the protection against myocardial stunning (28) and improvement of myocardial diastolic function during ischemia (29,30) in verapamil-treated patients with ischemic heart disease.

Explanatory Variables

The reduced event rates in the verapamil group might be related to the antihypertensive, anti-ischemic, and antiarrhythmic effects of verapamil.

Antihypertensive Effect

In patients with a history of systemic hypertension or with hypertension during admission, verapamil significantly prevented cardiovascular events (31). Of interest is that 10 patients in the placebo group stopped treatment with trial medication due to hypertension and no patients in the verapamil group stopped for that reason ($p < 0.01$) (Table 4). Fewer patients in the verapamil group were in treatment with antihypertensives at the follow-up visits (Table 3). The antihypertensive effect of verapamil is also demonstrated by the significantly lower blood pressure of 4 mmHg systolic and diastolic in the verapamil group compared to the placebo group (Table 3).

Antiarrhythmic Effect

It is noteworthy that significantly fewer patients in the verapamil group (0.8% vs. 2.5%, $p = 0.04$) were in antiarrhythmic treatment after 12 months (Table 3). The antiarrhythmic effect of verapamil was evaluated in the prospective ancillary Holter monitoring study

(32), which demonstrated that verapamil prevented supraventricular tachycardia and reduced ventricular premature contractions, a finding consistent with results from DAVIT-I (33).

Anti-Ischemic Effect

The anti-ischemic effect of verapamil is illustrated by the lower reported prevalence of angina pectoris at the follow-up visits (35.0% in the placebo group vs. 29.2% in the verapamil group $p < 0.05$) after 1 year (Table 3). Also, the cumulated first angina pectoris attack rate was significantly lower in the verapamil group (51.2%) compared with the placebo group (60.5%) after 18 months ($p = 0.0002$). Furthermore, Holter monitoring in a subgroup from DAVIT-II (34) demonstrated a significant reduction of ST-segment deviations during verapamil treatment both after one month (placebo 24%, verapamil 8%, $p = 0.04$) and after 1 year (placebo 26%, verapamil 4%, $p = 0.02$). The anti-ischemic effect might, apart from the coronary vasodilator effect of verapamil, also be explained by the lower blood pressure and heart rate in the verapamil compared to the placebo group (Table 3).

DAVIT-II demonstrated that (1) verapamil prevented major events, (2) the effect was concentrated in patients without congestive heart failure during the index infarction, (3) the effect was explained by prevention of sudden death and reinfarction, (4) verapamil treatment prevented angina pectoris, and (5) verapamil was associated with a lower use of diuretics.

CONCLUSION

Verapamil may be considered for secondary prevention after a myocardial infarction in patients without congestive heart failure and in patients who cannot tolerate beta-receptor blockade.

REFERENCES

1. Holzgreve H, Distler A, Michaelis J, Philipp T, Wellek S, VERDI Trial Research Group. Verapamil versus hydrochlorothiazide in the treatment of hypertension: results of long term double blind comparative trial. Br Med J 1989; 299:881–886.
2. Midtbø KA, Hals O, Lauve O, Van Der Meer J, Storstein L. Studies on verapamil in the treatment of essential hypertension: a review. Br J Clin Pharmacol 1986; 21:165S–171S.
3. Bachour G, Bender F, Hochrein H. Antiarrhythmische Wirkungen und hämodynamische Reaktionen unter Verapamil bei akutem Herzinfarkt. Herz/Kreislauf 1977; 9:89–95.
4. Hagemeijer F. Verapamil in the management of supraventricular tachyarrhythmias occurring after a recent myocardial infarction. Circulation 1978; 57:751–755.
5. Krikler DM, Spurrell RAJ. Verapamil in the treatment of paroxysmal supraventricular tachycardia. Postgrad Med J 1974; 50:447–453.
6. Livesley B, Catley PF, Campbell RC, Oram S. Double-blind evaluation of verapamil, propranolol, and isosorbide dinitrate against a placebo in the treatment of angina pectoris. Br Med J 1973; 1:375–378.
7. Mauritson DR, Johnson SM, Winniford MD, Gary JR, Willerson JT, Hillis LD. Verapamil for unstable angina at rest. A short-termed randomized, double blind study. Am Heart J 1983; 106:652–658.

8. Johnson SM, Mauritson DR, Willerson JT, Hillis LD. A controlled trial of verapamil for Prinzmetal's variant angina. N Engl J Med 1981; 304:862–866.

9. Nayler WG, Sturrock WJ. Inhibitory effect of calcium antagonists on the depletion of cardiac norepinephrine during postischemic reperfusion. J Cardiovasc Pharmacol 1985; 7:581–587.

10. Wallen NH, Held C, Rehnqvist N, Hjelmdal P. Platelet aggregability in vivo is attenuated by verapamil but not by metoprolol in patients with stable angina pectoris. Am J Cardiol 1995; 75:1–6.

11. Midtbø KA. Effect of long-term verapamil therapy on serum lipids and other metabolic parameters. Am J Cardiol 1990; 66:131–151.

12. Schulman SP, Weiss JL, Becker LC, Gottlieb SO, Woodruff KM, Weisfelt ML, Gerstenblith G. The effect of antihypertensive therapy on left ventricular mass in elderly patients. N Engl J Med 1990; 322:1350–1356.

13. Levy D, Garrison RJ, Savage DD, Kannel WB, Castelli WP. Prognostic implications of echocardiographically determined left ventricular mass in the Framingham Heart Study. N Engl J Med 1990; 322:1561–1566.

14. Messerli FH, Ventura OH, Elizardi DJ, Dunn FG, Frohlich ED. Hypertension and sudden death: increased ventricular ectopic activity in left ventricular hypertrophy. Am J Med 1984; 77:18–22.

15. McLenachan JM, Henderson E, Morris KI, Dargie HJ. Ventricular arrhythmias in patients with hypertensive left ventricular hypertrophy. N Engl J Med 1987; 317:787–792.

16. Parmley WW. Vascular protection from atherosclerosis: potential of calcium antagonists. Am J Cardiol 1990; 66:161–221.

17. The Danish Study Group on Verapamil in Myocardial Infarction. Verapamil in acute myocardial infarction. Eur Heart J 1984; 5:516–528.

18. The Danish Study Group on Verapamil in Myocardial Infarction. The effect of verapamil on mortality and major events after acute myocardial infarction (The Danish Verapamil Infarction Trial II—DAVIT II). Am J Cardiol 1990; 66:779–785.

19. The Danish Study Group on Verapamil in Myocardial Infarction. Secondary prevention with verapamil after myocardial infarction. Am J Cardiol 1990; 66:33I–40I.

20. Hansen JF, Danish Study Group on Verapamil in Myocardial Infarction. Treatment with verapamil after an acute myocardial infarction. Review of the Danish studies on verapamil in myocardial infarction (DAVIT I and II). Drugs 1991; 42(suppl 2):43–53.

21. Hansen JF, DAVIT Study Group. Review of postinfarct treatment with verapamil: combined experience of early and late intervention studies with verapamil in patients with acute myocardial infarction. Cardiovasc Drugs Ther 1994; 8:543–547.

22. The Norwegian Multicenter Study Group. Timolol-induced reduction in mortality and reinfarction in patients surviving acute myocardial infarction. N Engl J Med 1981; 304:801–807.

23. Rengo F, Carbonin P, Pahor M, De Caprio L, Bernabei R, Ferrara N, Carosella L, Acanfora D, Parlati S, Vitale D, CRIS Investigators. A controlled trial of verapamil in patients after acute myocardial infarction: results of the Calcium Antagonist Reinfarction Italian Study (CRIS). Am J Cardiol 1996; 77:365–369.

24. Nayler WG. Calcium antagonists and the ischemic myocardium. Int J Cardiol 1987; 15:267–285.

25. Opie LH. Calcium antagonists, ventricular arrhythmias, and sudden cardiac death: a major challenge for the future. J Cardiovasc Pharmacol 1991; 18(suppl 10):581–586.

26. The Multicenter Diltiazem Postinfarction Trial Research Group. The effect of diltiazem on mortality and reinfarction after myocardial infarction. N Engl J Med 1988; 319:385–392.

27. Goldstein RE, Boccuzzi SJ, Cruess D, Nattel S, Adverse Experience Committee, MDPIT Group. Diltiazem increases late-onset congestive heart failure in postinfarct patients with early reduction in ejection fraction. Circulation 1991; 83:52–60.

28. Przyklenk K, Kloner RA. Effect of verapamil on postischemic ''stunned'' myocardium: importance of timing of treatment. J Am Coll Cardiol 1988; 11:614–623.

29. Betocchi S, Piscione F, Perrone-Filardi P, Pace L, Cappilli-Bigazzi M, Alfano B, Ciarmiello A, Salvatore M, Condorelli M, Chiariello M. Effect of intravenous verapamil on left ventricular relaxation and filling in stable angina pectoris. Am J Cardiol 1990; 66:818–826.

30. Serato JF, Zaret BL, Schulman DS, Black HR, Soufer R. Usefulness of verapamil for congestive heart failure associated with abnormal left ventricular diastolic filling and normal left ventricular systolic performance. Am J Cardiol 1990; 66:981–986.

31. Jespersen CM, Hansen JF, DAVIT Study Group. Effect of verapamil on reinfarction and cardiovascular events in patients with arterial hypertension included in the Danish Verapamil Infarction Trial II. J Hum Hypertens 1994; 8:85–88.

32. Vaage-Nilsen M, Rasmussen V, Hansen JF, Hagerup L, Sørensen MB, Pedersen-Bjergaard O, Mellemgaard K, Holländer NH, Nielsen I, Sigurd B, DAVIT II Study Group. Effect of verapamil on arrhythmias and heart rate sixteen months following an acute myocardial infarction. Cardiovasc Drugs Ther 1994; 8:147–151.

33. The Danish Study Group on Verapamil in Myocardial Infarction. The Danish studies on verapamil in myocardial infarction. Br J Clin Pharmacol 1986; 21:197S–204S.

34. Vaage-Nilsen M, Rasmussen V, Holländer NH, Hansen JF, The DAVIT II Study Group. Prevalence of transient myocardial ischemia during the first year after a myocardial infarction. Effect of treatment with verapamil. Eur Heart J 1992; 13:666–670.

Section K
Heparin

Despite the widespread use of heparin administered intravenously or subcutaneously, there are few conclusive data that establish its efficacy as a generally applicable treatment for myocardial infarction. For some patients, particularly those treated with primary PTCA, intravenous heparin has a clear role. For other patients, such as those with large infarcts or evidence of left ventricular thrombi, heparin followed by a course of oral anticoagulants may reduce the frequency of secondary embolic events. For most other patients, however, there is little evidence of an additional benefit of heparin beyond that afforded by aspirin. Given the firmly held belief that many hold regarding the utility of heparin (especially in conjunction with fibrin-specific thrombolytic agents) as well as the development of newer antithrombotic therapies which may eclipse heparin because of their potency, ease of administration, or both, it is very unlikely that future large-scale clinical trials will clarify this issue.

32

GISSI-2

GIANNI TOGNONI and ALDO P. MAGGIONI

Gruppo Italiano per lo Studio della Sopravvivenza nell'Infarto Miocardico. GISSI-2: A factorial randomized trial of alteplase versus streptokinase and heparin versus no heparin among 12,490 patients with acute myocardial infarction. Lancet 1990;336:65–71.

BACKGROUND

The decision to go on with another trial on thrombolysis, after the results of the first study, was not so simple as the one that led to GISSI for various reasons (1). The pharmacological advantages of the tissue plasminogen activator (tPA, as it was still called at the time) appeared rather well established: Was it worthwhile to enter another major study with the aim being checking the degree of the transferability of such an advantage into a clinical one?

On the other side, it was rather puzzling to see that the claimed clot specificity of tPA was de facto contradicted by the mandatory addition of IV heparin. Further, the Italian cardiological community had become more interested in the epidemiological and public health implications of having a countrywide collaborative network. The concurrent interest in the role of SC heparin on coronary diseases suggested (together with the parallel planning of ISIS-3) a study strategy with a factorial design. The formulation of the study protocol around the questions listed in Table 1 reflects the spectrum of interests. It is worth underlining, in fact, that the third nonpharmacological aim was seen as possibly the most interesting one. The clinical focus of the study was also behind the decision to adopt a composite endpoint, with severe left ventricular dysfunction (2) included to provide important complementary information other than mortality on the "natural history" of acute myocardial infarction (AMI) patients in the thrombolytic era. The change of the spelling of the acronym, where SK was substituted with survival, was felt to be a symbolic indication of this focusing.

SETTING AND PROTOCOL DESIGN

The organization of the study reproduced closely the philosophy and the eligibility criteria of the first GISSI, as seen in the protocol summarized in Figure 1. An even higher number of Italian coronary care units (CCUs) (233 out of the registered 250) randomized 12,490

Table 1   Questions Addressed in GISSI-2

Does the pharmacologically more promising profile of alteplase translate
  into a clinically relevant advantage (higher efficacy, lower hemorrhagic
  risk) when compared directly with SK?
Does an anticoagulant prophylactic regimen with SC heparin add to the
  effect of aspirin, with respect to the incidence of early postinfarction
  ischemic events (and thus on the overall outcome)?
What is the yield of different prognostic tests at discharge?

patients over a period of 17 months (later the launching of an International Arm allowed
the inclusion of another 8000 patients). Patients were eligible for the 2×2 factorially
designed study: (a) if they had chest pain accompanied by ST segment elevation of 1 mm
or more in any limb lead of the electrocardiogram and/or of 2 mm or more in any precordial lead; (b) if they had been admitted to the CCU within 6 hours from the onset of
symptoms; and (c) if they had no clear contraindication to the fibrinolytic treatments or
to heparin.

RESULTS

According to the study aims, the results should be divided in two parts: findings related
to the pharmacological treatments and findings exploring the epidemiological characteristics of the overall study populations. The situation of no difference documented with
respect to the experimental treatments allowed the optimal use of the whole data base in
the latter direction [as this is not the place for discussing the main findings, the reader is
referred to some key references (3–6)]. The degree to which the results of treatment with

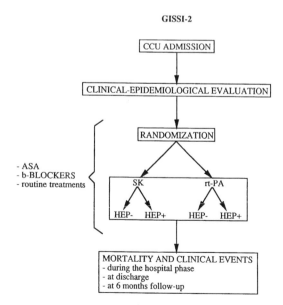

Figure 1   GISSI-2 protocol.

Table 2 GISSI-2: Effects of Randomized Treatment on Combined Endpoint

	tPA (n = 6182)	SK (n = 6199)	RR (95% CI)	Hep (n = 6175)	No hep (n = 6206)	RR (95% CI)	Total (n = 12,381)
Total events (%)	1428 (23.1)	1394 (22.5)	1.04 (0.95–1.13)	1403 (22.7)	1419 (22.9)	0.99 (0.91–1.08)	2822 (22.8)
Deaths	556 (9.0)	536 (8.6)		518 (8.3)	574 (9.3)		1092 (8.8)
Clinical heart failure	478 (7.7)	502 (8.1)		494 (8.0)	486 (7.8)		980 (7.9)
EF ≤ 35%	153 (2.5)	137 (2.2)		141 (2.3)	149 (2.4)		290 (2.4)
Myocardial segments injured ≥ 45%	106 (1.7)	90 (1.5)		108 (1.8)	87 (1.4)		196 (1.6)
QRS score > 10	135 (2.2)	129 (2.1)		141 (2.3)	123 (2.0)		264 (2.1)

EF = Ejection fraction; Hep = heparin; tPA = tissue plasminogen activator; SK = streptokinase; RR = relative risk.

the factorially tested drugs overlap is truly impressive (Table 2). No differences in outcome were seen between patients treated with SK or tPA, or between patients who were or were not given subcutaneous heparin. The cumulative evaluation of the GISSI-2 population and of the International Arm confirms the findings.

The absence of any clinical advantage in the tPA–treated group came as a surprise. It certainly was received as such, and correspondingly hotly debated (together with the similar findings of the bigger and blinded ISIS-3) (7). The similarity of clinical effects despite the documented pharmacological difference of the two thrombolytics was observed in all subgroup analyses. The only (not significant in GISSI-2; significant, as in ISIS-3, in the International Arm) difference was on the safety side (Table 3) (8).

The absence of a heparin-specific effect on reinfarction (expected to be one of the ways in which it also could influence mortality rates) could be attributed to the protection provided by aspirin, which had rapidly become a universally accepted treatment. The very impressive clinico-epidemiological survival profile of the GISSI-2 population as compared with the corresponding cohort of GISSI-1 (8.8% vs. 13%), which documented the overall benefit of thrombolysis, was ignored. The focus centered on the "explanation" of the unexplainable and unexpected equivalence. Many pointed to the way in which heparin had been used in the study, specifically with respect to tPA.

The "heparin controversy" was born and dominated the scene for years. Some authors (9,10) claimed that the expression of the full thrombolytic potential of tPA necessitated concomitant IV heparin rather than twice-daily SC treatment beginning after 12 hours. Data supporting such claims, however, derived from small series, where results regarding patency rates were clearly conflicting; one factor in this may be the various time intervals set for the assessment of coronary patency after thrombolysis (11–13). In any case, the "heparin controversy" was solved neither from the various "position papers" nor from GUSTO-I (14), as in this trial there was no direct comparison between tPA plus IV heparin (conventional administration) and tPA without IV heparin.

The adoption of a combined endpoint (mortality plus severe left ventricular dysfunction) appears to have been satisfactory from a methodological point of view, since it bridges two usually separate lines of evaluation of acute treatments in evolving myocardial

Table 3 Stroke Events: Comparison Between Different Thrombolytic Agents

A. GISSI-2/International Study

	SK (10,396)	tPA (10,372)	OR (95% CI)	RRCox (95% CI)
Etiology				
Overall	98 (0.94)	138 (1.33)	1.41 (1.09–1.83)	1.40 (1.08–1.82)
Hemorrhagic	30 (0.29)	44 (0.42)	1.47 (0.93–2.31)	1.39 (0.87–1.99)

B. ISIS-3 Study

	SK (13,607)	tPA (13,569)	OR (95% CI)
Overall	141 (1.0)	188 (1.4)	1.34 (1.08–1.66)
Hemorrhagic	32 (0.2)	89 (0.7)	2.58

infarction; in fact the GISSI-2 results, encouraging with respect to total in-hospital mortality rate, reliably documented the burden of chronic or long-term consequences of AMI, a problem faced by the subsequent GISSI-3 study (15).

REFERENCES

1. GISSI-2 Gruppo Italiano per lo Studio della Streptokinasi nell'Infarto Miocardico. A factorial randomised trial of alteplase versus streptokinase and heparin versus no heparin among 12,490 patients with acute myocardial infarction. Lancet 1990; 336:65–71.
2. De Vita C, Franzosi MG, Geraci E, et al. GISSI-2: mortality plus extensive left ventricular damage as "end-points." Lancet 1990; 335:289.
3. Volpi A, De Vita C, Franzosi MG, Geraci E, Maggioni AP, Mauri F, Negri E, Santoro E, Tabazzi L, Tognoni G, the Ad hoc working group of the Gruppo Italiano per lo Studio della Sopravvivenza nell'Infarto Miocardico (GISSI)-2 Data base. Determinants of 6-month mortality in survivors of myocardial infarction after thrombolysis. Results of the GISSI-2 data base. Circulation 1993; 88:416–429.
4. Maggioni AP, Zuanetti G, Franzosi MG, Rovelli F, Santoro E, Staszewsky L, Tavazzi L, Tognoni G on behalf of GISSI-2 Investigators. Prevalence and prognostic significance of ventricular arrhythmias after acute myocardial infarction in the fibrinolytic era. GISSI-2 results. Circulation 1993; 87:312–322.
5. Zuanetti G, Latini R, Maggioni AP, Franzosi MG, Santoro L, Tognoni G, for the GISSI-3 Investigators. Effect of the ACE inhibitor lisinopril on mortality in diabetic patients with acute myocardial infarction. Data from the GISSI-3 Study. Circulation 1997; 96:4239–4245.
6. Villella A, Maggioni AP, Villella M, Giordano A, Turazza FM, Santoro E, Franzosi MG, on behalf of the GISSI-2 Investigators. Prognostic significance of maximal exercise testing after myocardial infarction treated with thrombolytic agents: the GISSI-2 data-base. Lancet 1995; 346:523–529.
7. ISIS-3 (Third International Study of Infarct Survival Collaborative Group). ISIS-3: a randomised comparison of streptokinase vs tissue plasminogen activator vs anistreplase and of aspirin and heparin vs heparin alone among 41,299 cases of suspected acute myocardial infarction. Lancet 1992; 339:753–770.
8. Maggioni AP, Franzosi MG, Santoro E, White H, Van de Werf F, Tognoni G, the GISSI-2 and the International Study Group. The risk of stroke in patients with acute myocardial infarction after thrombolytic and antithrombotic treatment. New Engl J Med 1992; 327:1–6.
9. White HD. GISSI-2 and the heparin controversy. Lancet 1990; 336:297–298.
10. Sobel BE, Hirsh J. Principles and practice of coronary thrombolysis and conjunctive treatment. Am J Cardiol 1991; 68:382–388.
11. Ross AM, Hsia J, Hamilton W, et al. Heparin versus aspirin after recombinant tissue plasminogen activator therapy in myocardial infarction: a randomized trial. J Am Coll Cardiol 1990; 15 (suppl A):64A.
12. Topol EJ, George BS, Kereiakes DJ, et al. A randomized controlled trial of intravenous tissue plasminogen activator and early intravenous heparin in acute myocardial infarction. Circulation 1989; 79:281–286.
13. Bleich SD, Nichols T, Schumacher R, et al. The role of heparin following coronary thrombolysis with tissue plasminogen activator (tPA). Circulation 1989; 80:II-113.
14. The GUSTO Investigators. An international randomized trial comparing four thrombolytic strategies for acute myocardial infarction. N Engl J Med 1993; 329:673–682.
15. Gruppo Italiano per lo Studio della Sopravvivenza nell'Infarto Miocardico. GISSI-3: effects of lisinopril and transdermal glyceryl trinitrate singly and together on 6-week mortality and ventricular function after acute myocardial infarction. Lancet 1994; 343:1115–1122.

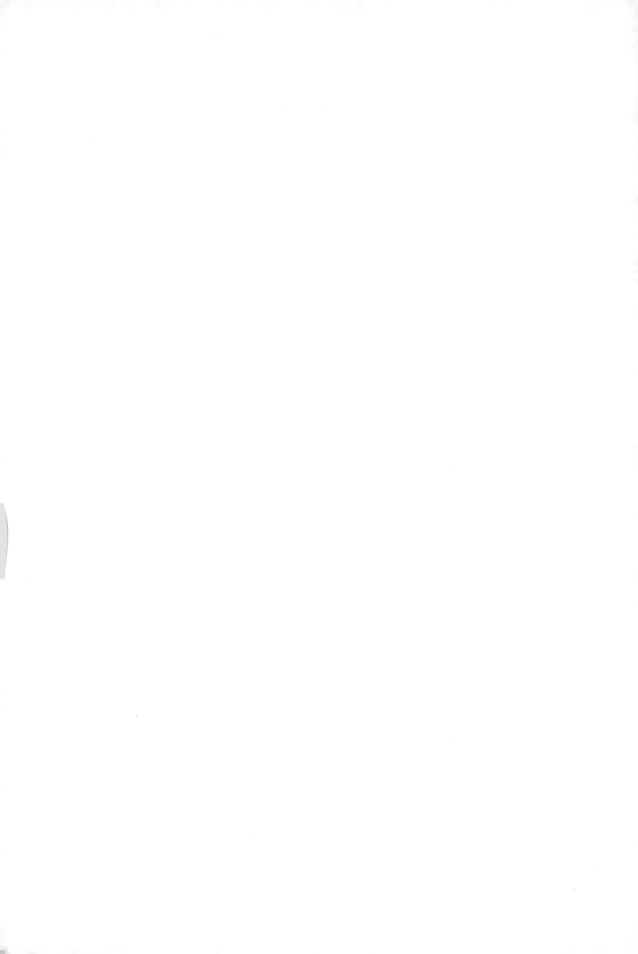

33

ISIS-3

PETER SLEIGHT

ISIS-3 (Third International Study of Infarct Survival) Collaborative
Group. ISIS-3: a randomised trial of streptokinase versus tissue
plasminogen activator versus anistreplase and of aspirin plus heparin
versus aspirin alone among 41,299 cases of suspected acute myocardial
infarction. Lancet 1992; 339:753–770.

INTRODUCTION

Although it is often considered axiomatic that the combination of an antiplatelet and an
antithrombin agent would be beneficial in acute myocardial infarction (MI), this has recently been questioned, particularly with the gradual realization that: (1) heparin is a difficult agent to control with a narrow therapeutic window; (2) aspirin alone or some other
antiplatelet agent is very effective in combating the tendency to coronary reocclusion,
particularly in the presence of fibrinolytic agents that activate platelets, as seen in ISIS-
2 (1), where the excess of reinfarction caused by streptokinase (SK) was completely reversed by 160 mg aspirin per day; (3) aspirin is also very effective in reducing mortality
in unstable angina (2); (4) the early benefit of aspirin in MI (which at 5 weeks resulted
in a 2.5% absolute reduction in mortality) holds out for many years (3); and (5) in the
presence of aspirin plus a fibrinolytic agent, the toxic (hemorrhagic) effects of heparin
might outweigh any benefit. Furthermore, other studies have shown that continuation of
long-term aspirin will approximately double the early benefit seen in ISIS-2, at least for
the first few years after an MI (2).

Because of the uncertainty of the risks and benefits of adding heparin to aspirin in the
presence of a fibrinolytic agent, ISIS-3 tested the effects of a widely practicable regimen of
25,000 units of subcutaneous heparin daily (12,500 units 12 hourly) added to adequate
oral aspirin, begun 4 hours after the start of aspirin plus fibrinolysis (4). The aspirin regimen used in ISIS-2, beginning with 160 mg of enteric-coated aspirin chewed for better
absorption, has a profound antiplatelet effect within 1 hour (5,6), whereas lower doses,
e.g., 75 mg, may take some days to exert a full effect (7,8).

ISIS-2 proved that aspirin added to heparin was better than heparin alone (1), but
did not test whether aspirin plus heparin was any better than aspirin alone. The benefit
of heparin was generally seen in the previous trials, which did not include aspirin, or later
trials where the dose of aspirin was inadequate for an early effect (9). One angiographic
trial (10), which used an adequate dose of aspirin, did find a modest (8%) increase in
patency but was too small to examine the risks or mortality benefit from this early small

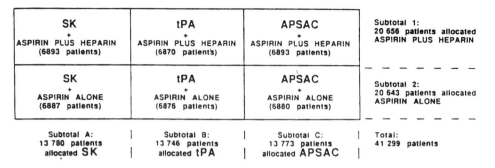

Figure 1 Factorial design of ISIS-3: 41,299 patients, 36,381 in whom the responsible clinician considered there to be a "clear indication" for fibrinolytic therapy, plus half of the 9475 in whom the indication was considered "uncertain."

increase in patency. This is important since several studies have shown a "rebound" increase in reocclusion after stopping heparin. The number of reocclusions that occur can be substantial, as shown by follow-up angiography in the APRICOT study (11).

For these reasons we chose a simple twice-daily subcutaneous injection of a high dose of unfractionated heparin beginning after a 4-hour period from the start of the thrombolytic comparison in order to avoid giving a long-acting heparin in the presence of potential bleeding from the thrombolytic [in GISSI-2 (12) this was after a delay of 12 hours]. Because the possibility of rethrombosis (and reinfarction) seemed highest for several days after onset, we chose to continue the 12,500 unit heparin injections b.i.d. for 7 days or until discharge, if earlier. We considered the use of control saline injections, but rejected this on the grounds of (1) patient comfort/compliance, and (2) difficulty in blinding, because of the bruising associated with active subcutaneous heparin. This regimen had been shown to have substantial antithrombotic effects in the absence of aspirin (13,14).

PATIENTS AND METHODS

The details of recruitment and randomization in the ISIS-3 trial are given in more detail in Chapter 4 and in the ISIS-3 report (4). Briefly, a total of 45,856 patients were randomized (by telephone) in 20 countries, with the participation of 914 hospitals, between September 1989 and January 1991. Mortality follow-up was through government records; in-hospital events were collected on a simple, single-page discharge form.

This report concerns the 41,299 patients who received thrombolytic therapy. This chapter deals only with the randomization between 7 days of aspirin alone or aspirin plus heparin. The trial also included separate (factorial) randomization to streptokinase, tPA, and anistreplase (anysolated plasminogen streptokinase activated complex, or APSAC). The design is shown in Figure 1.

RESULTS

Mortality

Nonvascular deaths during days 0–35 were evenly distributed (18 aspirin plus heparin vs. 18 aspirin alone), and subsequent analyses are of total mortality. Figure 2 shows the cumu-

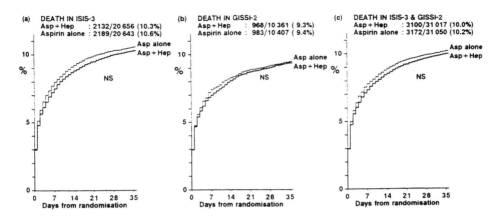

Figure 2 Cumulative percentage dead in days 0–35 in ISIS-3 and in GISSI-2: aspirin plus heparin versus aspirin alone. All patients allocated aspirin plus heparin (thicker line) versus all allocated aspirin alone in (a) ISIS-3; (b) GISSI-2; and (c) ISIS-3 and GISSI-2 combined. (From Ref. 4.)

lative mortality for ISIS-3, for GISSI-2, and the combined result in more that 60,000 randomized patients. No significant differences are shown. During the scheduled heparin treatment period, there were slightly fewer deaths in the aspirin group [i.e., days 0–7 in hospital: 1534 (7.4%) vs. 1633 (7.95); $p = 0.06$] with a slight convergence during further follow-up to day 35 [598 further deaths (3.1% of survivors) vs. 556 (2.9%)]. This analysis of mortality during the scheduled treatment period was, however, not prespecified, and there was no significant difference in terms of the prespecified endpoint of 35-day mortality [2132 (10.3%) aspirin plus heparin vs. 2189 (10.6%) aspirin alone], nor was there any significant difference in 6-month survival.

Side Effects and Other Clinical Features

Noncerebral bleeds (generally minor, such as oozing from puncture sites, microscopic hematuria, or blood-streaked vomit or sputum) were recorded more commonly among aspirin plus heparin–allocated patients (6.3% aspirin plus heparin vs. 3.9% aspirin alone; $p < 0.00001$). Half of this excess was during days 0–1 (4.1% vs. 3.0%; $p < 0.00001$). There was also a small excess of transfused or other major noncerebral bleeds (1.0% vs. 0.8%; 0.26% SD 0.09 excess; $p < 0.01$). The excess risk of any type of noncerebral bleed increased with age (<70 yr: 5.0% aspirin plus heparin vs. 3.4% aspirin alone; $\geq$ 70 yr: 9.8% versus 5.3%; $p < 0.00001$ for the difference between these excess risks).

No significant difference in the overall risk of stroke was observed [261 (1.28%) aspirin plus heparin vs. 240 (1.18%) aspirin alone (Fig. 3, top)]. A small but significant excess of strokes attributed to definite or probable cerebral hemorrhage among patients allocated aspirin plus heparin [114 (0.56%) vs. 82 (0.40%); 0.16% SD 0.07 excess; $p < 0.05$ (Fig. 3, bottom)] was counterbalanced by a nonsignificant shortfall of strokes attributed to infarct or unknown cause [147 (0.72%) vs. 158 (0.78%)]. The risk of stroke increased with age, but even among patients 70 years of age or over, the addition of subcutaneous heparin to aspirin was not associated with any significant excess of stroke (2.32% aspirin plus heparin vs. 2.23% aspirin alone) or of cerebral hemorrhage (0.90% vs. 0.79%). Reinfarctions were recorded in-hospital slightly less commonly among patients allocated

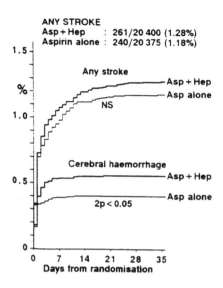

Figure 3 Cumulative percentage with any stroke (upper lines) and with (definite or probable) cerebral hemorrhage in hospital up to day 35 or prior discharge. All patients allocated aspirin plus heparin (thicker line) versus all allocated aspirin alone. (From Ref. 4.)

aspirin plus heparin [3.16% vs. 3.47%; 0.31% SD 0.18 difference; $p = 0.09$ (Fig. 4)]. This reduction arose during the scheduled heparin treatment period (reinfarctions during days 0–7: 2.39% aspirin plus heparin vs. 2.81% aspirin alone; 0.42% SD 0.16 difference; $p < 0.01$), with a very slight and nonsignificant excess of reinfarction thereafter (0.77% vs. 0.66%). There were no significant differences between these treatment groups in the reported incidence of other clinical events.

DISCUSSION

The ISIS-3 study showed (both for the thrombolytic and for the antithrombotic comparison) that regimens that aim for a more aggressive result in terms of coronary patency may incur risks (of hemorrhage or hemorrhagic stroke) that balance out the undoubted potential benefits of opening more vessels and keeping them open. A similar realization has more recently occurred in the field of coronary intervention, where heparin-based regimens have gradually been replaced by better antiplatelet regimens (15).

After the negative results of the ISIS-3 trial (particularly the lack of superiority of tPA), there was a great deal of criticism of the trial design, much of which focused on the "inadequacy" of subcutaneous heparin, and of the 4-hour delay in its administration. However, as shown above, and also in GISSI-2 (12), this relatively conservative regimen still resulted in a small excess of cerebral hemorrhage, which was particularly important in patients randomized to tPA rather than SK.

Although it is the rule that tPA is always accompanied by heparin plus aspirin, the randomized information on this is small and inadequate (very similar to the prior situation with PTCA/stent intervention). In fact, tPA might be considerably safer, especially in

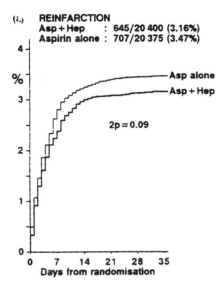

Figure 4 Cumulative percentage with reinfarction in hospital up to day 35 or prior discharge. All patients allocated aspirin plus heparin (thicker line) versus all allocated aspirin alone. (From Ref. 4.)

older subjects, if heparin were not used. Aspirin and/or IIb/IIIa receptor antagonists seem particularly promising and are undergoing larger-scale testing.

After ISIS-3 was published the GUSTO study investigators (16) incorporated an "ISIS-3" arm in their study. Ironically, in view of all the pre-GUSTO criticism of ISIS-3, the subcutaneous heparin regimen had the lowest reinfarction rate in GUSTO, better than the three intravenous heparin arms and with the lowest rate of cerebral hemorrhage of all four arms. In ISIS-3 there was a small and significant mortality advantage of added heparin during the treatment period, but as in GISSI-2 this was followed by a small excess of deaths after the treatment period so the net result was no significant difference in mortality (2 SD 2 fewer deaths from added heparin). It could be argued that a carefully controlled intravenous heparin regimen might be more effective than the high-dose subcutaneous regimen used in the ISIS and GISSI trials. However, the randomized data available are hopelessly inadequate to judge this (only about 1300 patients randomized to aspirin alone vs. aspirin plus intravenous heparin), and, as stated above, the direct comparison of intravenous and subcutaneous heparin was not promising for intravenous heparin, even for anterior MI. Certainly the use of more intensive heparin in one arm of GUSTO-II (17) and in two other studies (18,19) was stopped because of unacceptable cerebral bleeding.

In a recent systematic review of anticoagulant therapy in AMI, Collins et al. (20) concluded that in the absence of aspirin, anticoagulant therapy reduced mortality by 25% (SD 8%, CI 10–38%, $p = 0.002$) with a significant reduction in overall stroke. However, in the presence of aspirin there was only a marginal reduction in mortality (Fig. 5), but a significant excess of three major bleeds per 1000 patients treated. They again concluded that there was no evidence for adding any type of anticoagulant to aspirin in acute MI.

The use of additional heparin on top of aspirin does seem more promising in unstable angina (21).

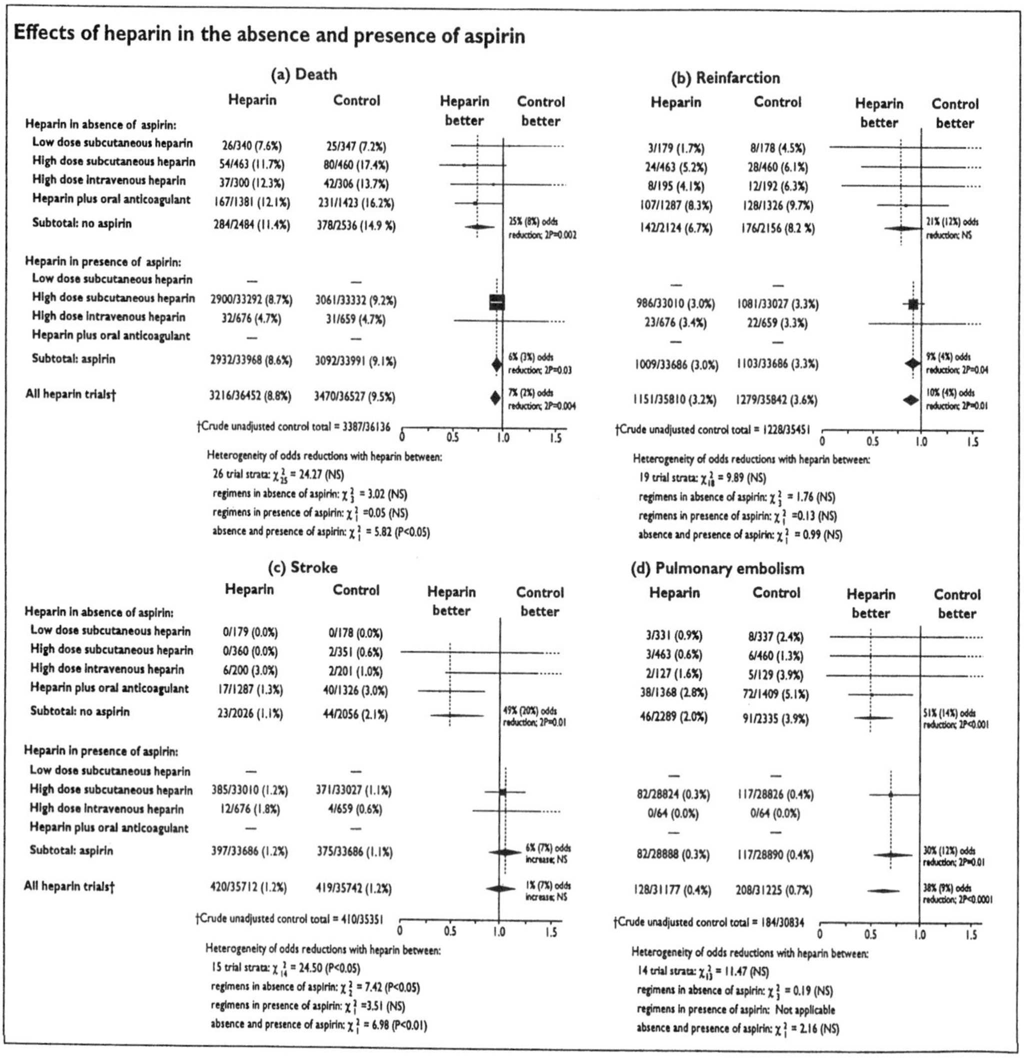

Figure 5 Effects of heparin in the absence and presence of aspirin. In most trials patients were allocated roughly evenly between treatment groups, but in some trials more patients were deliberately allocated to active treatment. To allow direct comparison between the percentages of patients in each group who had an event, adjusted totals have been calculated after conversion of any unevenly randomized trials to even ones by counting their control groups more than once. Statistical calculations are, however, based on the actual numbers from individual trials. Solid squares represent stratified odds ratios (heparin:control) for combinations of individual trials of particular anticoagulant regimens. Sizes of squares are proportional to the amount of "information" contributed; horizontal lines denote 99% confidence intervals. Diamonds represent stratified overviews (and 95% confidence intervals) of the results for all trials conducted in the absence and in the presence of routine aspirin; the difference in odds is given to the right of the solid vertical line. Black squares or diamonds to the left of the solid vertical line indicate additional benefit with heparin, but the result is significant ($p < 0.01$ for horizontal lines and $p < 0.05$ for diamonds) only when the entire confidence intervals lie to the left of the line. (From Ref. 20.)

CONCLUSION

Although intravenous heparin is still encouraged by some authorities (22,23), the evidence for its use in the presence of adequate aspirin is insufficient.

REFERENCES

1. ISIS-2 (Second International Study of Infarct Survival) Collaborative Group. Randomised trial of intravenous streptokinase, oral aspirin, both or neither among 17,187 cases of suspected acute myocardial infarction: ISIS-2. Lancet 1988; ii:349–360.
2. Antiplatelet Trialists' Collaboration. Collaborative overview of randomised trials of antiplatelet therapy—I: prevention of death, myocardial infarction, and stroke by prolonged antiplatelet therapy in various categories of patients. Br Med J 1994; 308:81–106.
3. Baigent C, Collins R, Appleby P, Parish S, Sleight P, Peto R on behalf of the ISIS-2 (Second International Study of Infarct Survival) Collaborative Group. ISIS-2: 10-year survival in a randomised comparison of intravenous streptokinase, oral aspirin, both, or neither among patients with suspected acute myocardial infarction. Br Med J 1998; 316:1337–1343.
4. ISIS-3 (Third International Study of Infarct Survival) Collaborative Group. ISIS-3: a randomised trial of streptokinase versus tissue plasminogen activator versus anistreplase and of aspirin plus heparin versus aspirin alone among 41,299 cases of suspected acute myocardial infarction. Lancet 1992; 339:753–770.
5. Gallus AS, Hirab J, Turtle RJ, Trebilcock R, O'Brien SE, Carroll JJ, et al. Small subcutaneous doses of heparin in prevention of venous thrombosis. N Engl J Med 1973; 288:545–551.
6. Warlow C, Terry G, Kenmore ACF, Beattie AG, Ogston D, Douglas AS. A double-blind trial of low doses of subcutaneous heparin in the prevention of deep-vein thrombosis after myocardial infarction. Lancet 1975; ii:934–936.
7. Roverson PA, Marke F. Preventing thromboembolism after myocardial infarction: effect of low dose heparin on smoking. Br Med J 1977; 1:18–20.
8. Cade JF, Andrews JT, Stubbs AE. Comparisons of sodium and calcium heparin in prevention of venous thromboembolism. Aust NZ J Med 1982; 12:501–504.
9. Bleich SD, Nichols TC, Schumacher RR, Cooke DH, Tate DA, Teichman SL. Effect of heparin on coronary arterial patency after thrombolysis with tissue plasminogen activator in acute myocardial infarction. Am J Cardiol 1990; 66:1412–1417.
10. De Bono DP, Simoons ML, Tijssen J, Arnold AER, Betriu A, Burgersdijk C, et al. for the European Co-operative Study Group. Effect of early intravenous heparin on coronary patency, infarct size, and bleeding complications after alteplase thrombolysis: results of a randomized double-blind European Co-operative Study Group trial. Br Heart J 1992; 67:122–128.
11. Meijer A, Verheught FWA, Werter CPJ, Lie KI, van der Pol JMJ, van Eenige MJ. Aspirin versus coumadin in the prevention of re-occlusion and recurrent ischaemia after successful thrombolysis: a prospective placebo-controlled angiographic study: results of the APRICOT Study. Circulation 1993; 87:1524–1530.
12. Gruppo Italiano per lo Studio della Streptochinasi nell'Infarto Miocardico (GISSI). GISSI-2: a factorial randomised trial of alteplase versus streptokinase and heparin versus no heparin among 12,490 patients with acute myocardial infarction. Lancet 1990; 336:65–71.
13. Collins R, Conway M, Alexopoulos D, Yusuf S, Sleight P, Brooks N, et al. for the ISIS pilot study investigators. Randomised factorial trial of high dose intravenous streptokinse, or oral aspirin and of intravenous heparin in acute myocardial infarction. Eur Heart J 1987; 8:634–642.
14. Bleich SD, Nicholls TC, Schumacher RR, Cooke DH, Tree DA, Teichman SL. Effect of hepa-

rin on coronary arterial patency after thrombolysis with tissue plasminogen activator in acute myocardial infarction. Am J Cardiol 1990; 66:1412–1417.

15. Karrillon GJ, Morice MC, Benveniste E, Bunouf P, Aubry P, Cattan S, et al. Intracoronary stent implantation without ultrasound guidance and with replacement of conventional anticoagulation by antiplatelet therapy. 30-day clinical outcome of the French Multicentre Registry. Circulation 1996; 94:1519–1527.

16. The GUSTO Investigators. An international randomized trial comparing four thrombolytic strategies for acute myocardial infarction. N Engl J Med 1993; 329:673–682.

17. The Global Use of Strategies to Open Occluded Coronary Arteries (GUSTO) IIa Investigators. Randomized trial of intravenous heparin versus recombinant hirudin for acute coronary syndromes. Circulation 1994; 90:1631–1637.

18. Antman EM. Hirudin in acute myocardial infarction: safety report from the Thrombolysis and Thrombin Inhibition in Myocardial Infarction (TIMI) 9A Trial. Circulation 1994; 90:1624–1630.

19. Neuhaus K-L, von Essen R, Tebbe U, et al. Safety observations from the pilot phase of the randomized r-Hirudin for Improvement of Thrombolysis (HIT-III) study. Circulation 1994; 90:1638–1642.

20. Collins R, MacMahon S, Flather M, Baigent C, Remvig L, Mortensen S, et al. Clinical effects of anticoagulant therapy in suspected acute myocardial infarction: systematic overview of randomized trials. Br Med J 1996; 313:652–659.

21. Lindahl B, Venge P, Wallentin L. Relation between troponin T and the risk of subsequent cardiac events in unstable coronary artery disease. The FRISC study group. Circulation 1996; 93:1651–1657.

22. Hirsh J, Fuster V. Guide to anticoagulant therapy. Part 1. Heparin. Circulation 1994; 89:1449–1468.

23. Ellerbeck EF, Jencks SF, Radford MJ, Kresowik TF, Craig AS, Gold JA, et al. Quality of care for Medicare patients with acute myocardial infarction. A four-state pilot study from the co-operative cardiovascular project. JAMA 1995; 273:1509–1514.

Section L
Nitrates

Oral, sublingual, and transdermal nitrates are useful agents for relieving symptoms and improving exercise tolerance in patients with angina. Intravenous nitroglycerin is useful for controlling ischemic symptoms in patients with unstable angina and in the treatment of hypertension and heart failure in the acute phase of a myocardial infarction. The two trials detailed here addressed the question of the efficacy of longer-term use of nitrates to improve prognosis in unselected patients with myocardial infarction. Neither topical (GISSI-3) nor oral (ISIS-4) therapy improved outcomes for these patients, about 70% of whom were treated with thrombolytics. Despite the frequent use of non-protocol nitrates in both studies, their extremely large size (combined enrollment of over 75,000 patients) makes it very unlikely that a positive benefit went undetected. These agents, then, should not be considered as part of the routine management of myocardial infarction patients.

34

GISSI-3

GIANNI TOGNONI and ALDO P. MAGGIONI

Gruppo Italiano per lo Studio della Sopravvivenza nell'Infarto Miocardico. GISSI-3: effects of lisinopril and transdermal glyceryl trinitrate singly and together on 6-week mortality and ventricular function after acute myocardial infarction. Lancet 1994; 343:1115–1122.

BACKGROUND AND QUESTIONS

Left ventricular dysfunction is known to be the strongest indicator of poor prognosis following myocardial infarction (1–3). The possibility of preventing such deterioration through very early intervention with angiotensin-converting enzyme (ACE) inhibitors (4,5), or nitrates (6) had been repeatedly emphasized mainly in relation to the theory of left ventricular remodeling (6–8). However, most studies on ACE inhibitors concentrated on selected groups of patients at higher risk of left ventricular dilation and dysfunction (9,10).

The results of a controversial meta-analysis (11) strongly supported a life-saving role for nitrates in patients with acute myocardial infarction (AMI): the widespread use of nitrates in coronary care units in the absence of definite data on their effects suggested the need for a formal evaluation. On the other hand, the unexpected and enforced termination of the CONSENSUS-II trial (12) suggested that early ACE inhibition was ineffective and possibly carried an excess risk for elderly patients.

SETTING

Between June 1991 and July 1993, a total of 43,047 patients were admitted to the 200 participating coronary care units (about two-thirds of such units in Italy). Of these patients, 19,394 (45%) were randomized (13).

PROTOCOL

The GISSI-3 protocol was explicitly designed not only to test the drug effects of ACE inhibitors and transdermal glyceryl trinitrate (GTN), but also to assess formally, with a classic 2×2 factorial design, the benefit-to-risk ratio of the combination of these drugs

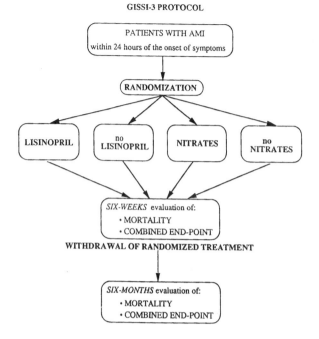

Figure 1   GISSI-3 protocol.

on the whole population of AMI patients and on elderly patients and women, who are at higher risk of AMI mortality, despite intensive use of recommended treatments.

As in GISSI-2, the main endpoint of the study included the combined outcome measure of mortality and severe ventricular dysfunction, which is highly predictive of poor outcome over the medium term (6 months).

Figure 1 shows the study protocol. Patients were elegible (1) if they had chest pain accompanied by elevation or depression of the ST segment of at least 1 mm in one or more peripheral leads of the EKG or of at least 2 mm in one or more precordial leads; (2) if they had been admitted to the participating CCUs within 24 hours of symptom onset; and (3) if they had no clear contraindications to the study treatments. The four treatment groups received lisinopril alone, transdermal GTN alone, combined therapy with lisinopril and transdermal GTN, or no trial medication. Study treatment was withdrawn at 6 weeks if there were no specific indications to continue, and patients were followed up for 6 months from randomization.

RESULTS

Systematic treatment with transdermal GTN to 6 weeks did not produce a significant benefit in terms of total mortality rate or combined endpoint rate. The survival curves showed a small but not significant benefit for GTN treatment (Fig. 2). Among both the group of patients aged over 70 and women, there was a significant reduction in the combined endpoint rate (9% and 10%, respectively; $2p = 0.048$). Nitrate treatment was discontinued mainly because of hypotension and headache (2.6% and 3.0%, respectively). There

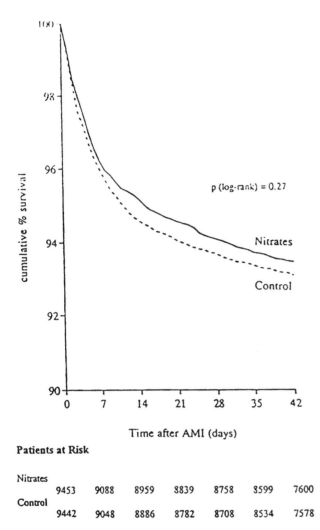

Patients at Risk

Nitrates
   9453   9088   8959   8839   8758   8599   7600
Control
   9442   9048   8886   8782   8708   8534   7578

Figure 2   GISSI-3: Six-week survival in nitrates group and control groups.

were no significant differences between GTN-allocated and control patients in rate of reinfarction, revascularization procedures, persistent hypotension, or renal dysfunction. The nitrate group had a slightly lower rate of postinfarction angina ($2p = 0.033$).

IMPLICATIONS

The absence of a statistically significant effect of transdermal GTN was probably unexpected by comparison with the available data on which the protocol was planned. The consistency of the GISSI-3 and ISIS-4 results (14) clearly showed that the systematic administration of transdermal GTN alone for 6 weeks after AMI does not produce any clinically relevant beneficial effect. However, these findings do not rule out the benefits of transdermal GTN for the treatment of anginal pain and/or cardiac failure in AMI.

REFERENCES

1.   Multicenter Post-Infarction Research Group. Risk stratification after myocardial infarction. N Engl J Med 1983; 309:331–336.
2.   Moss AJ, Bigger JT, Odoroff CL. Postinfarct risk stratification. Progr Cardiovasc Dis 1987; 29:389–412.
3.   White HD, Norris RM, Brown MA, et al. Left ventricular end-systolic volume as the major determinant of survival after recovery from myocardial infarction. Circulation 1987; 76:44–51.
4.   Oldroyd KG, Pye MP, Ray SG, et al. Effects of early captopril administration on infarct expansion, left ventricular remodeling and exercise capacity after acute myocardial infarction. Am J Cardiol 1991; 68:713–718.
5.   Sharpe N, Smith H, Murphy J, Greaves S, Hart H, Bamble G. Early prevention of left ventricular dysfunction after myocardial infarction with angiotensin-converting-enzyme inhibition. Lancet 1991; 337:872–876.
6.   Jugdutt BI, Warnica JJ. Intravenous nitroglycerin therapy to limit myocardial infarct size, expansion, and complications. Circulation 1988; 78:906–919.
7.   Eaton LW, Weiss JL, Bulkley BG, Garrison JB, Weisfeldt M. Regional cardiac dilation after acute myocardial infarction. N Engl J Med 1979; 300:57–62.
8.   Pfeffer MA, Braunwald E. Ventricular remodeling after myocardial infarction. Experimental observations and clinical implications. Circulation 1990; 81:1161–1172.
9.   Pfeffer MA, Kamas GA, Vaughan DE, Parisi AF, Braunwald E. Effect of captopril on progressive ventricular dilation after anterior myocardial infarction. N Engl J Med 1988; 319:80–86.
10. Sharpe N, Murphy J, Smith H, Hannan S. Treatment of patients with symptomless left ventricular dysfunction after myocardial infarction. Lancet 1988; i:255–259.
11. Yusuf S, Collins R, MacMahon S, Peto R. Effect of intravenous nitrates on mortality in acute myocardial infarction: an overview of the randomised trials. Lancet 1988; i:1088–1092.
12. Swedberg K, Held P, Kjekshus J, et al. Effects of the early administration of enalapril on mortality in patients with acute myocardial infarction: results of the Cooperative New Scandinavian Enalapril Survival Study II (CONSENSUS II). N Engl J Med 1992; 327:678–684.
13. Gruppo Italiano per lo Studio della Sopravvivenza nell'Infarto Miocardico. GISSI-3: effects of lisinopril and transdermal glyceryl trinitrate singly and together on 6-week mortality and ventricular function after acute myocardial infarction. Lancet 1994; 343:1115–1122.
14. ISIS Collaborative Group, Oxford, UK. ISIS -4: randomised study of oral isosorbide mononitrate in over 50,000 patients with suspected acute myocardial infarction. Circulation 1993; 88: I–394.

35

ISIS-4

PETER SLEIGHT

ISIS-4 (Fourth International Study of Infarct Survival) Collaborative
Group. ISIS-4: a randomized factorial trial assessing early oral captopril,
oral mononitrate, and intravenous magnesium sulfate in 58,050 patients
with suspected acute myocardial infarction. Lancet 1995; 345:669–685.

INTRODUCTION

Nitrates, such as inhaled amyl nitrate or sublingual trinitroglycerine, are one of the oldest
and most effective remedies for the relief of angina pectoris. They rapidly reduce cardiac
work by a combination of venous and arterial dilatation. The former reduces venous return
(preload) and pulmonary venous congestion, while the latter reduces afterload, and the
combined action reduces arterial pressure.

In both experimental and human studies, nitrates have been shown to reduce infarct
size, improve left ventricular (LV) function, and reduce remodeling (1). Although the
use of intermittent nitrate therapy is effective for symptom relief, continuous therapy,
particularly intravenous therapy, leads rapidly to pharmacological tolerance and reduced
or absent clinical benefit (2,3).

Despite this, several small trials of intravenous or oral nitrates suggested some overall benefit in patients with myocardial infarction, although most individual trials were too
small to be conclusive (3–7). As a result, early intravenous nitrates became routine treatment in many countries, although not in the United Kingdom. Because of the uncertainty,
and also because of growing evidence of the problems of tolerance, the nitrate arm of
ISIS-4 was designed as a study of an available mononitrate formulation or matching placebo [Imdur® Astra was designed to produce a sustained level of nitrate, but with a nitrate-
free period of some hours, in order to reduce the development of tolerance (8)]. Because
remodeling of the LV function is a slow process, taking days or weeks, the mononitrate/
placebo tablet was to be taken for 4 weeks.

PATIENTS AND METHODS

The details of the conduct of the ISIS-4 study have been outlined in earlier chapters (Chap.
21) and in the ISIS-4 publication (9). Briefly, 58,050 patients with suspected MI and
within 24 hours of onset were randomized to isosorbide mononitrate (Imdur® Astra) or

placebo between 1991 and 1993 in more than 1000 hospitals around the world (31 countries).

The median time to entry was 8 hours from onset of symptoms. About 80% had ST elevation on the initial ECG, about three quarters were male, and about 30% were over 70 years old. Infarction was later confirmed in 92% of all randomized patients.

Importantly, almost half of the patients received nontrial intravenous nitrates, and a further 8% received other short-term nitrates. This use varied strikingly from country to country, and it appeared that nontrial nitrate use was dictated more by coronary care unit policies for routine therapy than by the individual patient characteristics. Intravenous nitrates were used in about 75% of patients in the United States and Germany, but in less than a quarter in the United Kingdom, Sweden, and New Zealand. As expected in a blinded comparison, these nontrial nitrates were used equally in active and placebo nitrate groups.

Because we had concerns about the dangers of hypotension in a trial where three potentially hypotensive drugs were being tested together, we excluded patients with sustained entry systolic blood pressure (SBP) much below 100 mmHg; as a result only 4% developed cardiogenic shock, as opposed to 7% in ISIS-3 (10).

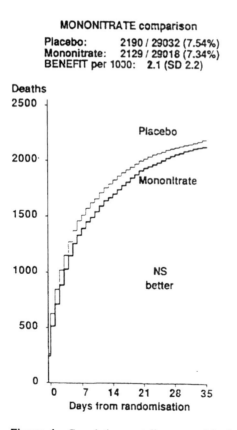

Figure 1 Cumulative mortality reported in days 1–35 for all patients allocated 1 month of oral controlled-release mononitrate (thicker line) versus all allocated matching placebo. (From Ref. 9.)

RESULTS

Effects of Oral Mononitrate on 5-Week Mortality and Later

There were nonsignificantly fewer deaths at 5 weeks (Fig. 1) on mononitrate compared with placebo (7.34% vs. 7.54%), with no divergence over the following year. In a post hoc analysis there was a significant reduction in mortality in the first 24–36 hours (from 2.16% on placebo to 1.77% on mononitrate, $p < 0.001$). If this effect were real one might have expected it to be more striking in those not receiving nontrial nitrate, but this was not the case. It does, however, mean that early nitrate treatment (e.g., for symptoms) is safe. Disappointingly there was no longer-term reduction in mortality with nitrate use, which might have been expected if reduction in LV dilatation (remodeling) had occurred.

In addition, there was no particular subgroup in which nitrates appeared to be more promising, including those with heart failure at entry. There did not appear to be any interaction between nitrates and other study treatments (Fig. 2).

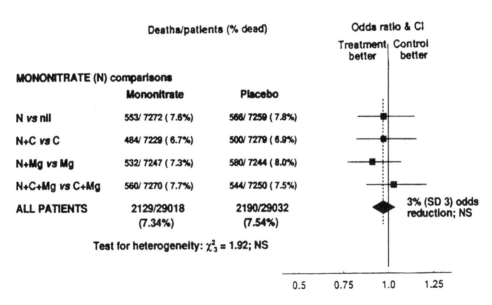

Figure 2 Nitrate result in ISIS-4. Mortality in days 0–35 subdivided by other randomly allocated study treatments. C = captopril, N = mononitrate; Mg = magnesium. Odds ratios (ORs: black squares with areas proportional to the amount of ''statistical information'' in each subdivision) comparing the mortality among patients allocated the study treatment to that among patients allocated the relevant control are plotted for each of the treatment comparisons, subdivided by the other randomly allocated study treatments, along with their 99% confidence intervals (CIs: horizontal lines). For the overall treatment comparison, the result and its 95% CI is represented by a diamond, with the overall proportional reduction (or increase) and statistical significance given alongside. Squares or diamonds to the left of the solid vertical line indicate benefit (significant at $2p < 0.01$ when the entire horizontal line is to the left of the vertical line). Chi-square tests for evidence of heterogeneity of the sizes of the ORs in the subdivisions are also given. (From Ref. 9.)

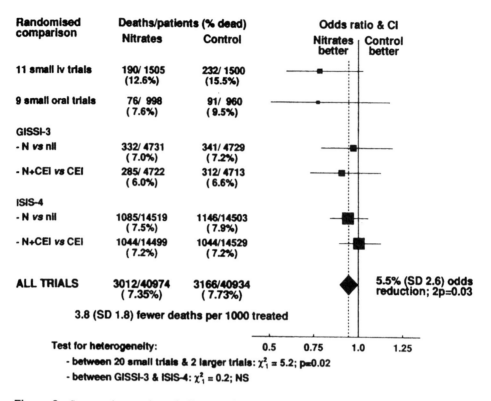

Figure 3 Systematic overview of effects on short-term mortality of starting nitrates early in acute myocardial infarction. Symbols as in Figure 2. (From Ref. 9.)

Effect of Mononitrate on Other Clinical Events

There was no evidence that 1 month of nitrate therapy reduced the number of patients who went on to develop proven infarction or later reinfarction. Nor, perhaps at first surprisingly, was there any reduction compared with placebo in reported postinfarction angina during the hospital stay. There was a small but significant excess of hypotension (8.1% vs. 6.7%, $p < 0.0001$). Headache was also significantly more common on active nitrate (2.31% vs. 0.44%, $p < 0.0001$).

DISCUSSION

Although the benefit from mononitrate was small and statistically nonsignificant, ISIS-4 demonstrated, as did GISSI-3 (11), that routine use of nitrates is safe in the early phase of acute MI. It does cause a small increase in side effects, and so the routine use of nitrates for patients with no clear need for them does not seem justified.

For patients with continued pain or with signs or symptoms of heart failure, ISIS-4 has shown that treatment with an oral preparation of isosorbide mononitrate is safe and likely to be effective. It may be argued that the study showed no evidence of reduction in reported anginal symptoms in hospital, but one must note that this trial was not designed to answer such a question reliably.

The overall result in ISIS-4 is similar to that of GISSI-3 (11) and of another large trial of a nitric oxide donor, ESPRIM (12), which randomized molsidomine in over 4000 patients, with a mortality at 2 weeks of 8.4% on active treatment versus 8.8% of controls (Fig. 3).

It is therefore clear that the previous small trials and their overview had given a falsely optimistic result, perhaps because of publication bias in favor of positive results. Egger et al. have published a funnel plot of the smaller nitrate trials versus one large trial (13), which shows that most of the point estimates for the former small studies are more positive than the large study, supporting a publication bias (Fig. 4).

Both the ISIS-4 and GISSI-3 trials have been criticized because of the large contamination by nonstudy use of other nitrates, particularly early intravenous nitrate, widely used as routine therapy in some countries. However, as pointed out above, such use of nonstudy nitrates did not seem to be guided by physician selection, but more by local protocol. The results of ISIS-4 in countries with high use of routine nontrial nitrates were no worse than those countries (like the United Kingdom) with no such large contamination. Further, the results were similar among patients who did not receive nonstudy nitrates.

Recent studies of other vasodilating drugs, particularly the nifedipine-like short-acting dihydropyridines, have shown no benefit either in the acute phase of MI or post-MI (14). It may be that short-acting vasodilators, which sometimes lower blood pressure sharply, produce baroreflex sympathetic activation, which may be harmful to some patients but beneficial to others.

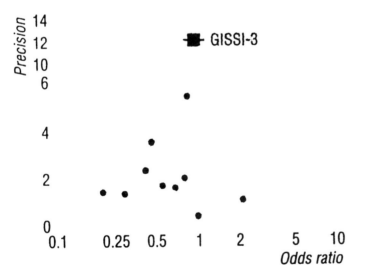

Figure 4 Funnel plot of nitrates smaller trials compared with the much larger GISSI-3. Filled circles indicate odd ratios from smaller trials. The square and horizontal line indicate odds ratio from GISSI-3 and 95% confidence interval. Note that almost all the points lie to the left of the large trial, perhaps indicating the results of publication bias. (From Ref. 13.)

CONCLUSION

Although 1 month of mononitrate in ISIS-4 was clearly safe, there seems no evidence for its routine use in otherwise complication-free patients.

REFERENCES

1. Jugdutt BI. Prevention of ventricular remodelling post myocardial infarction: timing and duration of therapy. Can J Cardiol 1993; 9:103–114.
2. Parker JO, Farrell B, Lahey KA, Moe G. Effect of intervals between doses on the development of tolerance to isosorbide dinitrate. N Engl J Med 1987; 316:1440–1444.
3. ISIS-4 (Fourth International Study of Infarct Survival) Pilot Study Investigators. Randomised controlled trial of oral captopril, of oral isosorbide mononitrate and of intravenous magnesium sulphate started early in acute myocardial infarction: safety and haemodynamic effects. Eur Heart J 1994; 15:608–619.
4. Latini R, Avanzini F, De Nicolao A, Rocchetti M, and the GISSI-3 Investigators. Effects of lisinopril and nitroglycerin on blood pressure early after myocardial infarction: the GISSI-3 pilot study. Clin Pharmacol Ther 1994; 56:680–692.
5. Jugdutt B, Tymchak W, Humen D, Gulamhusein S, Hales M. Prolonged nitroglycerin versus captopril therapy on remodelling after transmural myocardial infarction. Circulation 1990; 82: 111–142.
6. Yusuf S, Collins R, MacMahon S, Peto R. Effects of intravenous nitrates on mortality in acute myocardial infarction: an overview of the randomsied trials. Lancet 1988; i:1088–1092.
7. Jugdutt BI, Neiman JC, Michorowski BL, Tymchak WJ, Genge TJ, Fitzpatrick LK. Persistent improvement in left ventricular geometry and function by prolonged nitroglycerin therapy after anterior transmural acute myocardial infarction. J Am Coll Cardiol 1990; 15:214A.
8. Kendall MJ. Long-term therapeutic efficacy with once-daily isosorbide-5-mononitrate (Imdur®). J Clin Pharmacol Ther 1990; 15:169–185.
9. ISIS-4 (Fourth International Study of Infarct Survival) Collaborative Group. ISIS-4: a randomised factorial trial assessing early oral captopril, oral mononitrate, and intravenous magnesium sulphate in 58,050 patients with suspected acute myocardial infarction. Lancet 1995; 345:669–685.
10. ISIS-3 (Third International Study of Infarct Survival) Collaborative Group. ISIS-3: a randomised trial of streptokinase versus tissue plasminogen activator versus anistreplase and of aspirin plus heparin versus aspirin alone among 41,299 cases of suspected acute myocardial infarction. Lancet 1992; 339:753–770.
11. GISSI-3 (Gruppo Italiano per lo Studio della Streptochinasi nell'Infarto Miocardico). GISSI-3: effects of lisinopril and transdermal glyceryl trinitrate singly and together on 6-week mortality and ventricular function after myocardial infarction. Lancet 1994; 343:1115–1121.
12. European Study of Prevention of Infarct with Molsidomine (ESPRIM) Group. The ESPRIM trial: short-term treatment of acute myocardial infarction with molsidomine. Lancet 1994; 344: 91–97.
13. Egger M, Davey Smith G, Schneider M, Minder C. Bias in meta-analysis detected by a simple, graphical test. Br Med J 1997; 315:629–634.
14. Sleight P. Calcium antagonists during and after myocardial infarction. Drugs 1996; 51(2): 216–225.

Section M
Magnesium

In this section we present two randomized trials of the same intervention—intravenous infusion of magnesium sulfate—with differing outcomes. In LIMIT-2, there was a significant mortality benefit associated with treatment. In ISIS-4, there was not, and the large sample size of the latter trial (58,050) virtually excluded a beneficial effect. The authors offer differing interpretations of the discrepancy. Woods argues that there may have been subtle differences in the treatment protocol that diminished the likelihood of ISIS-4 detecting the treatment benefit seen in LIMIT-2. He also questions the primacy of large, simply designed trials (''mega-trials'') in resolving all questions of efficacy. Sleight argues that such large trials are, in fact, more reliable and more definitive, and that the disparate findings can be explained entirely on statistical grounds. Whichever interpretation one finds more compelling, we agree with both authors when they conclude that the role of intravenous magnesium in the care of patients with acute myocardial infarction is uncertain, and therefore cannot be recommended for routine use.

36

LIMIT-2

KENT L. WOODS

Woods KL, Fletcher S, Roffe C, Haider Y. Intravenous magnesium sulfate in suspected acute myocardial infarction: results of the second Leicester intravenous magnesium intervention trial (LIMIT-2). Lancet 1992;339:1553–1558.

BACKGROUND

The LIMIT-2 study was planned in response to the findings of several earlier clinical trials that had indicated that intravenous magnesium salts, administered in the acute phase of myocardial infarction, could reduce mortality (1). Two studies in particular, published almost simultaneously but conducted independently, had shown a striking similarity of design and outcome. Working in Leicester, Smith et al. had randomly assigned 400 patients admitted to a coronary care unit with suspected acute myocardial infarction to receive either a 24-hour intravenous infusion of magnesium sulfate or an equivalent volume of saline (2). In the first 24 hours there were 2 deaths among 92 patients with confirmed acute myocardial infarction in the magnesium group and 7 deaths among 93 patients with confirmed infarction in the saline group. Subsequent follow-up (3) showed a nonsignificantly lower mortality in the magnesium group over the following 2 years. Rasmussen et al. randomly allocated 273 patients with suspected acute myocardial infarction (AMI) to receive either a constant infusion of 62 mmol of magnesium chloride over 48 hours or an equivalent volume of saline (4). There were 56 patients with confirmed AMI among the 136 patients in the magnesium group, compared with 74 of the 137 patients in the saline group ($p < 0.05$). Among these, there were 7 deaths by 4 weeks in the magnesium group and 19 in the saline group ($p = 0.08$). The number of patients with clinically documented arrhythmias in the first week was lower in the magnesium group (21 vs. 47, $p = 0.004$). The difference was in supraventricular arrhythmias. Follow-up over the first year showed significantly lower all-cause mortality in the magnesium group ($p = 0.018$), which was entirely due to lower mortality from ischemic heart disease ($p = 0.006$) (5). Although both trials were too small to be conclusive, the similarities between them justified further research. There was in the literature some information on the cardiovascular effects of elevated levels of serum magnesium, which might be of benefit in the context of acute myocardial infarction (6). These reported effects included systemic and coronary vasodilatation, antiarrhythmic actions, inhibition of platelet function, and a concentration-dependent protection of myocardial contractile function during ischemia. However, it was clearly necessary to carry out a further study to test the hypothesis that intravenous magnesium salts improve the outcome of acute myocardial infarction, with the following design improvements:

1. Sufficient sample size to give adequate statistical power for a mortality endpoint using realistic assumptions of placebo group mortality and treatment effect.
2. A treatment regimen giving rapid elevation of plasma $[Mg^{2+}]$ to the target concentration at the earliest possible time in the evolution of AMI, i.e., a loading dose followed by a maintenance infusion. A constant infusion alone (as in both the earlier studies referred to above) takes some 6 hours to achieve steady state $[Mg^{2+}]$.
3. An intention-to-treat analysis using prespecified mortality endpoints.

DESIGN OF LIMIT-2

Entry Criteria

Patients were considered eligible if they were suspected of having AMI with onset in the preceding 24 hours. Exclusion criteria were as follows:

1. Inability or refusal to give verbal consent.
2. Complete heart block—a constraint applied because of the reported effect of raised Mg^{2+} on the AV node and the consequent possibility of delaying return of normal AV conduction.
3. Trial entry on a previous admission.
4. A clinical indication for therapeutic use of Mg^{2+}.
5. Serum creatinine > 300 μmol/liter in view of the renal excretion of Mg^{2+} and consequent risk of accumulation in the presence of substantial renal impairment.

Study Size

Descriptive historical information was available on the clinical population to be studied. The initial power calculation assumed that 60% of patients randomized would have AMI confirmed, that 28-day mortality would be 12.5% in these patients and zero in the remainder, and that the study should be able to detect a true reduction of approximately 30% in 28-day mortality with 80% probability at the two-sided 5% level of significance. This postulated treatment effect was based on the lower 95% confidence limit of a pooled analysis of available trial data. To detect any adverse outcome with minimum loss of study power, provision was made for up to 12 one-sided interim analyses at intervals of 4–6 months (7). The initial target size was 2000 patients, a total that made recruitment feasible with the clinical throughput of the Leicester Royal Infirmary coronary care unit. Particular advantages of single-center enrollment were the prior existence of a comprehensive clinical data system for all patients admitted to the unit, opportunity for consistent protocol adherence, and close control of data quality.

During the course of the study, aspirin and thrombolytic treatment were introduced into routine management in response to new trial evidence of their efficacy. Target study size was reestimated at 2500 to include 1500 patients with confirmed AMI, which was achieved during the period from September 1987 to February 1992.

Treatment Regimen

Trial treatments were provided in identical heat-sealed and numbered treatment packs of two syringes containing either magnesium sulfate solution 8 mmol in 4 ml for injection over 5 minutes and 65 mmol in 50 ml for infusion over the following 24 hours, or equal volumes of saline. A computer-generated blocked randomization schedule was used. Trial supplies were manufactured in the Sterile Production Unit of the Leicestershire District Pharmacy Service.

The infusion protocol for magnesium sulfate achieved an approximate doubling of serum magnesium concentration at the end of the loading injection (Fig. 1), sustained during the 24-hour infusion and returning to the physiological range for $[Mg^{2+}]$ at about 48 hours from randomization. This target $[Mg^{2+}]$ was chosen in the light of previous trial evidence, the reported pharmacological actions of Mg^{2+} on the cardiovascular system at this level (6), and the margin of safety provided before encountering any likelihood of Mg^{2+} toxicity.

Outcome Measures

Mortality

All-cause mortality at 28 days was used for power calculations and for interim safety analyses during the course of the trial. Long-term mortality (all causes and cause-specific) for the trial cohort was obtained by flagging the records of randomized patients in the

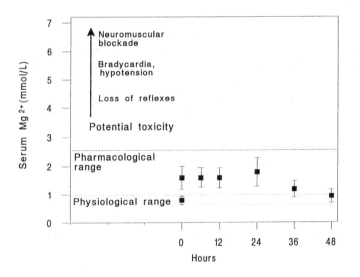

Figure 1 Serum $[Mg^{2+}]$ (mean $\pm$ SD) in a group of magnesium-treated patients ($n = 20$) in LIMIT-2 during 24 hours of trial treatment and the subsequent 24 hours. Also shown are the physiological range, the pharmacological range in which cardiovascular effects of Mg^{2+} have been reported in humans, and the range reported to be associated with risk of toxicity.

National Health Service Central Register. Death certificates were coded for cause by the Office of Population Censuses and Surveys and therefore blind to trial treatment allocation. To make possible timely interim analyses, early confirmation of each patient's survival status at 28 days from randomization was obtained from hospital and health authority records and from the general practitioner.

Morbidity

For all patients admitted to the cardiac care unit (CCU), whether entering the LIMIT-2 study or not, a standard data-set was captured giving information on medical history, presenting symptoms, clinical events, treatments, laboratory results, and final diagnosis. A discharge diagnosis of acute myocardial infarction was assigned on the basis of at least two of the following criteria: a clinical history of pain consistent with myocardial infarction; a doubling of serum cardiac enzymes (total creatinine kinase and hydroxybutyrate dehydrogenase); and ECG changes showing evolution consistent with AMI. Clinical events in the CCU and diagnosis at discharge from the CCU were recorded by staff unaware of the treatment allocation and were not subsequently revised.

Nested Substudies

Holter monitoring was performed in 70 patients within the trial for the first 24 hours after randomization. Blinded computer analysis of tapes was supplemented by visual verification of all detected abnormal rhythms (8).

Hemodynamic responses to trial treatment were studied in 44 patients using Doppler measurement of cardiac output velocity, simultaneous heart rate, and indirect blood pressure. Serum profiles of Mg^{2+} were studied in 20 randomized patients.

Results

Recruitment and Follow-Up

The interim analyses did not activate the stopping rule, and the study closed after 2316 patients had been recruited (1508 of whom had a discharge diagnosis of AMI). Mortality follow-up was 99.5% complete at one year from randomization. There was excellent balance of baseline characteristics of the patients in the magnesium and placebo groups. The major prognostic variables are shown in Table 1. In addition, analyses of the cumulative distribution of blood pressure and heart rate at baseline showed no evidence of a chance maldistribution of hemodynamically compromised patients to one or other treatment groups (Fig. 2). Median time to randomization in the study was 3 hours from symptom onset. Thrombolytic treatment was given to 35% of trial patients. In these, infusion of the thrombolytic drug (streptokinase in nearly all cases) was concurrent with the first hour of the trial infusion.

Mortality

All-cause mortality at 28 days was 7.8% in the magnesium group and 10.3% in the placebo group ($p = 0.04$), a relative reduction of 24% (95% CI 1–43%). There was no evidence of significant treatment effect modification by subgroups of age, sex, thrombolytic treatment, or aspirin treatment; the power of these subgroup analyses was, however, limited. After average follow-up of 2.7 years, cumulative all-cause mortality was 16% (2–29%) lower in the magnesium group relative to placebo ($p = 0.03$) (Fig. 3). This difference was entirely attributable to lower cumulative mortality from ischemic heart disease coded as ICD9 410–414. IHD mortality was 21% (5–35%, $p = 0.01$) lower in the magnesium

Table 1 Baseline Characteristics of Randomized Patients

	Magnesium	Placebo
Number	1159	1157
Male	855 (74%)	846 (73%)
Mean age in years (SD)	61.4 (11.4)	62.2 (11.5)
History		
Previous AMI	294 (25%)	302 (26%)
Previous angina	425 (37%)	454 (39%)
Known diabetes	116 (10%)	130 (11%)
Known hypertension	244 (21%)	222 (19%)
Current smoker	440 (38%)	439 (38%)
Ex-smoker	355 (31%)	345 (30%)
On beta-blocker	196 (17%)	191 (17%)
On diuretic	221 (19%)	224 (19%)
Cardiac arrest before trial entry	31 (3%)	31 (3%)
Elapsed time from symptom onset		
≤ 2 hr	328 (28%)	333 (29%)
≤ 4 hr	720 (62%)	742 (64%)
≤ 6 hr	863 (74%)	870 (75%)
≤ 9 hr	951 (82%)	946 (82%)
Final diagnosis		
AMI (Q-wave)	638 (55%)	631 (55%)
AMI (non–Q-wave)	116 (10%)	123 (11%)
Angina	313 (27%)	292 (25%)
Other	92 (8%)	111 (10%)
Infarct site		
Anterior	345 (46%)	381 (51%)
Inferior	348 (46%)	313 (42%)
Posterior	26 (3%)	15 (2%)
Uncertain	35 (5%)	45 (6%)
Thrombolytic/Antiplatelet treatment given on admission		
Thrombolysis	419 (36%)	402 (35%)
Aspirin	750 (65%)	767 (66%)
Prerandomization serum magnesium (mmol/liter)		
Mean (SD) serum Mg^{2+}	0.82 (0.12)	0.82 (0.12)

Source: Ref. 1.

group than in the placebo group (Fig. 4). The absolute difference in the probability of death from ischemic heart disease estimated by the Kaplan-Meier method was 2.5%, 3.0%, and 4.5% at 1, 2, and 3 years (1,56).

Morbidity

Recorded clinical events while in the CCU showed significant reduction in the occurrence of left ventricular failure, whether assessed clinically or radiologically ($p < 0.01$) (Table 2). This is supported by a lower use of diuretics and vasodilators for the treatment of heart failure in the magnesium group ($p = 0.03$). In contrast, recorded incidence of arrhythmias and the use of antiarrhythmic drugs in the unit showed no significant differences except for a slightly increased incidence of sinus bradycardia in the magnesium group,

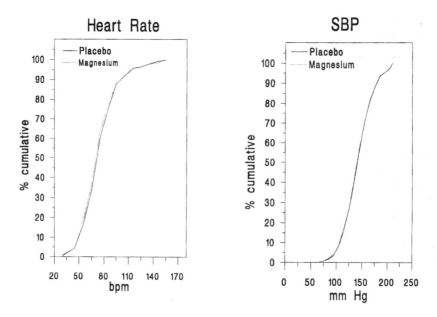

Figure 2 Cumulative distribution of prerandomization heart rate and systolic blood pressure in treatment groups of LIMIT-2.

accompanied by significantly greater use of atropine (Table 3). Since Mg^{2+} has the potential to block AV conduction at high concentrations in the laboratory, there was a reassuring lack of any significant excess of first, second, or third degree heart block or of the use of temporary pacemakers in the magnesium group. Data from the Holter monitoring substudy corroborated these findings, with no significant differences in any class of arrhythmia (8).

The hemodynamic effects of the magnesium regimen were a transient rise of 20% (SEM 5%, $p < 0.001$) in cardiac output, associated with a fall in blood pressure of 8

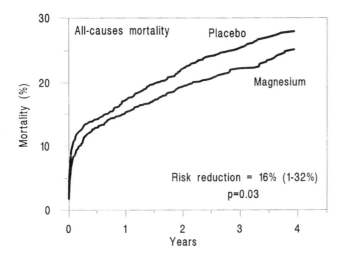

Figure 3 Cumulative all-cause mortality during long-term follow-up of patients randomized in LIMIT-2 by intention-to-treat analysis. (From Ref. 57.)

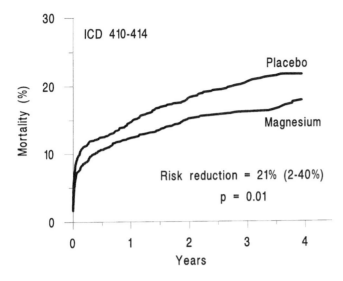

Figure 4   Cumulative mortality from ischemic heart disease (ICD9 410–414) during long-term follow-up of patients randomized in LIMIT-2 by intention-to-treat analysis. (From Ref. 56.)

mmHg plus (SEM 2.7 mmHg) systolic and 5 mmHg (SEM 1.8 mmHg) diastolic. These changes were attributable to the loading injection of magnesium and had subsided within 15 minutes.

LIMIT-2 FINDINGS IN THE CONTEXT OF OTHER EVIDENCE

Mechanism of Benefit of Mg^{2+}

Protection of Myocardial Pump Function

Impaired left ventricular function is strongly predictive of early mortality risk and poor long-term survival after AMI. The results of LIMIT-2 are internally consistent in that the

Table 2   Left Ventricular Dysfunction and Treatment in CCU

	Magnesium (n = 1159)	Placebo (n = 1157)	p-value
In-CCU events			
Clinical LVF	130 (11.2%)	172 (14.9%)	0.009
Radiological LVF	199 (17.2%)	255 (22.0%)	0.004
Hypotension	56 (4.8%)	56 (4.8%)	NS
Oliguria/anuria	26 (2.2%)	40 (3.5%)	0.08
Treatments received			
Loop diuretic	263 (22.7%)	307 (26.5%)	0.03
Sodium nitroprusside	24 (2.1%)	41 (3.5%)	0.03
Captopril	24 (2.1%)	34 (2.9%)	NS
Dopamine	28 (2.4%)	40 (3.5%)	NS
Dobutamine	32 (2.8%)	39 (3.4%)	NS

Source: Ref. 1.

Table 3 Arrhythmias and Treatment in CCU

	Magnesium ($n = 1159$)	Placebo ($n = 1157$)	p-value
In-CCU events			
Ventricular tachycardia	79 (6.8%)	93 (8.0%)	NS
Ventricular fibrillation	32 (2.8%)	44 (3.8%)	NS
Supraventricular tachycardia	21 (1.8%)	30 (2.6%)	NS
Atrial fibrillation	103 (8.9%)	111 (9.6%)	NS
Sinus bradycardia	125 (10.8%)	93 (8.0%)	0.02
Heart block	81 (7.0%)	70 (6.0%)	NS
Treatments received			
Lignocaine	53 (4.6%)	69 (6.0%)	NS
Amiodarone	48 (4.1%)	64 (5.5%)	NS
DC cardioversion	48 (4.1%)	47 (4.1%)	NS
Digoxin	71 (6.3%)	83 (7.2%)	NS
Atropine	128 (11.0%)	79 (6.8%)	0.0004
Temporary pacemaker	25 (2.2%)	19 (1.6%)	NS

Source: Adapted from Refs. 1 and 8.

incidence of clinical left ventricular failure in the CCU, 28-day mortality, and long-term mortality rate were each reduced by about a quarter in the magnesium group. The lack of any detectable difference in hemodynamic status at baseline supports the interpretation that the observed morbidity and mortality differences are treatment effects of Mg^{2+} and not due to a failure of effective randomization. There is now good evidence from a range of laboratory models of myocardial ischemia in several species, which demonstrate protection by Mg^{2+} (Table 4). Early models examining contractile function during global ischemia have been supplemented more recently by well-controlled studies measuring the effects of Mg^{2+} on contractile dysfunction and infarct size after regional ischemia, at concentrations similar to those reached in LIMIT-2.

At the level of the myocardial cell, possible mechanisms of protection by Mg^{2+} include limitation of cytoplasmic and mitochondrial calcium overload (9–11), conservation of intracellular ATP (12), and suppression of oxygen free radical production during reperfusion (13).

Antiplatelet Effects

An alternative mechanism of infarct limitation is suggested by recent work on the antiplatelet action of Mg^{2+}. Platelet activation and thrombus generation are important contributors to myocardial infarction, as indicated by the therapeutic effectiveness of antiplatelet agents such as aspirin in AMI. Mg^{2+} inhibits platelet activation in vitro and ex vivo in a dose-dependent fashion using a range of aggregants including collagen, thrombin, ADP, adrenaline, and arachidonic acid (14–16). Platelet inhibition by Mg^{2+} is synergistic with aspirin (15). In vivo, inhibition of platelet thrombus formation and embolization by intravenous Mg^{2+} has been demonstrated in experimental arterial injury (17).

Arrhythmias

Although intravenous Mg^{2+} has some antiarrhythmic effects in humans, the data from LIMIT-2 strongly indicate a lack of any antiarrhythmic action of Mg^{2+} in AMI (8). This

Table 4   Experimental Studies of Mg^{2+} Protection from Myocardial
Ischemia/Reperfusion Injury

Investigators (Ref.)	Species	Model	Effect measure	Mg^{2+} protection shown	Time window shown
Hearse et al., 1978 (49)	Rat	G	C	Yes	NE
Yano et al., 1985 (50)	Rat	G	C	Yes	Yes
Ferrari et al., 1986 (10)	Rabbit	G	C, M	Yes	NE
Borchgrevinck et al., 1989 (12)	Rat	G	C, M	Yes	NE
Hara et al., 1990 (51)	Rat	G	C, M	Yes	Yes
du Toit and Opie, 1992 (42)	Rat	G	C	Yes	Yes
Lareau et al., 1993 (52)	Human	T	C, M	Yes	NE
Ataka et al., 1993 (11)	Rabbit	G	C, M	Yes	NE
Atar et al., 1994 (53)	Pig	R	C	Yes	NE
Barros et al., 1995 (54)	Dog	R	I	Yes	NE
Christensen et al., 1994 (40)	Dog	R	I	Yes	Yes
Herzog et al., 1995 (41)	Pig	R	I	Yes	Yes
Schlack et al., 1995 (55)	Dog	R	I, C	No	NE
Leor and Kloner, 1995 (43)	Rat	R	I	Yes	Yes

G = Global ischemia; T = isolated trabeculae; R = regional ischemia; C = contractile dysfunction; I = infarct
size; M = metabolic indices; NE = not examined.

contrasts with the reports of a number of smaller studies, though it should be noted that
these have not themselves been consistent in the classes of rhythm disturbance which
appear to be modified by Mg^{2+} treatment (18–20). It is in any event unlikely that an
antiarrhythmic action of Mg^{2+} could explain a reduction in early mortality, since rhythm
disturbances are a rare cause of death in a coronary care unit. The slightly increased
incidence of sinus bradycardia in the magnesium group is consistent with the electrophysiological actions of Mg^{2+} (21,22) but affected only a minority of patients and was of no
clinical significance. Despite the potential for Mg^{2+} to delay conduction through the upper
part of the AV node, heart block was not precipitated by Mg^{2+} in LIMIT-2.

Vasodilatation

Mg^{2+} could in theory be of benefit in AMI through its vasodilator effect in the systemic
circulation, lowering peripheral resistance and reducing cardiac work (23). However, the
hemodynamic changes seen in the magnesium group of LIMIT-2 were minor and transient,
resolving quickly after the loading injection of trial treatment despite maintenance of elevated serum Mg^{2+} over the following 24 hours. It is likely that the coronary vasodilatation
produced by intravenous Mg^{2+} in humans is of similarly short duration and of no therapeutic importance.

Consistency of LIMIT-2 Results with Other Trial Evidence

Unpowered Trials

During the past decade or so, a number of relatively small randomized trials of intravenous
Mg^{2+} in AMI have been published (2,4,18,19,24–28). Recruiting up to a few hundred
patients each, their size had not been determined by appropriate power calculations though

several have shown statistically significant mortality reduction in Mg^{2+}-treated patients compared with placebo treated controls (5,25,28). Treatment protocols have varied, the total dose of Mg^{2+} ranging from 30 to 90 mmol infused over 24 to 96 hours following admission. However, the trials have been sufficiently similar in design to justify combining them in meta-analysis (29). Collectively, they indicate a highly significant reduction in short-term mortality ($p < 0.001$). Although the pooled estimate of effect is more extreme than the 28 day mortality result of LIMIT-2, there is no statistically significant heterogeneity when the LIMIT-2 data are included with them. However, the potential limitations of meta-analysis are well recognized, particularly the concern that selection bias may occur if studies with adverse or nonsignificant results are unpublished or unrecognized (30). This possibility can never be excluded with complete confidence though the lively debate which has occurred around the use of magnesium in AMI has not uncovered any overlooked trial results which would alter the outcome of meta-analysis. It should be noted that the small trials referred to here were conducted before the introduction of thrombolytic treatment or, in one case, was restricted to patients who were not considered suitable for thrombolytic treatment.

Fourth International Study of Infarct Survival (ISIS-4)

This large factorial trial of captopril, isosorbide mononitrate, and magnesium sulfate (31) is discussed elsewhere in this volume (see Chap. 37). It began recruitment while LIMIT-2 was in progress, and, like the latter, was designed to provide a properly powered test of the therapeutic effectiveness of Mg^{2+} in AMI, which had been suggested by the earlier small trials. ISIS-4 found no significant effect of intravenous magnesium sulfate on mortality, a result in striking contrast to that of LIMIT-2 and showing highly significant statistical heterogeneity with LIMIT-2 and all other trials ($p < 0.0001$). It is therefore important to examine whether there were any differences between ISIS-4 and LIMIT-2 that might have substantially modified any treatment effect.

The magnesium comparison within ISIS-4 was against open control. This is of no relevance to the mortality analysis, but raises the clear risk of reporting bias in the recording of common events such as hypotension or arrhythmias when there might be prior belief of a positive or negative association with Mg^{2+} treatment. This may account for the anomalous result that cardiogenic shock was reported more commonly in the magnesium group of ISIS-4 than in controls, but mortality was not increased.

Patients randomized into ISIS-4 had a lower baseline risk than those entering LIMIT-2, as indicated by control group mortality at 35 days of 7.2% in the former compared with placebo group mortality at 28 days in the latter of 10.3%. Contributing factors are likely to have included the selective nonrecruitment into ISIS-4 of hypotensive patients considered unsuitable for the vasodilator treatments included in the trial protocol, the higher rate of use of thrombolysis in ISIS-4 (70% vs. 35%), and late randomization in ISIS-4, which would exclude highest-risk patients dying within a few hours of admission. Although it has been reported that the mortality reduction seen with Mg^{2+} in the trials is inversely related to the baseline mortality risk, the relationship is not linear (32). There is no apparent mechanism to account for such a critical dependence of treatment effect on baseline risk, and the empirical association seems more likely to be a chance finding.

The intravenous magnesium regimen used in ISIS-4 differed only trivially from that of LIMIT-2; the loading infusion of 8 mmol was given over 15 minutes rather than 5 minutes, and the 24 hour maintenance infusion was 72 mmol (3 mmol/hour) rather than 65 mmol.

The factorial design of ISIS-4 is of no direct consequence for the magnesium comparison but was responsible for a protocol recommendation which with hindsight may have been unfortunate. Since all three active treatments in ISIS-4 are vasodilators, and since it was anticipated that most patients in the trial would also be receiving thrombolytic treatment with streptokinase, there was concern that simultaneous administration of trial treatments with streptokinase would cause a potentially hazardous degree of hypotension among those patients randomized to receive all three active trial drugs. For this reason, it was recommended that trial treatment should not be started until after thrombolysis had been carried out. Although the time interval between thrombolysis and the start of magnesium infusion was not recorded, indirect evidence suggests that it was typically 3 hours or more. It is known that the mean delay between symptom onset and randomization was 7 hours among thrombolyzed patients. According to the evidence from ISIS-3 (33), the typical delay from symptom onset to thrombolysis is likely to have been 3–4 hours. It must be concluded that thrombolyzed patients received Mg^{2+} after reperfusion and not before it, as in LIMIT-2. There may have been patients within ISIS-4 whose serum Mg^{2+} was raised before thrombolysis took effect, but they are likely to have been few in number in view of the protocol recommendation and cannot be retrospectively identified since the time of thrombolytic treatment was not recorded. The potential relevance of timing is discussed below in the light of experimental evidence now available.

Thrombolytic treatment was not given to 30% of patients randomized in ISIS-4—some 17,000 patients. The most likely reasons for nonuse of thrombolytic treatment are late presentation and diagnostic uncertainty; relatively few have a clinical contraindication (34). The nonthrombolyzed group was randomized to trial treatment an average of 12 hours from symptom onset. Therefore, despite its size, this subgroup would be of limited scope to detect treatment effects acting on early events in myocardial infarction or on spontaneous reperfusion. There would, for example, be only 57% power to detect a treatment effect having the same magnitude and time dependence as thrombolytic therapy (35).

Evidence from Other Trials

Cardiac surgery under bypass can be considered as a model of short-term ischemia and reperfusion of the human myocardium. Following the observation that plasma Mg^{2+} can fall quite markedly during bypass, several randomized trials have examined the effects of intravenous Mg^{2+} infusion on postoperative cardiac morbidity (36–38). Magnesium-treated patients have shown significantly better postoperative cardiac contractile function, lower cardiac enzyme release, and a reduction in ventricular arrhythmias compared with placebo controls.

Evidence for Critical Time Dependence of Mg^{2+} Effect

Timing of Mg^{2+} in Relation to Myocardial Reperfusion

ISIS-4 has clearly demonstrated that intravenous administration of Mg^{2+} after thrombolysis, or late after symptom onset in the absence of thrombolysis, is without therapeutic benefit. This is in striking contrast to the collective evidence from LIMIT-2 and the pooled data from 10 other smaller trials. Before dismissing this extreme diversity as random variation, it is important to examine the laboratory evidence shedding light on the effect of Mg^{2+} on early events in the pathogenesis of myocardial infarction. Recent laboratory models of myocardial reperfusion and of platelet activation on arterial endothelial lesions are relevant.

Early reperfusion of the infarct-related artery reduces infarct size and improves clinical outcome. However, reperfusion itself triggers myocardial injury, which has been attributed to the action of Ca^{2+}, the readmission of oxygen, and/or the generation of free radicals. In the clinical setting, reperfusion occurs not only after thrombolytic treatment; angiographic evidence has shown spontaneous reperfusion in at least a third of patients in the first 12–24 hours (39). Mg^{2+} protection of myocardium during ischemia and reperfusion has been shown experimentally in a wide range of laboratory models (Table 4).

Two recent studies in particular have demonstrated that the timing of Mg^{2+} administration relative to reperfusion substantially alters the treatment effect. In a dog model of coronary occlusion and reperfusion, Mg^{2+} was given to three groups of animals after 15 or 45 minutes of coronary occlusion or 15 minutes after the onset of reperfusion (40). In the first two groups, in which magnesium administration began before the onset of reperfusion, infarct size was significantly reduced by more than 60% in comparison with controls. In contrast, postreperfusion administration of Mg^{2+} did not significantly alter infarct size. In a swine model of regional ischemia and reperfusion, intracoronary Mg^{2+} started immediately at the onset of reperfusion significantly reduced infarct size by more than 50% but showed no protective effect when the administration of Mg^{2+} was delayed until one hour after the start of reperfusion (41). Other models have confirmed that supraphysiological Mg^{2+} in the perfusion medium produces myocardial contractile dysfunction (a phenomenon of stunning), but protection is lost if Mg^{2+} administration is delayed beyond the first 1–2 minutes of the onset of reperfusion (42,43).

These laboratory data indicate that the clinical effectiveness of intravenous Mg^{2+} will be powerfully modified by the timing of treatment in relation to the onset of myocardial reperfusion, whether spontaneous or induced by thrombolysis. Had the laboratory data been available at the time the Mg^{2+} trials were designed, it would have been apparent that the appropriate treatment regimen to test would achieve elevation of serum Mg^{2+} before the onset of action of any thrombolytic drug, and that raised Mg^{2+} should be maintained for as long as there was the likelihood of spontaneous reperfusion of still-viable myocardium. These conditions were met by all the early trials carried out in the prethrombolytic era and by LIMIT-2. They are unlikely to have been met for more than a small proportion of patients entering ISIS-4, and these cannot be retrospectively identified because the time delay between thrombolytic treatment and Mg^{2+} administration is not known for individual patients.

Timing in Relation to Platelet Thrombus Formation

The antiplatelet action of Mg^{2+} in vitro and ex vivo, even in the presence of aspirin, has already been referred to. Platelet activation and thrombus formation is a key early event in coronary occlusion. A recently reported experimental model has made it possible to study platelet thrombus formation and embolization at the site of an endothelial lesion in the rat femoral artery (17). Platelet thrombus formation was initiated by reperfusion of the artery after creation of the endothelial lesion and thrombus area was measured over time by in vivo microscopy. Intravenous Mg^{2+} started before reperfusion of the artery resulted in a significant 75% reduction in thrombus area; a third of the animals showed no thrombus formation at all. Intravenous infusion of Mg^{2+} beginning 10 minutes after reperfusion of the artery had no effect on the area of thrombus formed; thrombus was present in all animals in this group. These data suggest that supraphysiological Mg^{2+}

inhibits early events in the cascade of platelet activation following exposure of circulating platelets to thrombogenic subendothelial tissue. The implication for a clinical trial design is, again, that initiation of Mg^{2+} before reperfusion may be critically important if clinical outcome is to be modified.

INTERPRETATIONS OF THE LIMIT-2 DATA

The present state of the evidence in relation to the efficacy of Mg^{2+} in AMI is unsatisfactory, in that there are two widely divergent interpretations of the available data (31,35, 44–46). The issues that have been raised go beyond the specific therapeutic question of Mg^{2+}. Inability to reconcile the findings of three widely used research techniques—meta-analysis, a conventionally powered placebo-controlled trial, and a "mega-trial" (large, simple trial)—has important implications for their informativeness in other areas.

　　The first view is that ISIS-4, by virtue of its size, has shown definitively that intravenous Mg^{2+} has no effect on mortality of AMI. To support this argument it is necessary to accept the following propositions:

1. The meta-analyses of unpowered Mg^{2+} trials were sufficiently influenced by selection bias as to produce a strong positive bias in the pooled treatment effect estimate.
2. The positive result of LIMIT-2 arose from a type 1 error.
3. The various Mg^{2+} trials can be considered replicate experiments testing the same treatment effect, and empirical evidence of statistical heterogeneity between ISIS-4 and the other trials can be disregarded.
4. The experimental evidence for myocardial protection by Mg^{2+} during ischemia/reperfusion, and for Mg^{2+} inhibition of platelet function synergistic with aspirin, cannot be extrapolated to the pathophysiology of AMI.

An important corollary of this view is that the mega-trial must become the definitive test of therapeutic efficacy, and treatments cannot be confidently adopted on the evidence of meta-analysis supported by a hypothesis-testing trial of conventional design and power.

　　The alternative view is that the differing results of the trials reflect real (though unintentional) differences in the Mg^{2+} regimens that were actually tested. This conclusion requires that the following propositions be accepted:

1. A true treatment effect of Mg^{2+} was missed in the main analysis of ISIS-4.
2. All subgroup analyses permitted by the available data within ISIS-4 failed to include those treatment conditions under which Mg^{2+} could achieve a real effect on mortality or had insufficient power to demonstrate it.

The broader implication of such a view is that mega-trials have the potential to miss important treatment effects. Possible reasons include several sources of bias toward the null where data quality or protocol adherence are poor, and low power in retrospective subgroup analyses even when patient numbers are large (35). For example, the ISIS-4 captopril analysis failed to identify mortality reduction by captopril in a subgroup of over 8000 patients with heart failure at randomization (31); ACE inhibitors are now accepted to reduce mortality in such patients on the evidence of conventional trials recruiting around 2000 patients (47,48). The assumption that very large trials will not miss important treatment effects is thereby disproved.

In summary, a trials literature of more than 60,000 randomized patients has so far failed to define the place of intravenous Mg^{2+} in the early management of AMI. Laboratory research is now providing information on effect mechanisms that were inadequately understood when the trials were designed. Further work to resolve this controversy will help us to understand better the interdependence of empirical and mechanistic evidence and the strengths and weaknesses of different study designs. While the efficacy of intravenous Mg^{2+} continues to be debated, its safety, simplicity, and low cost are well established. If it is to be used, it should be started at the earliest opportunity with the aim of promptly doubling serum $[Mg^{2+}]$ and sustaining this level for as long as there is any likelihood of reperfusion of viable myocardium.

REFERENCES

1. Woods KL, Fletcher S, Roffe C, Haider Y. Intravenous magnesium sulphate in suspected acute myocardial infarction: results of the second Leicester Intravenous Magnesium Intervention Trial (LIMIT-2). Lancet 1992; 339:1553–1558.
2. Smith LF, Heagarty AM, Bing RF, Barnett DB. Intravenous infusion of magnesium sulphate after acute myocardial infarction: effects on arrhythmias and mortality. Int J Cardiol 1986; 12:175–180.
3. Woods KL, Fletcher S, Smith LFP. Intravenous magnesium in suspected acute myocardial infarction. Br Med J 1992; 304:119.
4. Rasmussen HS, Norregard P, Lindeneg O, McNair P, Backer P, Balsev S. Intravenous magnesium in acute myocardial infarction. Lancet 1986; i:234–236.
5. Rasmussen HS, Gronbaek M, Balslov CS, Nerregard P, McNair P. One-year death rate in 270 patients with suspected myocardial infarction, initially treated with intravenous magnesium or placebo. Clin Cardiol 1988; 11:377–381.
6. Woods KL. Possible pharmacological actions of magnesium in acute myocardial infarction. Br J Clin Pharmacol 1991; 32:3–10.
7. DeMets DL, Ware JH. Group sequential methods for clinical trials with a one-sided hypothesis. Biometrika 1980; 67:651–660.
8. Roffe C, Fletcher S, Woods KL. Investigation of the effects of intravenous magnesium sulphate on cardiac rhythm in acute myocardial infarction. Br Heart J 1994; 71:141–145.
9. White RE, Hartzell HC. Magnesium ions in cardiac function. Regulator of ion channels and second messengers. Biochem Pharmacol 1989; 38(6):859–867.
10. Ferrari R, Curello AS, Ceconi C, DiLisa F, Raddino R, Visioli O. Myocardial recovery during post-ischaemic reperfusion: effects of nifedipine, calcium and magnesium. J Mol Cell Cardiol 1986; 8:487–498.
11. Ataka K, Chen D, McCully J, Levitsky S, Feinberg H. Magnesium cardioplegia prevents accumulation of cytosolic calcium in the ischemic myocardium. J Mol Cell Cardiol 1993; 25:1387–1390.
12. Borchgrevink PC, Bergan AS, Bakoy OE, Jynge P. Magnesium and reperfusion of ischaemic rat heart as assessed by ^{31}P-NMR. Am J Physiol 1989; 256:H195–H204.
13. Dickens BF, Weglicki WB, Li YS, Mak IT. Magnesium deficiency in vitro enhances free radical-induced intracellular oxidation and cytotoxicity in endothelial cells. FEBS Lett 1992; 311:187–191.
14. Gawaz M, Ott I, Reininger AJ, Neumann FJ. Effects of magnesium on platelet aggregation and adhesion. Thrombosis Haemostasis 1994; 72(6):912–918.
15. Ravn HB, Vissinger H, Kristensen SD, Husted SE. Magnesium inhibits platelet activity—an in vitro study. Thrombosis Haemostasis 1996; 76:88–93.

16. Ravn HB, Vissinger H, Kristensen SD, Wennmalm A, Thygesen K, Husted SE. Magnesium inhibits platelet activity—an infusion study in healthy volunteers. Thrombosis Haemostasis 1996; 75:939–944.

17. Ravn HB, Kristensen SD, Hjortdal VE, Thygesen K, Husted SE. Early administration of intravenous magnesium inhibits arterial thrombus formation in rats. Circulation 1996; Suppl 94: I-461.

18. Ceremuzynski L, Jurgiel R, Kulakowski P, Gebalska J. Threatening arrhythmias in acute myocardial infarction are prevented by intravenous magnesium sulphate. Am Heart J 1989; 18: 1333–1334.

19. Abraham AS, Rosenmann D, Kramer M, Balkin J, Zion M, Farbstein H, Eylath U. Magnesium in the prevention of lethal arrhythmias in acute myocardial infarction. Arch Int Med 1987; 147:753–755.

20. Rasmussen HS, Suenson M, Norregard P, Balslev S. Magnesium infusion reduces the incidence of arrhythmias in acute myocardial infarction. A double-blind placebo-controlled study. Clin Cardiol 1987; 10:351–356.

21. Kulick DL, Hong R, Ryzen E, Rude RK, Rubin JN, Elkayam U, Rahimtoola SH, Bhandari AK. Electrophysiologic effects of intravenous magnesium in patients with normal conduction systems and no clinical evidence of significant cardiac disease. Am Heart J 1988; 115(2):367–373.

22. Rogiers P, Vermeier W, Kesteloot H. Effect of the infusion of magnesium sulfate during atrial pacing on ECG intervals, serum electrolytes, and blood pressure. Am Heart J 1989; 117:1278–1283.

23. Vigorito C, Giordano A, Ferraro P, Acanfora D, DeCaprio L, Naddeo C, Rengo F. Haemodynamic effects of magnesium sulphate on the normal human heart. Am J Cardiol 1991; 67: 1435–1437.

24. Feldstedt M, Bouchelouche P, Svenningsen A, Boesgaard S, Brooks L, Aldershvile J, Skagen K, Godtfredsen J, Lech Y. Failing effect of magnesium-substitution in acute myocardial infarction. Eur Heart J 1988; 9:226 (P1255).

25. Shechter M, Hod H, Marks N, Behar S, Kaplinsky E, Rabinowitz B. Beneficial effect of magnesium sulfate in acute myocardial infarction. Am J Cardiol 1990; 66:271–274.

26. Thögersen AM, Johnson O, Wester PO. Effects of intravenous magnesium sulphate in suspected acute myocardial infarction on acute arrhythmias and long-term outcome. Int J Cardiol 1995; 49:143–151.

27. Pereira D, Pereira TG, Rabaçal C, Carvalho E, Linder E, Afonso JS, Pereira JN, Halpern MJ, Fernandes JS. Efeito da administração de SO$_4$Mg por via intra-venosa na fase aguda do enfarte do miocárdio. Rev Port Cardiol 1990; 9:205–210.

28. Shechter M, Hod H, Chouraqui P, Kaplinsky E, Rabinowitz B. Magnesium therapy in acute myocardial infarction when patients are not candidates for thrombolytic therapy. Am J Cardiol 1995; 75:321–323.

29. Teo KK, Yusuf S, Collins R, Held PH, Peto R. Effects of intravenous magnesium in suspected acute myocardial infarction: an overview of the randomized trials. Br Med J 1991; 303:1499–1503.

30. Thompson SG, Pocock SJ. Can meta-analysis be trusted? Lancet 1991; 338:1127–1130.

31. ISIS-4 (Fourth International Study of Infarct Survival) Collaborative Group. ISIS-4: a randomised factorial trial assessing early oral captopril, oral mononitrate, and intravenous magnesium sulphate in 58,050 patients with suspected acute myocardial infarction. Lancet 1995; 345:669–685.

32. Antman EM, Lau J, Berkey C, McIntosh M, Chalmers TC, Mosteller F. Large versus small trials of magnesium for acute myocardial infarction: big numbers do not tell the whole story. Circulation 1994; 90 (suppl 1):325.

33. ISIS-3 (Third International Study of Infarct Survival) Collaborative Group. ISIS-3: a randomised comparison of streptokinase vs tissue plasminogen activator vs antistreplase and of aspirin

plus Xheparin vs aspirin alone among 41,299 cases of suspected acute myocardial infarction. Lancet 1992; 339:753–770.

34. European Secondary Prevention Study Group. Translation of clinical trials into practice: a European population-based study of the use of thrombolysis for acute myocardial infarction. Lancet 1996; 347:1203–1207.

35. Woods KL. Mega-trials and the management of acute myocardial infarction. Lancet 1995; 346:611–614.

36. England MR, Gordon G, Salem M, Chernow B. Magnesium administration and dysrhythmias after cardiac surgery. A placebo-controlled, double-blind, randomized trial. J Am Med Assoc 1992; 268(17):2395–2402.

37. Caspi J, Rudis E, Bar I, Safadi T, Saute M. Effects of magnesium on myocardial function after coronary artery bypass grafting. Ann Thorac Surg 1995; 59:942–947.

38. Karmy-Jones R, Hamilton A, Dzavik V, Allegreto M, Finegan BA, Koshal A. Magnesium sulfate prophylaxis after cardiac operations. Ann Thorac Surg 1995; 59:502–507.

39. de Wood MA, Spores J, Notske R, Mouser LT, Burroughs R, Golden MS, Lang HT. Prevalence of total coronary occlusion during the early hours of transmural myocardial infarction. N Engl J Med 1980; 303(16):897–902.

40. Christensen CW, Rieder MA, Silverstein EL, Gencheff NE. Magnesium sulfate reduces myocardial infarct size when administered before but not after coronary reperfusion in a canine model. Circulation 1995; 92:2617–2621.

41. Herzog WR, Schlossberg ML, MacMurdy KS, Edenbaum LR, Gerber MJ, Vogel RA, Serebruany VL. Timing of magnesium therapy affects experimental infarct size. Circulation 1995; 92:2622–2626.

42. du Toit EF, Opie LH. Modulation of severity of reperfusion stunning in the isolated rat heart by agents altering calcium flux at onset of reperfusion. Circ Res 1992; 70:960–967.

43. Leor J, Kloner RA. Does magnesium have a place in the therapy of acute myocardial infarction? Significance of early vs. late reperfusion. American College of Cardiology 44th Annual Scientific Session, New Orleans, LA, 1995, p. 189A.

44. Yusuf S, Flather M. Magnesium in acute myocardial infarction. ISIS-4 provides no ground for its routine use. Br Med J 1995; 310:751–752.

45. Baxter GF, Sumeray MS, Walker JM. Infarct size and magnesium: insights into LIMIT-2 and ISIS-4 from experimental studies. Lancet 1996; 348:1424–1426.

46. Antman EM. Magnesium in acute MI—timing is critical. Circulation 1995; 92:2367–2372.

47. The Acute Infarction Ramipril Efficacy (AIRE) Study Investigators. Effect of ramipril on mortality and morbidity of survivors of acute myocardial infarction with clinical evidence of heart failure. Lancet 1993; 342:821–827.

48. Pfeffer MA, Braunwald E, Moye LA, Basta L, Brown EJ, Cuddy TE, Davis BR, Geltman EM, Goldman S, Flaker GC, Klein M, Lamas GA, Packer M, Rouleau J, Rouleau JL, Rutherford J, Werthiemer JH, Hawkins CM, SAVE Investigators. Effect of captopril on mortality and morbidity in patients with left ventricular dysfunction after myocardial infarction. N Engl J Med 1992; 327:669–677.

49. Hearse DJ, Stewart DA, Braimbridge MV. Myocardial protection during ischaemic cardiac arrest. J Thorac Cardiovasc Surg 1978; 75(6):877–885.

50. Yano Y, Milam DF, Alexander JC. Terminal magnesium cardioplegia: protective effect in the isolated rat heart model using calcium accentuated ischemic damage. J Surg Res 1985; 39: 529–534.

51. Hara A, Matsumura H, Abiko Y. Beneficial effect of magnesium on the isolated perfused rat heart during reperfusion after ischaemia: comparison between pre-ischaemic and post-ischaemic administration of magnesium. Naunyn-Schmiedeberg's Arch Pharmacol 1990; 342:100–106.

52. Lareau S, Boyle A, Deslauriers R, Keon WJ, Kroft T, Labow RS. Magnesium enhances function of postischaemic human myocardial tissue. Cardiovasc Res 1993; 27:1009–1014.

53. Atar D, Serebruany V, Poulton J, Godard J, Schneider A, Herzog WR. Effects of magnesium supplementation in a porcine model of myocardial ischemia and reperfusion. J Cardiovasc Pharmacol 1994; 24:603–611.

54. Barros LFM, Chags ACP, da Luz PL, Pileggi F. Magnesium treatment of acute myocardial infarction: effects on necrosis in an occlusion/reperfusion dog model. Int J Cardiol 1995; 48: 3–9.

55. Schlack W, Bier F, Schäfer M, Uebing A, Schäfer S, Borchard U, Thämer V. Intracoronary magnesium is not protective against acute reperfusion injury in the regional ischaemic-reperfused dog heart. Eur J Clin Invest 1995; 25:501–509.

37

ISIS-4

PETER SLEIGHT

ISIS-4 (Fourth International Study of Infarct Survival) Collaborative Group. ISIS-4: a randomized factorial trial assessing early oral captopril, oral mononitrate, and intravenous magnesium sulfate in 58,050 patients with suspected acute myocardial infarction. Lancet 1995; 345:669-685.

INTRODUCTION

During the last 20 years there has been considerable experimental and clinical interest in the possible use of magnesium in acute myocardial ischemia (MI).

Magnesium has a number of potentially useful actions. First it appears to limit the harmful entry of calcium into ischemic cells, which may be cytoprotective and also anti-arrhythmic (1). Next, it acts as a coronary and general vasodilator, increasing coronary flow and reducing afterload and hence cardiac work (2–4). It also has an antiplatelet effect (5).

In experimental animals, magnesium given before or shortly after a coronary occlusion can limit infarct size, especially in magnesium-deficient animals (6). A recent epidemiological survey of 17 Swedish municipalities examining magnesium levels in local drinking water and death rates from myocardial infarction found an inverse relation, i.e., in those areas with the highest magnesium content there was a significantly reduced risk of death during myocardial infarction (approximately 35%) (7).

Because of earlier scientific work, clinical trials of magnesium as a treatment for MI began in humans. These culminated in a promising result in the Leicester Intravenous Magnesium Intervention Trial (LIMIT-2) (8,9), which showed a reduction in mortality of about 25%, albeit with wide confidence limits, approaching zero. As a result, magnesium was included as part of the ISIS-4 protocol (10), with the active design participation of Dr. Kent Woods, the chairman of the Leicester LIMIT Studies.

THE ISIS-4 TRIAL

The general outline of the ISIS-4 methodology is given in Chapter 21. Briefly, ISIS-4 (11) randomized by telephone 58,050 patients (no age limit) with suspected MI, within 24 hours of onset, in a 2 × 2 × 2 factorial design testing captopril, mononitrate, and magnesium. Patients with cardiogenic shock or low blood pressure (systolic blood pressure persistently <100 mmHg) were excluded. We encouraged the routine use of aspirin and fibrinolysis.

The study drugs were to be given immediately after the fibrinolytic, provided the blood pressure and circulation appeared stable. Streptokinase (SK) was the fibrinolytic in 90% of a 1000-patient sample. The magnesium was begun within 2 hours of the *start* of the fibrinolytic treatment, so a substantial number of arteries would have still been occluded at this time. For the subgroups randomized within 6 hours of onset of MI, 75% received magnesium within 2 hours of starting SK.

The patients received a regimen of intravenous magnesium sulfate very similar to that used in the LIMIT-2 trial [8 mmol (2 g) bolus + 72 mmol (18 g) infused over about 24 hours in 50 ml of water]. In the magnesium comparison we did not use a matching placebo infusion, since the characteristic flush and warm sensation from the magnesium infusion might have made blinding difficult.

RESULTS

After the promise of the earlier smaller studies and of LIMIT-2, the ISIS-4 magnesium result was unexpected and disappointing. During the first 5 weeks the mortality was 7.64% among the magnesium-allocated patients and 7.24% in the controls (NS), which is not compatible with the previous results (Fig. 1). One-year follow-up showed no further differences. Nor was there any indication of any significant interaction with the other treatments with captopril or mononitrate (Fig. 2). As can be seen in Figure 2, the overall result was on the "harm" side of the null effect line but overlaps the null effect and is thus not significant.

In no subgroup was there any evidence of a mortality reduction, whether one looks at the more than 23,000 patients randomized within 6 hours, or in patients who received magnesium soon after the start of lytic therapy or in the 17,000 patients who did not receive lytic therapy (as was the case for the majority of patients in the previous trials of magnesium). Importantly, in the 9000 patients who were randomized within 12 hours of onset (median 7 hours, similar to previous trials), there was also no evidence of benefit with magnesium (10.3% vs. 10.5%).

There was no evidence of any protective effect of magnesium in the prevention of confirmed infarction. There was a marginally significant reduction in ventricular fibrillation but a slight and greater increase in other arrests, with a marginally significant increase in second or third degree heart block while the infusion was being given and a highly significant increase in bradycardia.

There were more pronounced but small increases in heart failure (an excess of 12 per 1000 patients on magnesium $p < 0.001$) and cardiogenic shock (5 per 1000, $p < 0.01$), during or soon after the infusion.

DISCUSSION

After the results of ISIS-4 were presented, there was disappointment that this previously promising and simple treatment had not lived up to the prior expectations; there was also much discussion and debate in order to discover why the result in ISIS-4 differed so

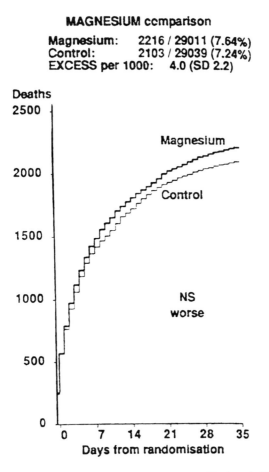

MAGNESIUM comparison

Magnesium: 2216 / 29011 (7.64%)
Control: 2103 / 29039 (7.24%)
EXCESS per 1000:   4.0 (SD 2.2)

Figure 1 Cumulative mortality reported in days 1–35 for all patients allocated magnesium sulfate infusion for 24 hours (thicker line) versus open control. There was a nonsignificant (NS) trend to a worse outcome with magnesium. (From Ref. 11.)

greatly from that of the earlier studies and LIMIT-2. Figure 3 from the ISIS-4 report shows the significant heterogeneity between these trials.

This was perhaps the most unexpected and most disappointing result of the ISIS-4 study. As in many other cases, the first studies gave unrealistic point estimates of 50% reduction in mortality—perhaps an unbelievable result for such an intervention—but with hugely wide confidence limits. Even in the LIMIT-2 trial with almost 2500 patients randomized, the lower confidence limit of the 25% point estimate was close to zero benefit.

As can be seen from Figure 3, the more conservative 99% confidence limits overlap the null effect line (and the result of ISIS-4). So on statistical grounds we should not be too surprised, particularly if one considers the influence of publication bias, favoring the submission only of positive results. A study by Egger et al. (12) used funnel plots (Fig. 4) from a number of trials to look for publication bias in meta-analyses of small trials and found evidence for this in several areas, including magnesium for MI.

Nevertheless, several criticisms of the design of ISIS-4 have been made in order to

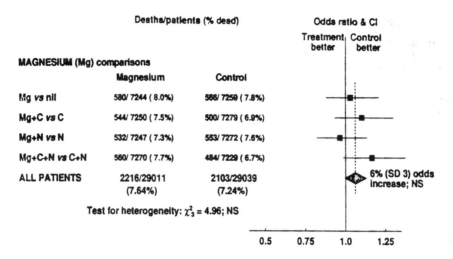

Figure 2 Magnesium result in ISIS-4. Mortality in days 0–35 subdivided by other randomly llocated study treatments. C = captopril; N = mononitrate; Mg = magnesium. Odds ratios (ORs: black squares with areas proportional to the amount of "statistical information" in each subdivision) comparing the mortality among patients allocated the study treatment to that among patients allocated the relevant control are plotted for each of the treatment comparisons, subdivided by the other randomly allocated study treatments, along with their 99% confidence intervals (CIs: horizontal lines). For the overall treatment comparison, the result and its 95% CI is represented by a diamond, with the overall proportional reduction (or increase) and statistical significance given alongside. Squares or diamonds to the left of the solid vertical line indicate benefit (significant at $2p < 0.01$ when the entire horizontal line is to the left of the vertical line). Chi-square tests for evidence of heterogeneity of the sizes of the ORs in the subdivisions are also given. (From Ref. 11.)

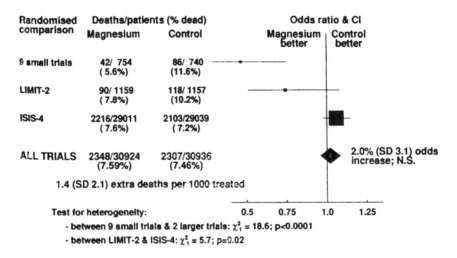

Figure 3 Systematic overview of the effects of early intravenous magnesium on short-term mortality in myocardial infarction. There is significant heterogeneity between these results. Symbols as in Figure 2. (From Ref. 11.)

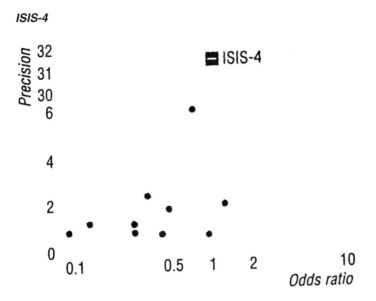

Figure 4 Funnel plot of magnesium smaller trials compared with the much larger ISIS-4. Filled circles indicate odd ratios from smaller trials. The square and horizontal line indicate odds ratio from ISIS-4 and 95% confidence interval. Note that almost all the points lie to the left of the large trial, perhaps indicating the results of publication bias. (From Ref. 12.)

seek a scientific rather than a statistical reason for this negative result. The reasons why many of these criticisms seem invalid have been outlined above.

As Woods (13) points out, clinical trials of new treatments are complicated by the need to give accepted medications such as aspirin, fibrinolysis, and beta-blockers and then show an incremental benefit on top of these. There is also the problem of heterogeneity in the patient population, although some would regard this as a strong point of large trials. Woods now believes that it would be important to have raised magnesium levels *before* reperfusion occurs and that perhaps in retrospect the infusion was given too late in ISIS-4 (13). However, as we argued in the ISIS-4 publication, even if we select out of the ISIS-4 population those patients who most resemble those in LIMIT-2, we have a much larger sample than LIMIT-2 itself and we still see no benefit. This point is often ignored by critics such as Woods (13) and Antman (14).

Antman (14) also makes the point [based on a complex meta-analysis of the earlier trials (15)] that he would not expect any benefit from magnesium in a patient population with a "low" early mortality of around 7%, as in ISIS-4. Again he ignores the lack of benefit seen in large high-mortality subgroups of ISIS-4. He also reiterates the point that it is necessary to have the calcium entry blockade caused by magnesium operative before reperfusion occurs. And yet we have no evidence of benefit in humans when any calcium blocker is given very early in acute MI (16). With regard to his meta-analysis (15), one should be wary of such analyses on trials with small numbers of events and with possible publication bias, as Egger et al. (12) point out.

A small study of magnesium in unstable angina (17) reported a significant reduction of ST changes seen on 48-hour Holter monitoring in 62 patients randomized to magnesium sulfate (80 mmol $MgSO_4$ over 24 hours) or matching placebo; urinary adrenaline and noradrenaline were somewhat reduced on magnesium. There were four hospital deaths on magnesium versus three on placebo (NS). The authors concluded that magnesium was worth further study in unstable angina.

There were two unexpected findings in the positive LIMIT-2 study of magnesium in acute MI: there was no antiarrhythmic effect and there was an unexpected reduction in heart failure. On the other hand, ISIS-4 did find an antiarrhythmic effect, balanced by some not unexpected increase in asystole. In keeping with the action of calcium entry blockade in acute MI there was an increase in cardiogenic shock with magnesium in ISIS-4.

CONCLUSIONS

ISIS-4 showed no benefit but nonsignificant harm from intravenous magnesium in acute MI. Until, and if, further evidence does emerge, this treatment cannot be recommended for routine use.

REFERENCES

1. du Toit EF, Opie LH. Modulation of severity of reperfusion stunning in the isolated rat heart by agents altering calcium flux at reperfusion. Circ Res 1992; 70:960–967.
2. Ferrari R, Albertini A, Curello S, et al. Myocardial recovery during post-ischaemic reperfusion: effects of nifedipine, calcium and magnesium. J Mol Cell Cardiol 1986; 18:487–498.
3. Altura BT, Altura BM. Endothelium-dependent relaxation in coronary arteries requires magnesium ions. Br J Pharmacol 1987; 91:449–451.
4. Woods KL. Possible pharmacological actions of magnesium in acute myocardial infarction. Br J Clin Pharmacol 1991; 32:3–10.
5. Berg RH, Vissinger H, Kristensen SD, Wennmalm A, Thygesen K, Husted SE. Magnesium inhibits platelet activity: an infusion study in healthy volunteers. Thrombosis Haemostasis 1996; 75:939–944.
6. Chang C, Varghese PJ, Downey J, Bloom S. Magnesium deficiency and myocardial infarct size in the dog. J Am Coll Cardiol 1985; 5:280–289.
7. Rubenowitz E, Axelsson G, Rylander R. Magnesium in drinking water and death from acute myocardial infarction. Am J Epidemiol 1996; 143:456–462.
8. Woods KL, Fletcher S, Roffe C, Haider Y. Intravenous magnesium sulphate in suspected acute myocardial infarction: results of the second Leicester Intravenous Magnesium Intervention Trial (LIMIT-2). Lancet 1992; 339:1553–1558.
9. Woods KL, Fletcher S. Long-term outcome after intravenous magnesium sulphate in suspected acute myocardial infarction: the second Leicester Intravenous Magnesium Intervention Trial (LIMIT-2). Lancet 1994; 343:816–819.
10. ISIS-4 Collaborative Group. Fourth International Study of Infarct Survival: protocol for a large simple study of the effects of oral mononitrate, of oral captopril, and of intravenous magnesium. Am J Cardiol 1991; 68:87D–100D.
11. ISIS-4 (Fourth International Study of Infarct Survival) Collaborative Group. ISIS-4: a randomised trial comparing oral captopril versus placebo, oral mononitrate versus placebo, and intravenous magnesium sulphate versus control among 58,050 patients with suspected acute myocardial infarction. Lancet 1995; 345:669–687.
12. Egger M, Davey Smith G, Schneider M, Minder C. Bias in meta-analysis detected by a simple, graphical test. Br Med J 1997; 315:629–634.
13. Woods KL. More on intravenous Mg^{2+} and the unstable coronary artery. Eur Heart J 1997; 18:1202–1203.

14. Antman EM. Magnesium in acute myocardial infarction: overview of available evidence. Am Heart J 1996; 132:487–494.

15. Antman EM, Seelig MS, Fleischmann K, Lau J, Kuntz K, Berkey CS, et al. Magnesium in acute myocardial infarction: scientific, statistical, and economic rationale for its use. Cardiovasc Drugs Ther 1996; 10:297–301.

16. Sleight P. Calcium antagonists during and after myocardial infarction. Drugs 1996; 51(2): 216–225.

17. Redwood SR, Bashir Y, Huang J, Leathem EW, Kaski J-C, Camm AJ. Effect of magnesium sulphate in patients with unstable angina: a double blind, randomised, placebo-controlled study. Eur Heart J 1997; 18:1269–1277.

Section N
Invasive or Conservative Management

Both trials discussed in this section provide support for the strategy of "watchful waiting" for signs of heart failure or recurrent ischemia before performing coronary angiography and subsequent revascularization in patients who have undergone thrombolysis for acute myocardial infarction. Some would challenge these findings as moot, because of the growing enthusiasm for primary angioplasty. Others have argued that in the current costconscious environment, early angiography may allow for more rapid risk stratification and shorter hospital stays, thereby paradoxically lowering overall costs despite more frequent catheterization. Nevertheless, most patients with acute infarction are admitted to hospitals without the capacity to perform primary angioplasty, so that this issue remains relevant. In addition, strict cost accounting studies may reach divergent conclusions based on their underlying assumptions, such as the cost of complications from "unnecessary" procedures or the value of avoiding later symptoms.

Studies of the variation of utilization of catheterization among regions of the U.S.[1] and between the U.S. and Canada[2] have highlighted striking regional and national differences in the use of coronary angiography following infarction without corresponding differences in patient outcomes. Indeed, the likelihood of a particular patient undergoing catheterization after infarction seems to depend as much on the availability of catheterization facilities and geographic location as it does on established clinical variables such as recurrent ischemic pain in the post-infarction period. These data lend further credence to a more selective use of these procedures and speak to the enduring importance of the studies presented here, which established the safety and clinical equivalence of this approach.

---

[1] Pilote L, Califf RM, Sapp S, Miller DP, Mark DP, Weaver D, et al. Regional variation across the United States in the management of acute myocardial infarction. N Engl J Med 1995;333:565–572.

[2] Tu JV, Pashos CL, Naylor CD, Chen E, Normand SL, Newhouse JP, et al. Use of cardiac procedures and outcomes in elderly patients with myocardial infarction in the United States and Canada. N Engl J Med 1997;336:1500–1505.

38

TIMI-IIB

CHRISTOPHER P. CANNON and EUGENE BRAUNWALD

The TIMI Study Group. Comparison of invasive and conservative strategies after treatment with intravenous tissue plasminogen activator in acute myocardial infarction. Results of the thrombolysis in myocardial infarction (TIMI) phase II trial. N Engl J Med 1989;320:618–627.

INTRODUCTION

Thrombolytic therapy has proven to be a major advance in the management of acute myocardial infarction. The benefit of thrombolytic therapy, as shown in the Thrombolysis in Myocardial Infarction (TIMI)-I Trial (1) and numerous other trials, is related to early achievement of patency of the infarct-related artery, whereby rapid coronary reperfusion limits infarct size, decreases left ventricular dysfunction, and improves survival (2–5). However, a residual stenosis in the infarct-related artery frequently remains following thrombolysis, which can lead to recurrent ischemia, reocclusion or reinfarction, and subsequently increased mortality.

An invasive strategy following thrombolysis (with mechanical revascularization, either catheter-based or surgical) was developed on the presumption that thrombolytic therapy may be effective in establishing reperfusion but could leave uncorrected a severe residual atherosclerotic narrowing of coronary artery responsible for the infarction (6,7). This "partially treated" condition could render the patient susceptible to reinfarction because of early reocclusion of the coronary artery as well as to recurrent ischemia related to persistent significant partial obstruction (6). Percutaneous transluminal coronary angioplasty (PTCA) or coronary artery bypass grafting (CABG) after thrombolytic therapy offered the potential benefit of relieving residual atherosclerotic narrowing and thus reducing the likelihood of recurrent ischemia-related events (7).

Thus, in the mid-1980s it was believed that following thrombolysis for acute MI, an invasive strategy of routine coronary angiography and revascularization might further improve clinical outcome. However, this hypothesis had not been tested, and the TIMI Investigators set out to address this important question, which had—and still has—implications for selection of management strategies, clinical outcome, and cost-effectiveness of cardiac care (8).

TIMI-IIB PROTOCOL

Eligibility Criteria

Between 1986 and 1988, 3339 patients were entered into the TIMI-IIB trial (8,9). Inclusion criteria for the trial were as follows: age < 76 years, chest discomfort suggestive of acute myocardial ischemia lasting 30 minutes or longer, ST segment elevation ≥ 0.1 mV in two contiguous electrocardiographic leads, and the feasibility of initiating treatment with recombinant tissue plasminogen activator (tPA) within 4 hours of the onset of chest pain. Exclusion criteria were a history of a bleeding disorder, surgery within the previous 2 weeks, recent prolonged cardiopulmonary resuscitation, PTCA or severe trauma within 6 months, previous CABG or prosthetic heart valve replacement, left bundle branch block, dilated cardiomyopathy, or other serious illness.

Two other major exclusion criteria were a history of cerebrovascular disease and acute hypertension, which were modified during the initial phase of the trial. Initially, patients with a history of stroke within 6 months were excluded, but because of concern regarding intracranial hemorrhage, patients with *any* history of stroke or transient ischemic attack (TIA) at any time were excluded (10,11). The blood pressure exclusion was changed from excluding patients with diastolic blood pressures of >120 mmHg on repeated measurements to excluding patients with *any* measurement more than either 180 systolic or 110 diastolic at *any* time during the current episode (8).

Thrombolytic Therapy

Patients were treated with tPA (Activase, Genentech, South San Francisco, CA). The first 520 patients received a 150 mg dose over 6 hours, administered intravenously as a 9 mg bolus, 81 mg infusion over the first hour, 20 mg over the second hour, and 10 mg/hour for the next 4 hours. Because of an unacceptably high rate of intracranial hemorrhage (see below), the dose was reduced to a total of 100 mg over 6 hours, administered as a 6 mg bolus, 54 mg infusion over the first hour, 20 mg over the second hour, and 5 mg/hour for the next 4 hours (8,10,11).

Heparin

Heparin was administered as a 5000 unit intravenous bolus, followed by an infusion of 1000 units per hour, subsequently adjusted to maintain an activated partial thromboplastin time (aPTT) of 1.5–2.0 times the control (8). The infusion was continued for 5 days and continued subcutaneously as 10,000 units twice daily until hospital discharge. For cardiac catheterization, the heparin infusion was reduced by 50% for 2–3 hours, and an additional 5000 unit bolus was administered after the arterial sheath was inserted. For patients undergoing PTCA, an additional 5000 units of heparin were administered.

Concomitant Therapy

Aspirin was administered at a dose of 80 mg daily beginning on day 1 in the first 328 patients and on day 2 in the remainder. On day 6, the dose was increased to 325 mg daily (8). Patients also received intravenous lidocaine for 24 hours. A substudy comparing intravenous beta-blockers followed by oral beta-blockade with delayed oral beta-blockade was also conducted, in which patients who were not already taking a beta-blocker, verapamil, or diltiazem and who did not have a contraindication to beta-blockade were randomly assigned to receive intravenous metoprolol or placebo (see Chap. 14). All patients were treated with oral metoprolol beginning on day 6.

Invasive Strategy

Patients randomly assigned to the invasive strategy were scheduled for coronary angiography and ventriculography between 18 and 48 hours after the initiation of the tPA infusion. PTCA (limited to the infarct-related artery) was performed during the same procedure unless (1) the infarct-related artery was occluded (TIMI grade 0 or 1 flow) and the patient had no recurrent ischemia; (2) the residual stenosis was less than 60%; (3) the lesion had unsuitable features, such as length $\geq$ 20 mm, involvement of an arterial bifurcation, or location in a distal position or beyond a tortuous proximal vessel; or (4) abrupt closure of the involved vessel was likely to cause catastrophic hemodynamic consequences (e.g., left main or equivalent anatomy) (8).

CABG was carried out in patients if there was a clinical indication, such as persistent ischemic pain, and there was coronary artery anatomy unsuitable for PTCA but well suited for surgery, such as stenosis of $\geq$70% in the left main coronary artery. CABG was also performed in some patients who had recurrent coronary occlusion after PTCA was attempted (8).

TIMI-IIA

As described in Chapter 40, the TIMI-IIA trial, conducted as a subset of TIMI-IIB, studied 586 patients who were randomized to one of three treatment strategies: (1) an early invasive strategy, involving immediate cardiac catheterization (within 2 hours) with PTCA when feasible, (2) a delayed invasive strategy with angiography and PTCA as appropriate at 18–48 hours, described above, or (3) a conservative strategy, as described below (12,13).

TIMI-IIB Operator Experience Requirement

To ensure that the operators performing PTCA in the TIMI trial were experienced and proficient, they were required to have personally performed at least 100 angioplasties, with a mortality rate below 2% and a success rate above 85% in their most recent 50 cases (8).

Conservative Strategy

In patients randomly assigned to the conservative strategy, the protocol specified that cardiac catheterization and PTCA/CABG be performed only if ischemia recurred at rest despite medical therapy during hospitalization or if ischemia was provoked during a prehospital discharge exercise test (8).

Endpoints

The primary endpoint was death or nonfatal MI occurring by 42 days. Secondary endpoints were death, MI and the combination at 1 and 3 years, exercise tolerance test results at 6 weeks, and left ventricular function at hospital discharge and 6 weeks. A prespecified subgroup was a "not-low-risk" group, defined as the presence of any one of the following: (1) prior MI, (2) anterior MI, (3) rales > one-third lung fields, (4) hypotension (systolic blood pressure < 100 mmHg) and sinus tachycardia, (5) atrial fibrillation or flutter, (6) age ≥ 70 years, (7) pulmonary edema, or (8) cardiogenic shock (8).

The success of angioplasty was evaluated at the clinical centers. "Full improvement" was defined as presence of TIMI grade 3 flow, or improvement in TIMI flow grade, and both an absolute reduction in the luminal stenosis by ≥20% and a final luminal stenosis of <60%. "Partial improvement" was defined as the development of only one of the anatomical improvements, unchanged or improved flow, and TIMI grade 2 or 3 flow (8).

RESULTS

Baseline Characteristics

A total of 1636 patients were randomly assigned to the invasive strategy group and 1626 patients to the conservative strategy group. The two groups were well matched (Table 1). Both groups were predominantly male, with a mean age of 57 years. Myocardial infarction was confirmed by electrocardiographic and/or enzymatic evidence in 95% of the patients in each group.

Catheterization and PTCA in the Invasive Strategy

In the invasive group, cardiac catheterization was carried out according to the protocol between 18 and 48 hours (mean 32.5 hours) after randomization in 93% of patients ran-

Table 1 Baseline Characteristics

	Invasive (%) (n = 1681)	Conservative (%) (n = 1658)
Age (mean, years)	57	57
Race (white)	88	89
Sex (male)	82	82
"Not low risk"	66	68
Age ≥ 70 years	12	11
Prior MI	14	14
Anterior MI	51	53
Rales ≥ 1/3 lung fields	4	4
Hypotension and sinus tachycardia	6	6
Atrial fibrillation or flutter	2	2
Pulmonary edema	1	1
Cardiogenic shock	2	1
Other risk factors:		
History of angina	55	53
History of CHF	3.2	2
History of hypertension	39	38
History of diabetes mellitus	13	13
Ongoing chest pain at tPA initiation	89	88
Time from onset of pain to study entry (mean, hours)	2.6	2.7

domized to the invasive group (8). An additional 66 patients (4%) required cardiac catheterization before 18 hours because of recurrent ischemia. The reasons that catheterization was not carried out as specified in the protocol in the remaining 109 patients assigned to the invasive strategy were as follows: death within 48 hours (35 patients); other clinical events, such as bleeding or hemodynamic instability (29 patients); refusal by the patient or physician (31 patients); miscellaneous reasons (14 patients).

In the patients assigned to the invasive strategy, PTCA was attempted during the specified interval in 878 of the 1636 patients (53.7%), representing 60.1% of the 1461 patients who underwent protocol-driven catheterization (8). The principal reasons for not attempting PTCA at this time were as follows: (1) an infarct-related artery unsuitable for PTCA in 13.4%; (2) no lesion of more than 60% in the infarct-related artery in 12.6%; (3) total occlusion of the infarct-related artery in 12.1%; and (4) other reasons in 2%. In an additional 50 patients (3.4%), PTCA was attempted on an emergency basis within 18 hours. Thus, a total of 928 of the 1636 patients (56.7%) randomly assigned to the invasive strategy underwent PTCA in the first 48 hours after randomization.

Outcome of PTCA

Of the 878 patients undergoing PTCA between 18 and 48 hours, 93.3% were judged by the angioplasty operator to have had immediate improvement (85.1% full, 8.2% partial) (8). PTCA was successful in 34 of 37 patients (91.9%) with occluded coronary arteries and ongoing myocardial ischemia. Of the 878 patients, 112 (12.8%) had one or more complications within 24 hours of attempted PTCA. Of these, 68 had total occlusion of the infarct-related artery or one of its branches; 47 had reinfarction; and 4 died. Thirty-six of the patients in whom PTCA was attempted according to the protocol went on to CABG within 14 days of randomization, which includes 21 patients in whom this operation was carried out within 24 hours of attempted PTCA.

The results were not as favorable in the 50 patients in whom emergency PTCA was performed within 18 hours; 40 had improvement (35 full, 5 partial), and 9 had one or more complications within 24 hours of attempted PTCA (8). Of the latter, 6 had total occlusion of the infarct-related artery or one of its branches; 3 had reinfarction; and 1 patient died. Twelve had CABG within 14 days, including 4 within 24 hours of PTCA.

Among the entire group of 1636 patients randomly assigned to the invasive strategy, 195 had CABG within 42 days, and 50 had CABG after PTCA, one half of the latter within 24 hours of the attempted PTCA.

Cardiac Catheterization and PTCA in the Conservative Strategy Group

Of the 1626 patients randomly assigned to the conservative strategy within the first 14 days after study entry, 26% developed recurrent ischemia, and 33% had cardiac catheterization. A total of 216 patients (13%) had PTCA (8). The PTCA was anatomically successful in 198 of them (92%, 86% full, 6% partial). Of the 216 patients, 48 had a complication within 24 hours of PTCA: 20 had total occlusion of the infarct-related artery, 25 had reinfarction, and 3 died. Of the 1626 patients, 108 (6.6%) had CABG within 14 days of randomization, either because of recurrent ischemia and appropriate anatomical findings

(91 patients) or after PTCA (17 patients). By 42 days, 16.1% of the cohort assigned to the conservative strategy had PTCA, and 10.5% had CABG.

Clinical Outcome

No significant difference was observed in the primary endpoint—death or nonfatal reinfarction—between the two groups: 10.9% for the invasive strategy versus 9.7% for the conservative strategy ($p = 0.25$) (8). Mortality to 42 days was 5.2% in the invasive group and 4.7% in the conservative group ($p = NS$) (Table 2) (8). Although reinfarction was higher in the invasive group *early* in the hospitalization ($p = 0.005$ by 1 week) (9), likely related to peri-procedural complications, rates were similar by 42 days: 6.4% in the invasive group versus 5.4% in the conservative group (8).

At hospital discharge, the exercise tests performed in conjunction with radionuclide angiography suggested myocardial ischemia in 12.8% of those assigned to the invasive strategy and 17.7% of those assigned to the conservative strategy ($p < 0.001$) (8). The higher incidence of ischemia in the conservative group led to cardiac catheterization and, if indicated, coronary revascularization according to the study protocol. Maximal exercise tests carried out at 6 weeks were positive for ischemia in 16.8% of the invasive group and 19.4% of the conservative group ($p = 0.09$) (8). At both the 6-week and 1-year follow-up visits, there was no difference in the proportion of patients experiencing angina or in the severity of angina based on the Canadian Cardiovascular Society Classification (9).

Table 2 Clinical Events to 42 Days

	Strategy group (%)		
Event	Invasive ($n = 1636$)	Conservative ($n = 1626$)	p-value
Death	5.2	4.7	0.49
Fatal or nonfatal reinfarction	6.4	5.8	0.45
Nonfatal reinfarction	5.9	5.4	0.57
Death or reinfarction	10.9	9.7	0.25
Any adverse end point[a]	13.0	10.6	0.04
All CABG	11.9	10.5	0.18
Any stroke (including ICH)	1.5	1.2	0.46
150 mg tPA	2.3	3.0	0.79
100 mg tPA	1.4	0.8	0.22
Any ICH	0.9	0.7	0.70
150 mg tPA	1.9	2.3	0.99
100 mg tPA	0.6	0.4	0.61
Positive exercise test at hospital discharge	12.8	17.7	<0.001
Positive exercise test at 6 weeks	16.8	19.4	0.09

[a] Defined as death, nonfatal reinfarction, intracranial hemorrhage, and coronary artery bypass surgery following percutaneous transluminal coronary angioplasty.
CABG = Coronary artery bypass grafting; ICH = intracranial hemorrhage; tPA = tissue plasminogen activator.

Hemorrhagic Events

Although intracranial hemorrhage was higher with the 150 mg dose of tPA, there was no major difference in its incidence in the invasive vs. conservative strategies: 0.6% vs. 0.4%, in patients who received the 100 mg dose ($p = 0.61$) (8). Blood transfusion was required in 15.5% of patients in the invasive group vs. 12.7% in the conservative group ($p = 0.02$) (8). Among patients receiving the 100 mg dose of tPA, nonsurgical hemorrhagic events were also more common in the invasive strategy ($p < 0.001$): the rate of major hemorrhage was 7.0% in the invasive strategy versus 4.2% in the conservative strategy, and of minor hemorrhage, 11.5% versus 8.7%, respectively (14).

Long-Term Follow-Up

Results at one year were similar: mortality was nearly identical for the invasive and conservative strategies, 8.2% versus 8.3% at one year, respectively (Table 3) (9). The endpoint of death or reinfarction was also not different in the two groups at one year (Fig. 1). The 2-year and 3-year mortality rates were also identical in the two groups; in the cohort of patients who were followed through 3 years, mortality was 11.5% and 11.0% in the invasive and conservative groups, respectively (15). Reinfarction similarly was identical between the two groups. The combination of death or MI to 3 years was 20.5% for the invasive strategy and 20.0% in the conservative strategy ($p = NS$) (15). During the first year of follow-up, however, more patients in the conservative group were rehospitalized for angina than in the invasive group (19.6% vs. 14.7%, respectively; $p < 0.001$) (9). Similarly, rehospitalization for cardiac reasons was observed more commonly in patients in the conservative arm (38.1%) than in patients in the invasive arm (29.6%, $p < 0.001$).

Table 3 Clinical Events Through 1-Year Follow-Up[a]

Event	Invasive (%) (n = 1681)	Conservative (%) (n = 1658)	p-value
Death (all causes)			
21 days	4.9	4.1	0.25
6 weeks	5.2	4.6	0.43
1 year	6.9	7.4	0.59
Reinfarction (fatal and nonfatal)			
21 days	6.7	6.1	0.43
6 weeks	7.0	6.7	0.67
1 year	9.4	9.8	0.81
Death and reinfarction			
21 days	10.5	9.2	0.18
6 weeks	11.1	10.1	0.31
1 year	14.7	15.2	0.83
Recurrent ischemia			
Recurrent chest pain in hospital during first 10 days	25.5	29.8	0.05
21 days	13.0	13.5	0.81
6 weeks	14.7	16.8	0.14
1 year	24.3	27.6	0.04

[a] Cumulative event rates (Kaplan-Meier estimates).

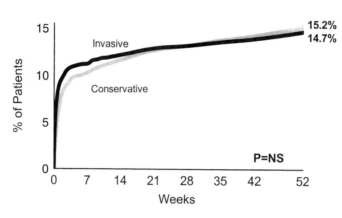

Figure 1 Rates of death or MI through 1 year of follow-up for patients following an invasive versus conservative strategy. (Adapted from Ref. 9.)

On the other hand, there was no difference in the total days of rehospitalization between the two groups (9). The incidence of stroke during follow-up in the two groups was the same (2.0%) at 1 year (9).

Non–Q-Wave Versus Q-Wave MI

Because of differences observed in the prethrombolytic era in the prognosis and rate of recurrent MI following non–Q-wave MI compared with Q-wave MI, these two groups of patients were compared in TIMI-II (16). To avoid confounding, the analysis was restricted to patients with their first MI as the qualifying MI for TIMI-II. Of these ST elevation MI patients treated with tPA, 71% developed Q-waves. By 18–48 hours, non–Q-wave MI patients compared with Q-wave MI patients had a higher rate of TIMI grade 3 flow in the infarct-related artery (72.2% vs. 62.6%, $p < 0.01$), a higher percentage with normal left ventricular function, EF > 55% (43.4% vs. 24.1%, $p < 0.001$), a lower rate of congestive heart failure (11.6% vs. 18.9%), and a tendency, although not statistically significantly, toward lower 1-year mortality (3.4% vs. 4.4%, $p = 0.25$) (16).

These observations are all consistent with the hypothesis that early, more complete reperfusion leads to absence of Q-waves on the ECG and improved left ventricular function. On the other hand, as observed in previous trials in the prethrombolytic era (17,18), the incidence of reinfarction was higher in patients with non–Q-wave MI, 9.4% versus 7.4% by 1 year ($p = 0.07$) (16). Furthermore, in patients with non–Q-wave MI, the rate of recurrent MI was not lower in the early invasive strategy compared with the conservative strategy. Although it was hoped (and still sometimes recommended) (19) that an invasive approach would prevent reinfarction in patients with non–Q-wave MI, this was not observed in TIMI-IIB. Similar findings, i.e., that an invasive strategy did not prevent recurrent MI in non–Q-wave MI, were observed in TIMI-IIIB (20), which enrolled patients with non–Q-wave MI presenting without ST segment elevation, and in the VANQWISH trial (21). Thus, with a goal of preventing recurrent MI, attention has again focused on more potent antithrombotic therapy, such as low molecular weight heparin (22,23) and oral platelet IIb/IIIa inhibitors (24) in the management of these patients.

Results in Community Versus Tertiary Hospitals

In patients assigned to the conservative arm, a comparison of practice in community hospitals (without available on-site cardiac catheterization facilities) versus tertiary care hospitals (with such facilities) was carried out (25). At community hospitals, patients in the conservative strategy were referred for cardiac catheterization less often, 32% by 6 weeks, compared with 45% of patients at tertiary care hospitals with on-site cardiac facilities ($p < 0.001$) (25). Similarly, PTCA was used less often in community hospitals, 11% versus 18% at tertiary care hospitals by 6 weeks ($p < 0.01$); CABG was performed in 12% versus 18% of patients, respectively ($p < 0.05$) (25). Clinical outcome on the other hand was similar: death or MI to 42 days was 9.5% in community and 9.8% in tertiary hospitals ($p = NS$). Similarly, death or MI at 1 year, as well as angina class, were identical in the two types of hospitals in the conservative arm (25). At 1 year, only 1.5% of patients in the conservative arm at each type of hospital had Canadian Class 3 or 4 angina. The findings from this analysis provide further support for the excellent outcomes that can be obtained with the ''watchful waiting'' strategy.

The difference in the rate of cardiac catheterization and revascularization between the two types of hospitals may have been due to more intensive monitoring for recurrent ischemia and a lower threshold for referral for angiography when ischemia recurs. Similar findings of increased use of cardiac procedures at hospitals with on-site facilities have subsequently been reported by numerous investigators (26–28). Similar observations have also been made when comparing patients in Canada with patients in the United States: many fewer procedures are performed in Canada, but overall mortality for patients in the United States and Canada is similar (29). One analysis from the GUSTO trial showed similar mortality but a potentially improved quality of life for patients in the United States, where angiography was performed much more often (30). However, a more recent study of over 233,700 patients again found no difference in mortality between the two countries, despite striking lower rates of angiography and revascularization in Canada (31). These registry findings lend further support to the findings from TIMI-IIB that coronary angiography can be reserved for patients who demonstrate recurrent ischemia post-MI and need not be applied to all patients. In the current era of cost containment, close scrutiny of the indications for cardiac catheterization, with more strict adherence to its need in patients with true recurrent ischemia post-MI, may allow reductions in the use of cardiac procedures (and thus costs) without any loss of clinical benefit.

Costs/Use of Revascularization

With no difference in clinical outcome, one looks to the difference in revascularization as a major expenditure in health care resources. The rate of revascularization in the two strategies was vastly different: 72.3% of patients in the invasive strategy group underwent PTCA or CABG by 1 year, compared to only 35.5% in the conservative strategy group ($p < 0.001$) (Fig. 2) (9,32). This difference was due to a three times higher rate of PTCA in the invasive group, 61.2% by 1 year compared with 20.5% in the conservative group (9). Interestingly, the rate of CABG was similar in both groups: 17.5% and 17.3% by one year in the invasive and conservative strategies, respectively. This indicates that the patients who ultimately need CABG (e.g., severe three-vessel disease and reduced left ventricular function) can be identified by the conservative strategy (32).

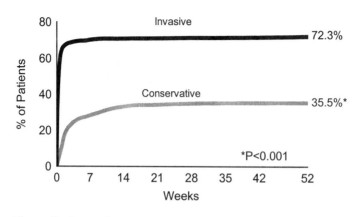

Figure 2 Rates of revascularization with PTCA or CABG by 1 year.

DANAMI Trial

A recent trial, DANAMI, established that the TIMI-IIB conservative approach, with cardiac catheterization and revascularization for recurrent ischemia at rest or on exercise testing, is greatly superior to a *very* conservative approach, in which revascularization of post-MI of patients is reserved for those with severe recurrent ischemia that cannot be controlled by medication. In the DANAMI trial, patients following a strategy identical to the TIMI-IIB conservative strategy had a significantly lower rate of death, MI, or unstable angina requiring rehospitalization during long-term follow-up (15.4%) than those treated even more conservatively (29.5%, $p < 0.001$) (33). It thus appears that being extremely conservative is harmful to patients, whereas the TIMI-IIB "conservative" strategy with angiography and revascularization only for recurrent ischemia is the most cost-effective strategy for management of patients following thrombolytic therapy.

Public Health Considerations

This trial has public health implications for the care of patients with acute MI. Given the favorable results of either strategy, beginning with intravenous thrombolytic therapy, patients with acute MI can be treated in community hospitals with well-staffed and well-equipped coronary care units, but without the more specialized personnel, equipment, or facilities required for cardiac catheterization, PTCA, and CABG. Had the invasive strategy led to an outcome distinctly superior to that resulting from the conservative strategy, it would have pointed to the need for a greater number of experts in angioplasty and to the expansion of cardiac catheterization laboratories, as well as "standby" surgical facilities and personnel, thus greatly complicating the care of acute MI and increasing its costs. Such a debate now rages with the advent of primary angioplasty, where some physicians advocate primary angioplasty for all patients, regardless of what type of hospital they are admitted to. Future trials will help clarify whether emergent transfer of patients or wide-scale expansion of the number of facilities in which primary angioplasty for acute MI can be performed will be beneficial. In patients treated with thrombolytic therapy, however, the TIMI-IIB trial has firmly established that this is not necessary.

Outcome of PTCA

The overall results with PTCA were quite favorable in the TIMI-II trial (34). Procedural success was achieved in 89% of patients undergoing PTCA. Acute complications were also low, with 0.7% mortality and 4.0% MI rate within 24 hours. It should be recalled that to participate in the TIMI-II trial, angioplasty physicians had to be experienced and have low complication rates (8). A specified volume of procedures was necessary in order to qualify as a participating center. This experience of the angioplasty operators in the TIMI-II trial may explain the favorable results of angioplasty in this relatively high-risk angioplasty population. Subsequent analyses have shown that the requirements prospectively established for TIMI-II were wise: physicians with low caseloads have higher complication rates (35). Based on data such as these, the American College of Cardiology and American Heart Association have established guidelines similar to those used in TIMI-II for operator (and catheterization laboratory) volume.

Would the PTCA Results Be Different Today?

In the invasive arm of TIMI-IIB, PTCA was actually carried out within 48 hours in only 56.7%. Of the remainder, a small percentage of patients had died before coronary arteriography could be carried out. There were three reasons (of equal frequency) why one-third of the patients had cardiac catheterization but not PTCA: the infarct-related artery did not have a critical residual stenosis, the artery was deemed anatomically unsuitable for PTCA, or it was totally occluded (not to be dilated according to protocol). Given the advances in angioplasty technique and the widespread use of stents, it is quite possible that the majority of the total occlusions and the "anatomically unsuitable" lesions might be approachable by PTCA. This could potentially improve outcomes with an invasive strategy, but this hypothesis would need to be tested in future trials.

The procedural success rate was very high overall (93%), and was also high (92%) among patients with occluded coronary arteries and ongoing myocardial ischemia. However, the success rate for emergency procedures was lower (80%) and the complication rate was high (18% total; 12% abrupt closure, 6% reinfarction, and 2% deaths). Similarly, during the initial hospitalization, reinfarction was more common in the invasive group. With the use of platelet glycoprotein IIb/IIIa inhibitors and of stents and other new devices, the incidence of complications may be lower, and a benefit of the invasive strategy might become evident.

ADDITIONAL LESSONS FROM TIMI-II

Intracranial Hemorrhage

Intracranial hemorrhage is one of the most serious complications of thrombolytic therapy. In TIMI-II, a 150 mg dose of tPA was initially given, but this led to a 1.5% rate of intracranial hemorrhage (8). The dose was then reduced to 100 mg, which resulted in a 0.5% rate of intracranial hemorrhage (8,11). Two important risk factors for developing intracranial hemorrhage were identified: age > 60 years (especially >70 years) and a prior history of cerebrovascular disease (either transient ischemic attack or stroke). When data from TIMI-II were combined with those from other major thrombolytic trials (44), four independent risk factors for intracranial hemorrhage were found: age > 65, body weight < 70 kg, hypertension at presentation with BP $\geq 170/95$, and treatment with tPA (36). Knowing these four risk factors should help to identify patients at increased risk for intracranial hemorrhage who might benefit from a less aggressive thrombolytic regimen or an alternate means of reperfusion, e.g., primary catheter-based revascularization.

It should be noted, however, that in other thrombolytic trials [e.g., ISIS-2 (37) or GUSTO (4)], the overall clinical benefit for the elderly in reduction of cardiovascular mortality outweighed the increased risk of intracranial hemorrhage. In addition, although intracranial hemorrhage is often a devastating complication, it is not uniformly fatal or disabling: in TIMI-II, mortality for patients suffering an intracranial hemorrhage was 61% at 1 year, with 31% of patients having either a full recovery or left with only a partial residual neurologic deficit (11).

Major Hemorrhage and Relationship of Heparin Dose and aPTT to Bleeding

One potential means of reducing the rate of intracranial hemorrhage and major bleeding is to reduce the dose of heparin and/or the level of anticoagulation given in conjunction with thrombolytic therapy. In TIMI-IIB, patients received the "standard" dose of heparin: 5000 U bolus and 1000 U/hr infusion titrated to an activated partial thromboplastin time (aPTT) of 1.5–2.0 times control. Using a time-dependent Cox proportional hazard model, a comparison was made between aPTT and the risk of hemorrhage during the first 5 days of treatment: patients with an aPTT of >90 seconds had a relative risk of 1.7 for major hemorrhage compared with patients who had lower aPTT values ($p < 0.01$) (14). Subsequent analyses in TIMI-IV and TIMI-V trials revealed that among patients who received tPA, aspirin, and heparin, an aPTT of >90 seconds led to a more than doubling of the risk of hemorrhage (38), with similar results in the GUSTO-I trial (39). These results from TIMI-IIB were further corroborated by findings from TIMI-IXA/B (40,41) and GUSTO-IIa/b (42,43).

Relationship of aPTT to Patency

Intravenous heparin has been demonstrated in several studies to be important in preventing reocclusion following tPA (44,46). Because of the known variability of the effect of heparin, the level and consistency of anticoagulation were examined in TIMI-IIB with regard to achieving patency of the infarct-related artery. The degree of activated partial thromboplastin time (aPTT) prolongation was important for patency. In patients with a patent infarct-related artery at 18–48 hours, the 8-hour mean aPTT was higher—77 seconds—compared to 70 seconds for patients with an occluded artery ($p < 0.01$) (47). In addition, the stability of the aPTT over the first 48 hours was found to be important: Patients with a patent infarct-related artery had therapeutic aPTT values more frequently than patients with an occluded artery (47). These data, together with those from TIMI-IV (48), underscore the need for frequent monitoring of the aPTT and adjustment of the heparin dose in order to optimize anticoagulation following thrombolytic therapy (48).

Time to Treatment

The importance of early treatment with thrombolytic therapy was first suggested by the GISSI-1 trial, in which patients treated with streptokinase within one hour of symptom onset exhibited a 47% reduction in mortality compared with placebo, whereas the entire

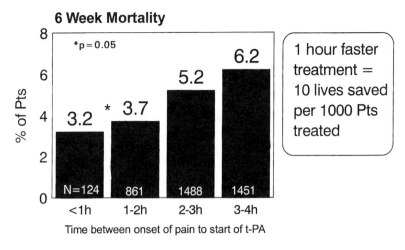

6 Week Mortality

Figure 3 TIMI-II: effect of time to treatment on 42-day mortality. For each hour earlier that patients were treated, there was an absolute 1% lower mortality, which translates into 10 lives saved for every 1000 patients treated. (From Ref. 51.)

group of patients in the trial, treated within 12 hours, had a 19% reduction in mortality (49). The TIMI-II trial also found a benefit of treatment within the first hour on left ventricular function (50). More importantly, it was observed in TIMI-II that for each hour earlier that a patient received thrombolytic therapy, there was a decrease in the absolute mortality by 1% (Fig. 3) (8,50). These findings have helped focus current attention on developing strategies to rapidly identify and treat patients with acute MI (51,52).

CONCLUSION

The TIMI-IIB trial examined the relative benefits of two treatment strategies following thrombolysis for acute MI: routine angiography and coronary revascularization versus selective angiography used only for recurrent ischemia. There was no difference in short- or long-term mortality or nonfatal outcomes, but there was a much lower rate of use of cardiac procedures in the conservative arm, thus establishing the ''watchful waiting'' strategy as the most cost-effective management strategy post-MI. In the current era of cost reductions and managed care with ''evidence-based'' guidelines, the TIMI-IIB trial provides strong support for a selected use of angiography following thrombolysis. In addition, with the wealth of data from TIMI-IIB, many other insights described above may improve the care of patients with acute MI.

ACKNOWLEDGMENTS

We acknowledge with appreciation the very important contributions made by Dr. Genell Knatterud and her staff at the Maryland Medical Research Institute, by Drs. Eugene Passamani and Patrice Desvigne-Nickens at the National Heart, Lung and Blood Institute, and by the TIMI-IIB investigators and research coordinators, who are listed in Ref. 8.

REFERENCES

1. TIMI Study Group. The Thrombolysis in Myocardial Infarction (TIMI) Trial; phase I findings. N Engl J Med 1985; 312:932–936.

2. Braunwald E. Myocardial reperfusion, limitation of infarct size, reduction of left ventricular dysfunction, and improved survival: Should the paradigm be expanded? Circulation 1989; 79: 441–444.

3. The GUSTO Angiographic Investigators. The comparative effects of tissue plasminogen activator, streptokinase, or both on coronary artery patency, ventricular function and survival after acute myocardial infarction. N Engl J Med 1993; 329:1615–1622.

4. The GUSTO Investigators. An international randomized trial comparing four thrombolytic strategies for acute myocardial infarction. N Engl J Med 1993; 329:673–682.

5. Braunwald E. The open-artery theory is alive and well—again. N Engl J Med 1993; 329: 1650–1652.

6. Harrison DG, Ferguson DW, Collins SM, et al. Rethrombosis after reperfusion with streptokinase: importance of geometry of residual lesions. Circulation 1984; 69:991–999.

7. Williams DO, Ruocco NA, Forman S, and the TIMI Investigators. Coronary Angioplasty after recombinant tissue-type plasminogen activator in acute myocardial infarction: a report from the Thrombolysis in Myocardial Infarction (TIMI) Trial. J Am Coll Cardiol 1987; 10:45B–50B.

8. TIMI Study Group. Comparison of invasive and conservative strategies after treatment with intravenous tissue plasminogen activator in acute myocardial infarction. Results of the Thrombolysis in Myocardial Infarction (TIMI) phase II trial. N Engl J Med 1989; 320:618–627.

9. Williams DO, Braunwald E, Knatterud G, et al. One-year results of the Thrombolysis in Myocardial Infarction Investigation (TIMI) phase II trial. Circulation 1992; 85(2):533–542.

10. TIMI Operations Committee: Braunwald E, Knatterud GL, Passamani ER, Robertson TL. Announcement of protocol change in Thrombolysis in Myocardial Infarction (TIMI) trial (letter). J Am Coll Cardiol 1987; 9:467.

11. Gore JM, Sloan M, Price T, et al. Intracerebral hemorrhage, cerebral infarction, and subdural hematoma after acute myocardial infarction and thrombolytic therapy in the Thrombolysis in Myocardial Infarction Study. Thrombolysis in Myocardial Infarction, Phase II, pilot and clinical trial. Circulation 1991; 83:448–459.

12. TIMI Research Group. Immediate vs delayed catheterization and angioplasty following thrombolytic therapy for acute myocardial infarction. TIMI II A results. JAMA 1988; 260:2849–2858.

13. Rogers WJ, Baim DS, Gore JM, et al. Comparison of immediate invasive, delayed invasive, and conservative strategies after tissue-type plasminogen activator. Results of the Thrombolysis in Myocardial Infarction (TIMI) phase II-A trial. Circulation 1990; 81:1457–1476.

14. Bovill EG, Terrin ML., Stump DC, et al. Hemorrhagic events during therapy with recombinant tissue-type plasminogen activator, heparin, and aspirin for acute myocardial infarction. Results of the Thrombolysis in Myocardial Infarction (TIMI) phase II trial. Ann Intern Med 1991; 115:256–265.

15. Terrin ML, Williams DO, Kleiman NS, et al. Two- and three-year results of the Thrombolysis in Myocardial Infarction (TIMI) phase II clinical trial. J Am Coll Cardiol 1993; 22:1763–1772.

16. Aguirre FV, Younis LT, Chaitman BR, et al. Early and 1-year clinical outcome of patients' evolving non-Q wave versus Q-wave myocardial infarction after thrombolysis: results from the TIMI II study. Circulation 1995; 91:2541–2548.

17. Gibson RS. Non-Q wave myocardial infarction: prognosis, changing incidence, and management. In: Gersh BJ, Rahimtoola SH, ed. Acute Myocardial Infarction. New York: Elsevier, 1991:284–307.

18. Schechtman KB, Capone RJ, Kleiger RE, et al. Differential risk patterns associated with 3

month as compared with 3 to 12 month mortality and reinfarction after non-Q wave myocardial infarction. J Am Coll Cardiol 1990; 15:940–947.

19. Ryan TJ, Anderson JL, Antman EM, et al. ACC/AHA guidelines for the management of patients with acute myocardial infarction: a report of the American College of Cardiology/ American Heart Association Task Force on Practice Guidelines (Committee on Management of Acute Myocardial Infarction). J Am Coll Cardiol 1996; 28:1328–1428.

20. The TIMI IIIB Investigators. Effects of tissue plasminogen activator and a comparison of early invasive and conservative strategies in unstable angina and non-Q-wave myocardial infarction: Results of the TIMI IIIB trial. Circulation 1994; 89:1545–1556.

21. Boden WE, O'Rourke RA, Crawford MH, et al. Outcomes in patients with acute non-Q-wave myocardial infarction randomly assigned to an invasive as compared with a conservative strategy: The multicenter VA Non-Q-Wave Infarction Strategies in-Hospital (VANQWISH) trial.

22. Cohen M, Demers C, Gurfinkel EP, et al. A comparison of low-molecular-weight heparin with unfractionated heparin for unstable coronary artery disease. N Engl J Med 1997; 337:447–452.

23. The Thrombolysis in Myocardial Infarction (TIMI) IIA Trial Investigators. Dose-ranging trial of enoxaparin for unstable angina: results of TIMI IIA. J Am Coll Cardiol 1997; 29:1474–1482.

24. Cannon CP, McCabe CH, Borzak S, et al. A randomized trial of an oral platelet glycoprotein IIb/IIIa antagonist, sibrafiban, in patients after an acute coronary syndrome: Results of the TIMI 12 trial. Circulation 1998; 97:340–349.

25. Feit F, Mueller HS, Braunwald E, et al. Thrombolysis in Myocardial Infarction (TIMI) phase II trial: Outcome comparison of a ''conservative strategy'' in community versus tertiary hospitals. J Am Coll Cardiol 1990; 16:1529–1534.

26. Every NR, Larson EB, Litwin PE, et al. The association between on-site cardiac catheterization facilities and the use of coronary angiography after acute myocardial infarction. N Engl J Med 1993; 329:546–551.

27. Every NR, Parson LS, Fihn SD, et al. Long-term outcome in acute myocardial infarction patients admitted to hospitals with and without on-site cardiac catheterization facilities. Circulation 1997; 96:1770–1775.

28. Blustein J. High-technology cardiac procedures. The impact of service availability on service use in New York state. JAMA 1993; 270:344–349.

29. Rouleau JL, Moye LA, Pfeffer MA, et al. A comparison of management patterns after acute myocardial infarction in Canada and the United States. N Engl J Med 1993; 328:779–784.

30. Mark DB, Naylor CD, Hlatky MA, et al. Use of medical resources and quality of life after acute myocardial infarction in Canada and the United States. N Engl J Med 1994; 331:1130–1135.

31. Tu JV, Pashos CL, Naylor D, et al. Use of cardiac procedures and outcomes in elderly patients with myocardial infarction in the United States and Canada. JAMA 1997; 336:1500–1505.

32. Cannon CP, McCabe CH, Braunwald E. The Thrombolysis in Myocardial Infarction (TIMI) trials. In: Becker RC, ed. The Modern Era of Coronary Thrombolysis. Boston: Kluwer Academic Publishers, 1994:53–67.

33. Madsen JK, Grande P, Saunamaki K, et al. Danish multicenter randomized study of invasive versus conservative treatment in patients with inducible ischemia after thrombolysis in acute myocardial infarction (DANAMI). Circulation 1997; 96:748–755.

34. Baim DS, Diver DJ, Feit F, et al. Coronary angioplasty performed within the Thrombolysis in Myocardial Infarction (TIMI II) Study. Circulation 1992; 85:93–105.

35. Jollis JG, Peterson ED, DeLong ER, et al. The relation between the volume of coronary angioplasty procedures at hospitals treating medicare beneficiaries and short-term mortality. N Engl J Med 1994; 331:1625–1629.

36. Simoons ML, Maggioni AP, Knatterud G, et al. Individual risk assessment for intracranial hemorrhage during thrombolytic therapy. Lancet 1993; 342:1523–1528.

37. ISIS-2 (Second International Study of Infarct Survival) Collaborative Group. Randomised trial of intravenous streptokinase, oral aspirin, both, or neither among 17,187 cases of suspected acute myocardial infarction: ISIS-2. Lancet 1988; 2:349–360.

38. Cannon CP, Becker RC, Loscalzo J, et al. Usefulness of APTT to predict bleeding for hirudin (and heparin) (abstr). Circulation 1994; 90[Pt. 2]:I-563.

39. Granger CB, Hirsh J, Califf RM, et al. Activated partial thromboplastin time and outcome after thrombolytic therapy for acute myocardial infarction: results from the GUSTO-I Trial. Circulation 1996; 93:870–878.

40. Antman EM, for the TIMI 9A Investigators. Hirudin in acute myocardial infarction: Safety report from the Thrombolysis and Thrombin Inhibition in Myocardial Infarction (TIMI) 9A trial. Circulation 1994; 90:1624–1630.

41. Antman EM, for the TIMI 9B Investigators. Hirudin in acute myocardial infarction: Thrombolysis and Thrombin Inhibition in Myocardial Infarction (TIMI) 9B trial. Circulation 1996; 94: 911–921.

42. The Global Use of Strategies to Open Occluded Coronary Arteries (GUSTO) IIa Investigators. A randomized trial of intravenous heparin versus recombinant hirudin for acute coronary syndromes. Circulation 1994; 90:1631–1637.

43. The Global Use of Strategies to Open Occluded Coronary Arteries (GUSTO) IIb Investigators. A comparison of recombinant hirudin with heparin for the treatment of acute coronary syndromes. N Engl J Med 1996; 335:775–782.

44. Hsia J, Hamilton WP, Kleiman N, et al. A comparison between heparin and low-dose aspirin as adjunctive therapy with tissue plasminogen activator for acute myocardial infarction. N Engl J Med 1990; 323:1433–1437.

45. Bleich SD, Nichols T, Schumacher RR, Cooke DH, Tate DA, Teichman SL. Effect of heparin on coronary patency after thrombolysis with tissue plasminogen activator in acute myocardial infarction. Am J Cardiol 1990; 66:1412–1417.

46. de Bono DP, Simoons MI, Tijssen J, et al. Effect of early intravenous heparin on coronary patency, infarct size, and bleeding complications after alteplase thrombolysis: results of a randomized double blind European Cooperative Study Group trial. Br Heart J 1992; 67:122–128.

47. Tracy RP, Kleiman NS, Thompson B, et al. Relationship of coagulation parameters to patency and recurrent ischemia in the Thrombolysis in Myocardial Infarction (TIMI) phase II trial. Am Heart J 1998; 135:29–37.

48. Flaker GC, Bartolozzi J, Davis V, McCabe CH, Cannon CP. Use of a standardized nomogram to achieve therapeutic anticoagulation after thrombolytic therapy in myocardial infarction. Arch Intern Med 1994; 154:1492–1496.

49. Gruppo Italiano per lo Studio della Streptochinasi nell'Infarto Miocardico (GISSI). Effectiveness of intravenous thrombolytic treatment in acute myocardial infarction. Lancet 1986; 1: 397–401.

50. Timm TC, Ross R, McKendall GR, Braunwald E, Williams DO, and the TIMI Investigators. Left ventricular function and early cardiac events as a function of time to treatment with t-PA: a report from TIMI II (abstr). Circulation 1991; 84:II-230.

51. Cannon CP, Antman EM, Walls R, Braunwald E. Time as an adjunctive agent to thrombolytic therapy. J Thromb Thrombolysis 1994; 1:27–34.

52. National Heart Attack Alert Program Coordinating Committee—60 Minutes to Treatment Working Group. Emergency department: rapid identification and treatment of patients with acute myocardial infarction. Ann Emerg Med 1994; 23:311–329.

53. Cannon CP, Braunwald E, McCabe CH, Antman EM, for the TIMI Investigators. The Thrombolysis in Myocardial Infarction (TIMI) trials—the first decade. J Intervent Cardiol 1995; 8: 117–135.

39

SWIFT

DAVID P. de BONO

SWIFT (Should We Intervene Following Thrombolysis?) Trial Study
Group. SWIFT trial of delayed elective intervention versus conservative
treatment in acute myocardial infarction. Br Med J 1991;302:555–560.

The SWIFT (Should We Intervene Following Thrombolysis?) trial, conducted between
1986 and 1988, was an attempt to find out whether early, but not immediate, intervention
by angioplasty or coronary bypass grafting would improve outcome in patients with acute
myocardial infarction initially treated with thrombolytic therapy (1). This chapter attempts
to reassess the SWIFT study in the light of subsequent experience with thrombolysis and
revascularization following myocardial infarction, to identify its strengths and weaknesses,
and to draw lessons for current research and clinical practice.

When the SWIFT trial was designed, the concept of thrombolytic therapy for coronary thrombolysis had already been current for some 25 years, but evidence that it actually
improved survival was only just becoming available (2,3). The concept that the main
mechanism by which thrombolytic therapy worked was by restoring coronary patency
was only just beginning to be generally accepted after years of controversy. It was accepted
that a high proportion of patients would be left with a severe residual stenosis following
thrombolysis, and there was concern that such patients would rethrombose as soon as
intensive anticoagulation was discontinued (4). The adverse and sometimes catastrophic
consequences of recurrent thrombosis were well recognized. Concern over rethrombosis
was not allayed by knowledge of the structure of the ruptured atheromatous plaque provided by the work of Davies, Falk, and their colleagues (5,6).

At the same time, the rapid expansion of the use of coronary angioplasty appeared to
provide a straightforward means of dealing with residual stenosis. An important question at
the time the trial was designed was: In patients in whom thrombolysis has been successful
in restoring coronary flow but has left a significant residual coronary stenosis, is it safe
to leave well enough alone, or would it be better to perform an early intervention? Whether
in retrospect that was the best question to have asked is discussed below.

The SWIFT trial was designed within the constraints of the British and Irish health
care systems, where access to coronary angiography is both restricted and centralized.
The vast majority of patients with acute myocardial infarction are admitted to hospitals
that do not have angiography facilities. The concept the trial wished to test was whether
patients who had received thrombolytic therapy needed to be transferred to an angiography

center for further evaluation. This determined the time scale of 24–48 hours for angiography.

TRIAL DESIGN

Trial design and entry criteria for the SWIFT study are shown in Figure 1. Patients fulfilling clinical and ECG criteria for acute infarction were scheduled to receive thrombolytic therapy with anistreplase followed by heparin. Telephone randomization allocated patients either to continuing conservative management in the form of heparin followed by warfarin or to angiography. Angiography was to be performed 24–48 hours after thrombolysis. Intervention following angiography was at the operators' discretion, but the protocol specified guidelines, shown in Table 1. The intent was to treat patients with a significant residual stenosis in the infarct-related artery by angioplasty or coronary bypass grafting. The trial protocol did not specify that attempts should be made to open or bypass an occluded infarct-related artery.

First acute MI;Symptoms < 3 hours; ST elevation

Exclusions: Cardiogenic shock, major CI to thrombolysis

Thrombolysis: anistreplase 30u + heparin

Randomize within 24 hours

Conservative Management:
Heparin, Warfarin, Timolol
Intervene only for clinical
indication

Intervention:
Angiography within
48 hours with view to
intervention

Endpoints: Death + nonfatal reinfarction within 12 months

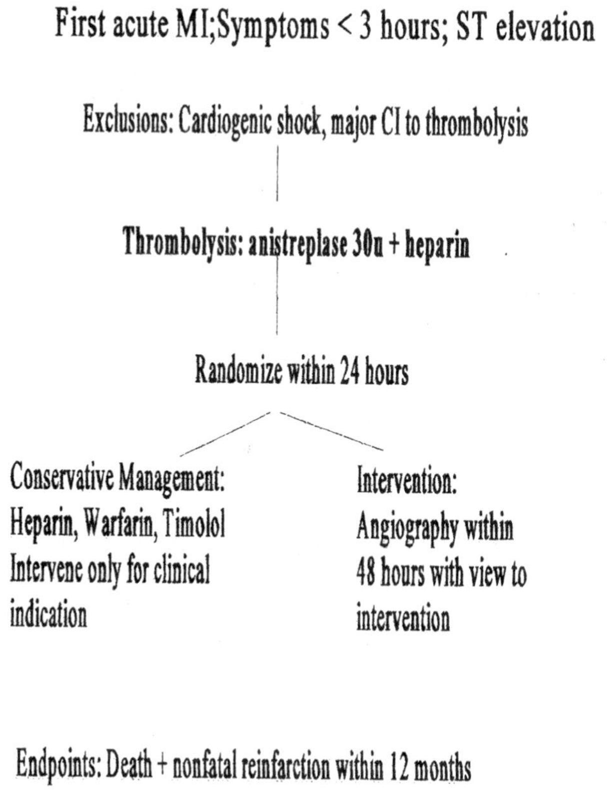

Figure 1   The design and entry criteria for the SWIFT study.

Table 1 Guidelines for Intervention in SWIFT

Angioplasty is the preferred mode of treatment.

The index or culprit segment is the primary target.

The prime indication for intervention is "any antegrade flow through a main target artery judged still to be compromised by a narrow segment."

The degree of narrowing that indicates vulnerability is a diameter stenosis > 50%.

Attempted recanalization of an occluded vesssel is not required.

Coronary bypass grafting is allowed if angioplasty is not feasible or unlikely to be successful, if multiple lesions are present, or if angioplasty is unsuccessful.

RESULTS

Nine hundred and ninety-three patients entered the study and received thrombolytic therapy, of whom 800 were randomized to either early angiography ($n = 397$) or conservative management ($n = 403$). One hundred and ninety-three patients were not randomized, roughly half for procedural reasons, such as failure to secure informed consent, and half for medical reasons, such as death, cardiogenic shock, or pulmonary edema. Early angiography and conservative management groups were well matched for baseline characteristics. In the group randomized to early angiography, 95% of patients actually had an angiogram performed; 70% of the angiograms were performed within 48 hours. In the intervention group, 169 patients (42%) underwent angioplasty, 58 patients (16%) had coronary bypass surgery, and 169 patients (42%) had no intervention. Blood flow in the infarct-related vessel at the time of initial angiography was TIMI grade 3 in 58%, grade 2 in 10%, and grade 1 or 0 in 32%. Revascularization was attempted in 180 of 255 (71%) patients with TIMI 2 or 3 flow and 45 of 118 (38%) patients with TIMI 0 or 1 flow. The allocation of patients to angioplasty, surgery, and medical management is shown in Figure 2.

The major outcomes of the trial are given in Table 2. The composite measure of death and nonfatal myocardial infarction was more frequent in the intervention group at 30 days, but there was no significant difference at 1 year. There was no significant difference in the prevalence of angina at 1 year. Patients in the conservative management group were more likely to have had a subsequent angiogram or intervention between leaving hospital and the 1-year follow-up (Table 3). The in-hospital death rate was low in both

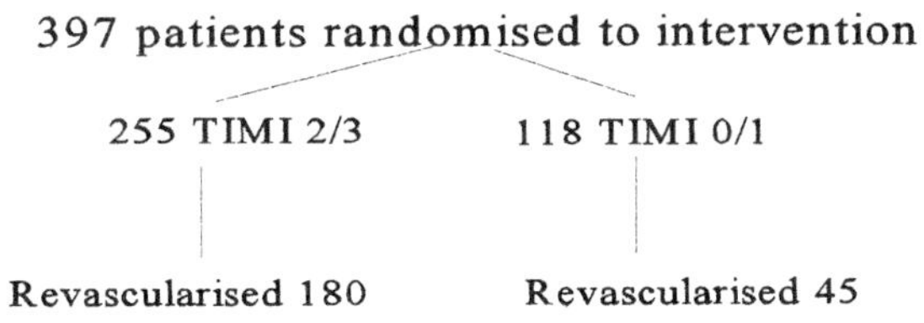

397 patients randomised to intervention

255 TIMI 2/3   118 TIMI 0/1

Revascularised 180   Revascularised 45

Figure 2 Revascularization and TIMI flow status at initial angiography.

Table 2 Major Outcomes

	Intervention	Conservative	Odds ratio
In-hospital death	13/397 (3.3%)	11/403 (2.7%)	1.20 (0.53–2.72)
Death at 12 months	23/390 (5.8%)	20/393 (5.0%)	1.18 (0.64–2.10)
Reinfarction at 12 months	60/320 (15.1%)	52/326 (12.9%)	1.16 (0.77–1.75)
Angina at 12 months	69/357 (19.3)	92/365 (25.2)	0.71 (0.50–1.01)
Ejection fraction	51.7% (SD 15.4)	50.7% (SD 14.2)	ns

Table 3 Late Interventions[a]

	Intervention group (n = 384)	Conservative group (n = 392)	*p*-value
Diagnostic angiogram	20 (5.2%)	57 (14.5%)	<0.001
Angioplasty	4 (1.0%)	16 (4.0%)	0.011
Bypass graft	10 (2.6%)	24 (6.1%)	0.022

[a] Hospital discharge to 12 months.

the intervention (3.3%) and conservative management (2.7%) groups but considerably higher in patients given thrombolysis but not subsequently randomized (13%), particularly if the nonrandomization was for medical reasons. The incidence of major bleeding complications was low in both groups.

DISCUSSION

The principal outcome of the SWIFT trial was the finding that there was no benefit, in terms of survival or recurrent infarction at 30 days, as a result of a strategy of early angiography followed by intervention when compared with a strategy of conservative management with angiography and intervention only if indicated by symptoms or other clinical findings. Broadly similar results were obtained in each of the other major trials that evaluated early elective intervention following thrombolysis (7,8). There seems to be no reason to believe that the thrombolytic agent used in SWIFT, anistreplase, had any influence on the outcome, and similar results have been reported in trials where alteplase was used instead.

Some of the "disbenefit" seen at 30 days in the elective intervention group related to the morbidity and mortality of the revascularization procedures. The increased risk of abrupt vessel closure in angioplasty procedures carried out in the context of unstable angina or following thrombolysis is now well recognized. It may relate both to exposure of thrombogenic material from the atheromatous plaque and to lack of support for vessel wall dissections, particularly after removal of thrombus by thrombolytic therapy. The latter may be particularly important in the context of the apparent paradox of good results from primary angioplasty (9,10). Although the thrombolysis protocol for SWIFT did not specify the use of aspirin, the angioplasty protocol allowed operators to use their own medication regimen and virtually all operators premedicated with aspirin. All of the angioplasty operators in SWIFT were experienced, and the centralization of invasive cardiology in the United Kingdom and Ireland facilitated this. However, the imaging equipment and angioplasty hardware used at the time of the SWIFT trial were primitive by contemporary standards, and stents were not available. In this context the results of angioplasty in the SWIFT study were actually surprisingly good. There were only three procedure-related deaths, of which two were related to angioplasty and one to coronary bypass surgery. The immediate success rate of angioplasty in the intervention group was 87%.

The question SWIFT was designed to answer focused on the relief of residual stenosis. Was this the right question? Should we have been more interested in flow than in stenosis? Should we have made more effort to recanalize occluded vessels? There is now good evidence that coronary flow, as assessed by TIMI criteria and/or an angiographic frame count, is a better predictor of outcome following thrombolysis than the degree of residual stenosis (11,12). This information was not, of course, available at the time of the SWIFT study. Most of the studies on the influence of flow on outcome have been based on angiograms performed early after giving thrombolytic therapy; there are few data linking flow in later angiograms to outcome. The message is probably that patients with good flow but a severe residual stenosis have a better medium-term prognosis than we had anticipated in designing the SWIFT study and should have been left alone. The question about late elective recanalization of occluded or virtually occluded vessels is as yet unanswered. There are observational data and data from animal studies showing that late patency of an infarct-related vessel has a beneficial effect on ventricular remodeling (13). Clinical data from trials of rescue angioplasty show a trend toward improved outcome, but no trial has yet reported the effect of elective late recanalization of an occluded vessel in terms of improved ventricular function or survival, although several anecdotal reports have shown it to be effective in relieving angina. To put all this in perspective, it should be remembered that although more than 40% of patients in the intervention arm of SWIFT had unsatisfactory (i.e., less than TIMI grade 3) flow at the time of angiography, and this was presumably also the case in the conservative management group, 1-year mortality in both groups was equally low at 5.8% and 5.0%, respectively. It would require a very large trial indeed to show a significant survival difference from late intervention on occluded vessels. If anything, the most important message of SWIFT has been that patients who survive for 24 hours or so after a myocardial infarct without developing cardiogenic shock or pulmonary edema have already selected themselves into a high-survival group.

What effect has SWIFT had on cardiological practice in Britain and Ireland? Paradoxically, one effect has been to encourage the increasingly widespread use of thrombolysis in acute myocardial infarction by helping to remove the worry that optimum results would be dependent on subsequent intervention. Coronary angiography and intervention facilities remain centralized, and most patients who develop severe complications after infarction need to be transferred to a tertiary center. Early rescue angioplasty for patients with severe hemodynamic disturbance despite thrombolysis is commonly performed, but overall survival in this group remains unsatisfactory. Results are better in patients with recurrent ischemia but well-deserved ventricular function. Current guidelines emphasize risk stratification in postinfarct patients based on clinical factors and noninvasive testing, with angiography and intervention indicated for persistent, recurrent, or provocable ischemia (14).

REFERENCES

1. SWIFT (Should We Intervene Following Thrombolysis?) Trial Study Group. SWIFT trial of delayed elective intervention conservative treatment after thrombolysis with anistreplase in acute myocardial infarction. Br Med J 1991; 302:555–560.

2. ISIS-2 (Second International Study of Infarct Survival). Randomised trial of intravenous streptokinase, oral aspirin, both or neither among 17,187 cases of suspected acute myocardial infarction: ISIS 2. Lancet 1988; ii:349–360.

3. AIMS Trial Study Group. Effect of intravenous APSAC on mortality after acute myocardial infarction: preliminary report of a placebo-controlled clinical trial. Lancet 1988; 1:545–549.

4. Harrison DG, Ferguson DW, Collins SM, et al. Rethrombosis after reperfusion with streptokinase: importance of geometry of residual lesions. Circulation 1984; 69:991–999.

5. Davies MJ, Thomas A. Thrombosis and acute coronary artery lesions in sudden ischaemic cardiac death. N Engl J Med 1984; 310:1137–1140.

6. Falk E. Plaque rupture with severe pre-existing thrombosis precipitating coronary thrombosis. Characteristics of coronary atherosclerotic plaques underlying fatal occlusive thrombi. Br Heart J 1983; 50:27–134.

7. TIMI Study Group. Comparison of invasive and conservative strategies after treatment with intravenous tissue plasminogen activator in acute myocardial infarction. Results of the thrombolysis in myocardial infarction (TIMI) phase II trial. N Engl J Med 1989; 320:618–627.

8. TIMI (Thrombolysis in Myocardial Infarction) Research Group. Immediate v. delayed catheterisation and angioplasty following thrombolytic therapy for acute myocardial infarction. TIMI-IIA results. JAMA 1988; 260:2849–2858.

9. Zijlstra F, de Boer M, Hoorntje JCA, Reiffers S, Reiber JHC, Suryapranata H. A comparison of immediate coronary angioplasty with intravenous streptokinase in acute myocardial infarction. N Engl J Med 1993; 328:680–684.

10. Grines CL, Browne KF, Marco J, et al. A comparison of immediate angioplasty with thrombolytic therapy for acute myocardial infarction. N Engl J Med 1993; 328:673–679.

11. Anderson JL, Karagounis L, Lewis CB, Sorensen SG, Menlove RL for the TEAM-3 investigators. TIMI perfusion grade 3 but not grade 2 results in improved outcome after thrombolysis for myocardial infarction. Circulation 1993; 87:1829–1839.

12. Simes RJ, Topol EJ, Holmes DR, White HD, Rutsch WR, Vahanian A, Simoons ML, Morris D, Betriu A, Califf RM, Ross AM for the GUSTO investigators. Link between the angiographic substudy and mortality outcomes in a large randomized trial of myocardial reperfusion. Importance of early and complete reperfusion. Circulation 1995; 91:1923–1928.

13. Lamas GA, Flaher GC, Mitchell G, Smith SC, Gersh BJ, Wun CC, et al. Effects of infarct artery patency on prognosis after acute myocardial infarction. Circulation 1995; 92:1101–1109.

14. The Task Force on the Management of Acute Myocardial Infarction of the European Society of Cardiology. Acute myocardial infarction: pre hospital and in hospital management. Eur Heart J 1996; 17:43–63.

Section O
Thrombolysis and PTCA

These final two chapters illustrate quite well the rapidly changing field of defining the optimum modality for achieving the primary goal in the treatment of patients with myocardial infarction—the prompt, safe, complete, and durable restoration of coronary blood flow. Giugliano and Braunwald review the lessons of the TIMI-IIA Trial, which evaluated the role of immediate PTCA in the setting of thrombolytic therapy. Is its primary finding of no advantage, and possible harm from immediate PTCA after thrombolysis still relevant? The authors are careful to point out the sensitivity of this conclusion to advances in the drugs used to achieve reperfusion as well as the techniques (particularly stents) available for angioplasty. O'Neill traces the history of the interplay of PTCA and thrombolysis as therapies sometimes applied together, sometimes separately, and comes down in favor of the use of acute PTCA without antecedent thrombolysis.

Perhaps the simplest conclusion to draw from these studies is that coronary reperfusion should remain the primary treatment goal for patients with myocardial infarction. The use of thrombolytic agents, as discussed in the first section of this book, is of clear benefit. Acute angioplasty (with or without stenting) is also beneficial, and is likely to meet with greater success if used directly, as opposed to being used as an adjunct to thrombolysis. The selection of thrombolysis or acute angioplasty is likely to be driven by local factors such as the availability of PTCA facilities and operators. Whether this should be the case, or whether the data compel us to make acute angioplasty more available, is a broader social question, analogous perhaps to the availability of advanced trauma services at some, but not all, hospitals. It is also predictable that the efficacy of both thrombolysis and acute angioplasty will benefit from the use of newer antithrombotic strategies now being evaluated.

40

TIMI-IIA

ROBERT P. GIUGLIANO and EUGENE BRAUNWALD

Rogers WJ, Baim DS, Gore JM, Brown BG, Roberts R, Williams DO, et al. Comparison of immediate invasive, delayed invasive, and conservative strategies after tissue-type plasminogen activator. Results of the thrombolysis in myocardial infarction (TIMI) phase II-A trial. Circulation 1990; 81:1457–1476.

DeWood's (1) recognition that total coronary occlusion by a fresh thrombus is the primary mechanism responsible for acute myocardial infarction (AMI) paved the way for aggressive therapeutic advances. Subsequently, coronary angiography with intracoronary streptokinase was shown to be safe and efficacious (2). However, angiographic trials in AMI demonstrated that the culprit vessel frequently remains stenotic or occluded despite thrombolytic treatment; furthermore, recovery of left ventricular function after thrombolysis appeared to be linked to restoration of adequate flow (3). Since many of the early investigations of thrombolytics entailed coronary artery catheterization either to deliver the lytic agent or to assess its results, it was a logical next step to perform a mechanical revascularization following thrombolysis. Thus, within 3 years of Gruntzig's (4) initial description of percutaneous transluminal coronary angioplasty (PTCA), the first report of immediate PTCA after intracoronary streptokinase in a small series of patients with acute myocardial infarction appeared (5). A more aggressive approach to residual coronary artery disease after successful early thrombolysis was deemed promising, and as early as 1982 some authors even suggested considering routine early PTCA for noncritical occlusions (6).

Several other studies of PTCA performed very early in the course of AMI treated with thrombolytics soon followed (7–12). Although this strategy was not universally accepted and significant practice variation existed in the mid-1980s, it became quite popular with some cardiologists despite the lack of any single large experience. One investigator even entitled his paper on this subject ''Is transluminal coronary angioplasty mandatory after successful thrombolysis?'' (7).

Whether the benefits observed with an open artery with normal flow following immediate angioplasty outweighed the risks associated with immediate intervention was unknown. The American College of Cardiology/American Heart Association Task Force Guidelines for PTCA (13) published in 1988 reflected the clinical equipoise that existed at the time regarding routine immediate angioplasty following myocardial infarction and considered PTCA in this setting a Class II indication—one in which there was divergence of opinion with respect to its justification in terms of value and appropriateness. Thus, the stage was set in the late 1980s for larger randomized clinical trials to address the issue of whether improved clinical outcomes could be realized with the use of routine immediate PTCA following thrombolysis (14–19).

THE TIMI-IIA TRIAL

Objectives

The primary objective of the TIMI-IIA trial was to establish the feasibility and optimal timing of PTCA in patients with AMI treated with tPA. The primary study endpoint was resting global left ventricular ejection fraction as measured by contrast ventriculography prior to hospital discharge. Secondary endpoints included (1) value and success of protocol PTCA; (2) predischarge infarct-vessel patency as assessed by angiography; (3) exercise test performance; need for nonprotocol procedures including coronary angiography, (re) PTCA, and coronary artery bypass surgery (CABG); and (4) frequency of complications.

Trial Design

The TIMI-IIA trial was nested in the much larger TIMI-II trial of 3534 patients (Fig. 1). Between April 11, 1986, and June 30, 1988, 586 patients were enrolled at one of seven hospitals with expertise in angioplasty participating in the TIMI-IIA substudy. Patients were less than 76 years of age, within 4 hours of the onset of ischemic chest discomfort lasting at least 30 minutes in association with $\geq$1.0 mm ST elevation. Patients were ex-

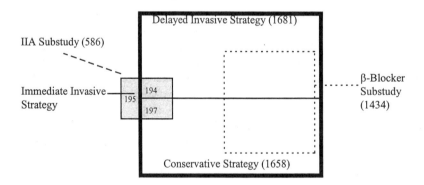

Figure 1 Design of the TIMI-II Main Trial and Substudies. Diagram showing interrelation of TIMI-II studies. The TIMI-II trial included 3534 patients. There were three studies as follows: (1) TIMI-II main study (large square, $n = 3339$) in which patients were randomized between delayed invasive strategy ($n = 181$) and conservative strategy groups ($n = 1658$); (2) TIMI-IIA substudy (hatched rectangle, $n = 586$), overlapping with main study but including immediate invasive strategy treatment group; and (3) beta-blocker substudy ($n = 1434$), a component of main study in which patients eligible for immediate intravenous beta-blocker were randomized (in a 2 $\times$ 2 factorial design) between immediate and delayed beta-blocker therapy as well as between delayed invasive strategy and conservative strategy groups. (From Ref. 17.)

cluded if they had prior CABG, PTCA within 6 months, or were at increased risk for stroke or bleeding.

Medications

All patients received tPA over 6 hours. In the first 195 patients 150 mg tPA was administered as a constant infusion over 6 hours at a rate of 25 mg/hr. Due to an unacceptable frequency of hemorrhage, the dose of tPA was decreased to 100 mg (391 patients) administered as an intravenous bolus of 6 mg and a constant infusion of 54 mg during the first hour, 20 mg during the second hour, and 5 mg during each of the next 4 hours. Aspirin (81 mg for 5 days, then 325 daily) was administered at day 1 (first 127 patients) or day 2 (subsequent patients), along with 5 days of intravenous heparin (5000 U bolus followed by 1000 U/hr initial infusion) titrated to maintain a therapeutic aPTT followed by subcutaneous heparin beginning on day 6. All patients received sublingual nitroglycerin, prophylactic lidocaine, morphine at presentation, and nifedipine 10–20 mg three times daily for the first 4 days unless a contraindication existed. In all patients without contraindication to beta-blockade, oral metoprolol was initiated prior to discharge and continued for one year in all patients without contraindication.

Management Strategies

Patients were randomly allocated to the immediate invasive strategy, delayed invasive strategy, or conservative strategy group (Fig. 2). Patients assigned to the immediate invasive strategy underwent coronary arteriography and ventriculography within 120 minutes of tPA initiation, while those randomized to the delayed invasive strategy were catheterized between 18 and 48 hours following tPA initiation. In the immediate invasive strategy, PTCA was performed while tPA was still being infused, whether the infarct-related artery was open or closed, except when the coronary anatomy was unsuitable. Unsuitable features included lesions that were associated with <60% residual stenosis, ≥20 mm in length, involved a bifurcation, located distally or beyond a tortuosity, or left-main functional equivalents. In contrast, in the delayed invasive strategy, PTCA was performed between 18 and 48 hours *only* if the infarct-related artery was open *and* the artery was suitable. Patients assigned to the conservative strategy underwent routine medical management; angiography was discouraged until immediately prior to hospital discharge (usually day 8–10) unless refractory recurrent ischemia developed despite stepwise augmentation of the antiischemic regimen. In all groups, CABG was limited to high-risk patients with anatomy unsuitable for PTCA (e.g., >70% left-main stenosis) or patients with urgent clinical indications such as refractory angina.

Pre- and Postdischarge Evaluation

Resting and bicycle-exercise radionuclide ventriculography was performed in all patients between days 8 and 10 to assess left ventricular function and clinical response to submaximal exercise. Following these studies, coronary angiography and ventriculography were performed in all patients. In patients assigned to the conservative strategy, medical therapy was advised unless there was evidence of left-main stenosis ≥70% or resting or exercise-induced ischemia on predischarge testing.

At 6 weeks, resting and exercise radionuclide ventriculography was repeated. Exer-

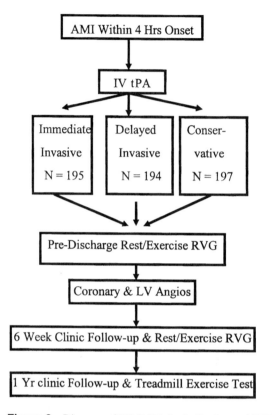

Figure 2 Diagram of TIMI-IIA Study Design and PTCA Outcomes. Diagram of TIMI-IIA study design. AMI, acute myocardial infarction; IV, intravenous; tPA, recombinant tissue-type plasminogen activator; RVG, radionuclide ventriculogram; LV, left ventricular; angios, angiograms. (From Ref. 17.)

cise was continued until the age-adjusted maximal predicted heart rate was achieved or symptoms occurred. At 1 year, a maximum symptom-limited treadmill exercise test was performed using the standard Bruce protocol. Clinical events including procedures were recorded at both postdischarge evaluations.

Results

Rates of angiography and PTCA were different for each of the three groups as expected per protocol (Fig. 3). In the immediate invasive strategy group, 99% of patients underwent angiography within 2 hours of tPA initiation; PTCA was attempted in 72% of the patients catheterized. Improvement in stenosis as assessed by the TIMI Core Radiographic Laboratory was observed in 77% of the patients undergoing PTCA within 2 hours, with a higher rate of improvement observed for patients with still-occluded arteries compared to those with patent but stenotic infarct-related arteries (90% vs. 73% $p = 0.06$).

In the delayed invasive strategy group, angiography was performed between 18 and 48 hours in 90% of patients, with 62% of these undergoing PTCA. Of the 19 patients who did not undergo angiography at the specified timepoint, 5 had died and 12 had urgent

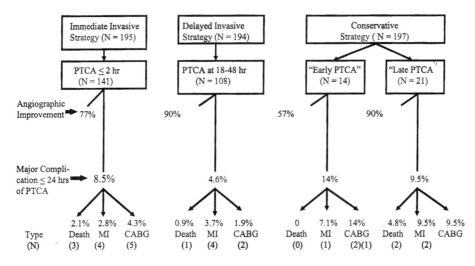

Figure 3 Diagram Showing Outcome of Patients Having PTCA. Angiographic improvement was more likely with delayed invasive strategy group as compared with immediate invasive strategy (90% vs. 77%), and major complications were fewer (8.5% vs. 4.6%). Among patients in conservative strategy group, only a small number of patients underwent either "early PTCA" (before scheduled predischarge coronary arteriogram) or "late PTCA" (after predischarge coronary arteriogram); however, more angiographic improvement and fewer complications were also evident in the "late PTCA" groups compared with the "early PTCA group." (From Ref. 17.)

angiography prior to 18 hours. Compared to the immediate invasive group, significantly more patients in the delayed invasive strategy were judged by the core laboratory to have an improvement in stenosis (90% vs. 77%, $p < 0.01$)

In the conservative strategy group, 35 patients (18%) underwent "early" angiography prior to the scheduled predischarge catheterization; of these, the majority underwent revascularization (40% PTCA, 17% CABG). In the conservative group, 14 patients had an urgent PTCA performed "early" due to clinical indications. In 8 (57%) of these cases, PTCA resulted in an improvement of stenosis. In contrast, of the 21 patients in the conservative strategy group who underwent elective PTCA predischarge (i.e., "late PTCA"), 19 (90%) had an improvement in stenosis. Furthermore, "late PTCA" was associated with a slightly lower rate of major complications (9.5% vs. 14%), although small numbers (21 "late PTCA," 14 "early PTCA") and the selected nature of the "early PTCA" patients limit the ability to make a useful comparison.

A key observation in the TIMI-IIA trial was that the performance of PTCA early following thrombolysis was associated with a relatively higher rate of complication. Major complications (death, reinfarction, or need for emergent CABG) within 24 hours of PTCA occurred in 12 patients (8.5%) in the immediate invasive strategy compared to 5 patients (4.6%) in the delayed invasive strategy ($p = 0.31$). Among patients in the conservative strategy group, only 14 patients underwent early PTCA and 21 late PTCA; 2 patients in each group experienced a major complication within 24 hours. Thus the trend toward more complications and poorer angiographic outcomes when PTCA was performed early was also observed within the conservative strategy group.

Bypass surgery was performed in 67 of the 586 patients (11%) within 21 days of enrollment, with over one-third of the total immediately following an attempted PTCA and the remainder for anatomic reasons. While the use of CABG for anatomic findings was similar across the three management strategies, there was a significantly greater use of CABG after attempted PTCA in the immediate invasive strategy group compared to the delayed invasive and conservative strategy groups (7.7, 2.1 and 2.5%, respectively; p = 0.01). The mortality rate for CABG after attempted PTCA was 16.7% (4 of 24 patients), sevenfold higher than the 2.3% (one of 43 patients) mortality rate observed when CABG was performed for anatomic considerations (p = 0.05). Furthermore, all of the periopera- tive infarctions occurred in the attempted PTCA-CABG group, resulting in a perioperative infarct rate of 25% (6 of 24 patients) compared to a perioperative infarction rate of 0% for the unfavorable anatomy–CABG group (p = 0.01).

Patency of the infarct-related artery at the protocol-mandated catheterization within 2 hours for the immediate invasive and at 18–48 hours in the delayed invasive strategy groups were similar (81% vs. 83%, respectively). Likewise, predischarge assessment of patency did not differ among the three groups (81, 84, and 86%).

Quantitative coronary angiography demonstrated differences among the groups that were of uncertain clinical significance. On initial angiography, patients in the immediate invasive strategy group had a greater degree of stenosis of the infarct-related artery com- pared to delayed invasive patients (80% vs. 75%, p = 0.01), and had fewer nonobstructive (i.e., <60% diameter stenosis) lesions (6.2% vs. 14.4%, p = 0.01) This likely reflects the earlier timepoint for angiography in the immediate invasive group. Prior to discharge, the mean degrees of stenosis in the two invasive strategies were significantly lower than that for the conservative strategy group (51, 48, and 67%, respectively; $p < 0.001$) and more patients in the invasive groups had nonobstructive lesions of ≤60% diameter stenosis (68, 75, and 31%, respectively; $p < 0.001$).

Despite the higher degree of stenosis and lower rates of revascularization in the conservative group, efficacy endpoints did not favor either invasive strategy. The mean ejection fraction measured by contrast left ventriculography (primary endpoint) was nearly identical across the groups (0.50, 0.49, 0.49). The percentage of patients with either normal EF (≥50%) or severely impaired EF (<30%) were also not statistically different among the three groups. Furthermore, other more sensitive assessment of ventricular function including end-systolic and end-diastolic volume indices, cardiac index, and measurement of wall motion in the infarct and noninfarct zones were similar among the three groups. Rest and exercise ejection fractions at 6 weeks postdischarge were also not different across the groups. Nor were there consistent differences in the rate of positive exercise tests predischarge and 6 weeks postdischarge across the three treatment strategies. Of the clini- cal outcome events not dictated by protocol, only CABG rates at 21 days (due to higher CABG post–attempted PTCA in the immediate invasive strategy group) differed across the groups (see Fig. 3) at 21 days, 6 months, or 1 year. As expected, PTCA rates in the conservative strategy group postdischarge increased at a greater rate compared to the immediate invasive and delayed invasive strategy groups, with the percentage of patients in the conservative strategy group undergoing a PTCA at 21 days and 1 year increasing from 18.3 to 23.9%, while the rate of PTCA changed little between 21 days and 1 year in the immediate invasive and delayed invasive strategy groups (75.2 to 75.8% and 63.2 to 64.3%, respectively).

Discussion of TIMI-IIA Results

The immediate invasive strategy, in which routine catheterization and angioplasty (if feasi- ble) were performed within 2 hours, was the least desirable approach as it resulted in more complications, no net improvement in survival, left ventricular function, or exercise performance at 6 weeks, and did not reduce the risk of reinfarction.

Criticisms of the study included a slightly higher risk profile in the immediate invasive group, a delay of aspirin therapy until 24 hours after randomization in some patients, and the routine use of lidocaine and nifedipine, which were without proven benefit. These criticisms seem unlikely to have invalidated the trial's main findings; this was borne out in subsequent studies in which these criticisms did not apply (18,19). Unlike several other contemporary studies in AMI, patients with pulmonary edema or cardiogenic shock were eligible for TIMI-IIA provided they had not received prolonged CPR. These more critically ill patients would, however, be expected to bias against a conservative strategy.

Experience of the angioplasty operator is an important predictor of success. Angioplasty operators in TIMI-IIA were required to have performed at least 200 procedures, of which at least 20 were in patients with complete occlusion. These requirements were stricter than the existing 1988 ACC/AHA guidelines for PTCA (13), which required only 75 procedures as the primary operator. If the study had been restricted to operators with even greater experience, attempted angioplasty in the invasive strategy would have likely increased and more patients with the most difficult lesions and/or those who subsequently underwent bypass surgery would have then undergone high-risk angioplasty. Although we cannot make any firm conclusions about the impact of such an increase in high-risk angioplasty attempts, the European Cooperative Study Group (15) performed PTCA on nearly all (92%) patients in the immediate invasive strategy following thrombolysis and found increased morbidity and mortality at 14 days compared to the conservative strategy.

LITERATURE POST–TIMI-IIA

After commencement of the enrollment phase of TIMI-IIA, evidence from other quarters began to mount that foreshadowed the eventual trial results. Experimental deep vessel wall injury induced by balloon trauma was demonstrated to expose thrombogenic substrates to circulating blood resulting in new thrombus formation and arterial reocclusion (20). A review of autopsies carried out on 19 patients following myocardial infarction treated with thrombolysis and/or PTCA revealed severe hemorrhage at the angioplasty site in patients treated with thrombolysis and PTCA; in contrast, none of the patients treated with PTCA alone had intraplaque bleeding (21). Finally, two other clinical trials, the TAMI-I trial (14) and the European Cooperative Group Trial (15) reported their results within 6 months of the TIMI-IIA trial, and both concluded that immediate angiography and PTCA following thrombolysis conferred no additional benefit over more conservative management; in fact, immediate PTCA in unselected patients who had just received thrombolytic therapy appeared to be potentially harmful. Thus it was concluded on the basis of three separate trials, which included TIMI-IIA, and involved a total of 1339 patients, that the immediate invasive strategy of routine early PTCA postthrombolysis produced no benefit (and possible harm) compared with strategies that utilized PTCA later or more selectively.

As a result of the accumulating evidence in favor of a conservative strategy, by the early 1990s most physicians considered immediate catheterization and immediate intervention following thrombolysis appropriate only when required for clinical indications. This message was repeatedly voiced in editorials and reviews (22–37). Despite some heterogeneity in the patient populations (e.g., TAMI-I randomized only patients with patent arteries while the TIMI-IIA and European Cooperative Study Group enrolled patients regardless of perfusion status) and medical treatment (dose and administration of tPA, use of adjunctive aspirin), there was remarkable consistency in the results favoring a conservative approach. Furthermore, an experimental model in dogs in which residual critical stenosis following reperfusion was compared to full reperfusion without stenosis revealed that restoration of normal coronary flow did not influence infarct size or early left ventricular functional recovery (38). This finding was used to support the idea that total reperfusion with immediate angioplasty following thrombolysis may not add immediate clinical benefit (26). In sum, routine, immediate angioplasty was considered to offer little benefit with the potential for resulting in harm. The "Blitzkrieg strategy" (23) had suffered a severe blow, and the "reperfusion momentum" (24) in which early angiography yielded a more frequent documentation of high-grade stenosis and resultant increase in early intervention ["oculostenotic reflex" (39)] had been slowed.

Subsequently the AHA/ACC Task Force Committees on PTCA (40) concluded that "data from a number of important randomized clinical trials all suggest that angioplasty should be deferred and performed as clinically indicated following successful thrombolysis" and now considered dilation of borderline residual lesions in the absence of ischemia to be a class III situation (angioplasty not ordinarily indicated) (40,41). The AHA/ACC guideline for management of AMI noted that "immediate catheterization of all patients following thrombolytic therapy to identify those with an occluded infarct-related artery is impractical, costly, and often associated with bleeding complications" (41). Thereafter, attention turned to possible subgroups (e.g., patients with persistent occlusion and hemodynamic compromise) that might benefit from early intervention.

Finally, in the most comprehensive research synthesis in this area completed to date, Michels and Yusuf reviewed 23 clinical trials of PTCA in acute myocardial infarction (35). They found that when mortality at 6 weeks was analyzed for PTCA as an adjunct to thrombolytic therapy, four of the five different approaches to angioplasty (immediate PTCA vs. no PTCA, early PTCA vs. no PTCA, delayed PTCA vs. no PTCA, and immediate PTCA vs. delayed PTCA) demonstrated trends toward increased risk for the more aggressive treatment strategy. Furthermore, no benefit from PTCA following thrombolysis was apparent if the combined endpoint of death and nonfatal MI at 6 weeks was considered. In conclusion, the addition of various strategies of PTCA to thrombolytic therapy did not convincingly indicate a clinically different outcome compared to a more conservative strategy, in which angioplasty is used only when it is clinically indicated.

EVOLUTION OF AMI MANAGEMENT SINCE TIMI-IIA—IMPLICATIONS

The treatment of acute myocardial infarction has continued to evolve at an increasing pace with the development of new thrombolytics, adjunctive antithrombins and antiplatelet agents, mechanical interventional techniques, and greater appreciation of the importance of aspirin, lower doses of heparin, and shortened time to treatment. Lessons learned from the TIMI-IIA experience and the other similar trials discussed above may or may not apply to current and future treatment regimens. In particular, the reduction in death and MI observed in clinical trials with glycoprotein IIb/IIIa inhibitors (42–46) in association with percutaneous interventions, if also present during interventions postthrombolysis, has the potential to make immediate angioplasty more desirable. In fact, the combination of glycoprotein IIb/IIIa inhibitors with thrombolytics is currently being investigated in several clinical trials and is being closely followed with great interest. Also, advances in interventional cardiology, in particular, the availability of a "bailout" stent, has reduced the need for emergent bypass surgery in complicated or failed percutaneous interventions. Even a simple measure, such as minor reductions in the amount of heparin administered in conjunction with thrombolytics and intervention, has resulted in dramatic reductions in hemorrhagic complications. Thus, it may be reasonable in the near future to resurrect a clinical trial similar to that of TIMI-IIA, taking advantage of these new advances in the field.

UNRESOLVED ISSUES

While the TIMI-IIA trial answered the question of which treatment strategy—conservative, immediate invasive, or delayed invasive—is preferable, it resulted in the generation of many more questions. Current and future trials are investigating a number of these issues, such as determining which subgroups of patients may benefit from immediate intervention, whether faster flow leads to improved outcome, and if noninvasive markers (serum, ECG) can accurately predict failure to reperfuse and thus identify individuals who might benefit from an early invasive strategy. While mortality has declined dramatically since the institution of proactive treatment for acute MI in the late 1970s, AMI remains the most common cause of in-hospital death in industrialized nations, and both mortality rates and morbidity in survivors are unacceptable high. General acceptance over the past decade of the "open-artery hypothesis" (47), which advances the notion that a patent infarct-related artery and myocardial reperfusion results in benefit exceeding that attributed to the salvage of ventricular function alone, has continued the drive to discover alternative methods to open the infarct artery quickly and completely. In this search for the optimum approach to restoration of normal flow, it is quite possible that in the near future we will have come full circle and need to readdress the question posed by TIMI-IIA, albeit with different thrombolytic and antiplatelet regimens.

REFERENCES

1. DeWood MA, Spores J, Notske R, et al. Prevalence of total coronary occlusion during the early hours of transmural myocardial infarction. N Engl J Med 1980; 303:897–902.
2. Kennedy JW, Ritchie JL, Davis KB, Fritz J. Western Washington randomized trial of intracoronary streptokinase in acute myocardial infarction. N Engl J Med 1983; 309:1477–1482.
3. Sheehan FH, Mathey DG, Schofer J, Dodge H, Bolson EL. Factors that determine recovery of left ventricular function after thrombolysis in patients with acute myocardial infarction. Circulation 1985; 71:1121–1128.
4. Gruntzig AR, Senning A, Siegenthaler WE. Nonoperative dilatation of coronary-artery stenosis. N Engl J Med 1979; 301:61–68.
5. Meyer J, Merx W, Schmitz H, et al. Percutaneous transluminal coronary angioplasty immediately after intracoronary streptolysis of transmural myocardial infarction. Circulation 1982; 66:905–913.
6. Swan HJC. Thrombolysis in acute myocardial infarction: treatment of the underlying coronary artery disease. Circulation 1982; 66:914–916.
7. Serruys PW, Wijns W, Van Den Brand M, et al. Is transluminal coronary angioplasty mandatory after successful thrombolysis? Br Heart J 1983; 50:257–265.
8. Papapietro SE, MacLean WA, Stanley Jr. AW, et al. Percutaneous transluminal coronary an-

gioplasty after intracoronary streptokinase in evolving acute myocardial infarction. Am J Cardiol 1985; 55:48–53.

9. Topol EJ, Eha JE, Brin KP, et al. Applicability of percutaneous transluminal coronary angioplasty to patients with recombinant tissue plasminogen activator mediated thrombolysis. Cathet Cardiovasc Diagn 1985; 11:337–348.

10. Erbel R, Pop T, Henrichs KJ, et al. Percutaneous transluminal coronary angioplasty after thrombolytic therapy: a prospective controlled randomized trial. J Am Coll Cardiol 1986; 8: 485–495.

11. Williams DO, Ruocco NA, Forman S. Coronary angioplasty after recombinant tissue-type plasminogen activator in acute myocardial infarction: a report from the Thrombolysis in Myocardial Infarction (TIMI) trial. J Am Coll Cardiol 1987; 10(5 suppl B):45B–50B.

12. Guerci AD, Gerstenblith G, Brinker JA, et al. A randomized trial of intravenous tissue plasminogen activator for acute myocardial infarction with subsequent randomization to elective coronary angioplasty. N Engl J Med 1987; 317:1613–1618.

13. Ryan TJ, Faxon DP, Gunnar RM, et al. Guidelines for percutaneous transluminal coronary angioplasty: a report of the American College of Cardiology/American Heart Association task force on assessment of diagnostic and therapeutic cardiovascular procedures (subcommittee on percutaneous transluminal coronary angioplasty). Circulation 1988; 78:486–502.

14. Topol EJC, George BS, et al. A randomized trial of immediate versus delayed elective angioplasty after intravenous tissue plasminogen activator in acute myocardial infarction. N Engl J Med 1987; 317:581–588.

15. Simoons ML, Arnold AER, Betriu A, et al. Thrombolysis with tissue plasminogen activator in acute myocardial infarction: no additional benefit from immediate percutaneous coronary angioplasty. Lancet 1988; 1:197–203.

16. TIMI Research Group. Immediate vs delayed catheterization and angioplasty following thrombolytic therapy for acute myocardial infarction. JAMA 1988; 260:2849–2858.

17. Rogers WJ, Baim DS, Gore JM, et al. Comparison of immediate invasive, delayed invasive, and conservative strategies after tissue-type plasminogen activator: results of the Thrombolysis in Myocardial Infarction (TIMI) phase II-A trial. Circulation 1990; 81:1457–1476.

18. TIMI Study Group. Comparison of invasive and conservative strategies after treatment with intravenous tissue plasminogen activator in acute myocardial infarction: results of the Thrombolysis in Myocardial Infarction (TIMI) phase II trial. N Engl J Med 1989; 320:618–627.

19. SWIFT Trial Study Group. SWIFT trial of delayed elective intervention vs conservative treatment after thrombolysis with anistreplase in acute myocardial infarction. Br Med J 1991; 302: 555–560.

20. Fuster V, Badimon L, Cohen M, Ambrose JA, Badimon JJ, Chesebro J. Insights into the pathogenesis of acute ischemic syndromes. Circulation 1988; 77:1213–1220.

21. Waller BF, Roghbaum DA, Pinkerton CA, et al. Status of the myocardium and infarct-related coronary artery in 19 necropsy patients with acute recanalization using pharmacologic (streptokinase, r-tissue plasminogen activator), mechanical (percutaneous transluminal coronary angioplasty) or combined types of reperfusion therapy. J Am Coll Cardiol 1987; 9:785–801.

22. Ryan TJ. Angioplasty in acute myocardial infarction: Is the balloon leaking? N Engl J Med 1987; 317:624–626.

23. Cheitlin MD. The aggressive war on acute myocardial infarction: Is the blitzkrieg strategy changing? JAMA 1988; 260:2894–2896.

24. Holmes DR, Topol EJ. Reperfusion momentum: lessons from the randomized trials of immediate coronary angioplasty for myocardial infarction. J Am Coll Cardiol 1989; 14:1572–1578.

25. Guerci AD, Ross RS. TIMI II and the role of angioplasty in acute myocardial infarction. N Engl J Med 1989; 320:663–665.

26. Salem DN, Desnoyers MR, Berman AD, Konstam MA. Coronary angioplasty and thrombolysis for acute myocardial infarction: Is two a crowd? Am J Med 1989; 86:259–261.

27. Sleight P. Do we need to intervene after thrombolysis in acute myocardial infarction? Circulation 1990; 81:1707–1709.

28. Baim DS, Braunwald E, Feit F, et. al. The thrombolysis in myocardial infarction (TIMI) trial phase II: additional information and perspectives. J Am Coll Cardiol 1990; 15:1188–1192.

29. Mueller HS. Reperfusion therapy in acute myocardial infarction: Present status and controversy. Clin Cardiol 1990; 3:239–246.

30. Ryan TJ. Revascularization for acute myocardial infarction: strategies in need of revision. Circulation 1990; 1990:II-110–II-116.

31. Coplan NL. Evolving strategy for managing patients following thrombolytic therapy. Am Heart J 1990; 120:464–466.

32. Geltman EM. Conservative management after thrombolysis: the strategy of choice. J Am Coll Cardiol 1990; 16:1535–1537.

33. Grech ED, Ramsdale DR. Percutaneous transluminal coronary angioplasty and acute myocardial infarction. Br J Hosp Med 1994; 52:35–41.

34. de Marchena E. Tang S. The role of percutaneous transluminal coronary angioplasty in acute myocardial infarction. Clin Cardiol 1994; 17(suppl. I):17–19.

35. Michels K, B., Yusuf S. Does PTCA in acute myocardial infarction affect mortality and reinfarction rates?: a quantitative overview (meta-analysis) of the randomized clinical trials. Circulation 1995; 91:476–485.

36. Anderson HV. Role of Angiography. Cardiol Clin 1995; 13:407–419.

37. Bates DW, Miller E, Bernstein SJ, Hauptman PJ, Leape LL. Coronary angiography and angioplasty after acute myocardial infarction. Ann Intern Med 1997; 126:539–550.

38. Lefkowitz CA, Pace DP, Gallagher KP, Buda AJ. The effects of a critical stenosis on myocardial blood flow, ventricular function, and infarct size after coronary reperfusion. Circulation 1988; 77:915–926.

39. Topol EJ. Coronary angioplasty for acute myocardial infarction. Ann Intern Med 1988; 109: 970–980.

40. Ryan RJ, Bauman WB, Kennedy JW, et al. Guidelines for percutaneous transluminal coronary angioplasty: a report of the American College of Cardiology/American Heart Association task force on assessment of diagnostic and therapeutic cardiovascular procedures (committee on percutaneous transluminal coronary angioplasty). J Am Coll Cardiol 1993; 22:2033–2054.

41. Ryan TJ, Anderson JL, Antman EM, et al. ACC/AHA guidelines for the management of patients with acute myocardial infarction. J Am Coll Cardiol 1996; 28:1328–1428.

42. EPIC Investigators. Use of a monoclonal antibody directed against the platelet glycoprotein IIb/IIIa receptor in high-risk coronary angioplasty. N Engl J Med 1994; 330:956–961.

43. EPILOG Investigators. Platelet glycoprotein IIb/IIIa receptor blockade and low-dose heparin during percutaneous coronary revascularization. N Engl J Med 1997; 336:1689–1696.

44. CAPTURE Investigators. Randomised placebo-controlled trial of abciximab before and during coronary intervention in refractory unstable angina: the CAPTURE study. Lancet 1997; 349: 1429–1435.

45. RESTORE Investigators. The effects of platelet glycoprotein IIb/IIIa blockade with tirofiban on adverse cardiac events in patients with unstable angina or acute myocardial infarction undergoing coronary angioplasty. Circulation 1997; 96(5):1445–1453.

46. IMPACT-II Investigators. Randomised placebo-controlled trial of effect of eptifibatide on complications of percutaneous coronary intervention: IMPACT-II. Lancet 1997; I:1422–1428.

47. Kim CB, Braunwald E. Potential benefits of late reperfusion of infarcted myocardium: the open artery hypothesis. Circulation 1993; 88: 2426–2436.

41

TAMI and PAMI

WILLIAM W. O'NEILL

Topol EJ, Califf RM, George BS, Kereiakes DJ, Abbottsmith CW, Candela RJ et al. and the Thrombolysis and Angioplasty in Myocardial Infarction Study Group. A randomized trial of immediate versus delayed elective angioplasty after intravenous tissue plasminogen activator in acute myocardial infarction. N Engl J Med 1987;317:581–588

Grines CL, Browne KF, Marco J, Rothbaum D, Stone GW, O'Keefe, et al. for the Primary Angioplasty in Myocardial Infarction Study Group. A comparison of immediate angioplasty with thrombolytic therapy for acute myocardial infarction. N Engl J Med 1993;328:673–679.

The role of catheterization and mechanical reperfusion techniques in the management of acute myocardial infarction (AMI) has been the subject of enormous controversy for over two decades (1). This controversy is ironic since the modern era of reperfusion therapy was actually initiated by Rentrop's attempt at guidewire recanalization of freshly occluded vessels during AMI catheterization (2). This quickly led to his pioneering observations on the value of intracoronary streptokinase therapy (3). Kennedy shortly thereafter demonstrated a survival advantage for patients treated with intracoronary streptokinase (4) and provided the first strong (5) data validating the open artery hypothesis. These interventional studies performed in the early 1980s were incredibly exciting because they suggested that for the first time the devastating effects of abrupt thrombotic coronary occlusion could be ameliorated.

In the early 1980s, the main focus of clinical investigation centered on catheterization-based studies. The catheterization-based findings of a high prevalence of total occlusion and scientific demonstration of the ability of intracoronary streptokinase to lyse thrombus and reestablish coronary blood flow (6) were crucial in establishing the mechanistic underpinnings for thrombolytic therapy.

By 1985, we were convinced of the value of mechanical reperfusion strategies. Although we first demonstrated that intracoronary streptokinase was superior to placebo in establishing arterial patency (7), we were disappointed in the impact of this therapy on ventricular function (8). Hartzler suggested that balloon angioplasty might more effectively preserve ventricular function (9). From a mechanistic standpoint this appeared logical because angioplasty not only could recanalize coronary arteries, it could also relieve the underlying obstruction, which invariably persisted after thrombolytic therapy. This concept led us to initiate a randomized trial of primary angioplasty versus intracoronary streptokinase therapy (10). The results of this study (Table 1) were greatly in favor of primary angioplasty in terms of relief of the underlying obstruction, improvement of ejection fraction and regional wall motion, and a decrease of postinfarction ischemia. These observations led us to become advocates of mechanical strategies. It also placed us in an uphill battle with the advocates of intravenous thrombolytic therapy.

In the early 1980s balloon angioplasty therapy of acute MI was largely confined to a few research institutions worldwide. Both angioplasty and intracoronary streptokinase therapy were greatly limited by the obligatory requirements for skilled personnel and catheterization facilities. In 1985, the landmark GISSI trial (11) demonstrated that intravenous reperfusion therapy could be offered as a broad-based reperfusion strategy. Shortly after publication of this trial, tPA became available as an even more potent thrombolytic agent (12). Many investigators and clinicians fervently hoped that intravenous reperfusion therapy would do away with the need for catheterization-based treatments.

Unfortunately, before 1985, intracoronary streptokinase therapy was the only scientifically validated therapy for acute MI. In fact, intracoronary streptokinase received FDA approval around that time. With publication of the GISSI trial, the comparative efficacy of intravenous versus intracoronary streptokinase therapy was questioned. Because of the debate about the efficacy of intravenous lytic therapy, an initial RFP from the NHLBI was proposed to compare intravenous to intracoronary streptokinase. This NHLBI-sponsored trial was named the Thrombolysis in Myocardial Infarction (TIMI) trial. Although the original proposal sought to compare intravenous to intracoronary streptokinase therapy, the emphasis of the trial shifted to a comparison of intravenous streptokinase to tPA. It is fascinating in retrospect to reconstruct the logic employed in testing these three competing reperfusion strategies (Fig. 1).

Intracoronary streptokinase was the first scientifically validated effective reperfusion strategy. We next demonstrated that coronary angioplasty was superior to intracoronary streptokinase. Logic should have dictated that any new reperfusion strategy (either intravenous streptokinase or intravenous tPA) should be compared to the existing gold standard. This comparison, in fact, never occurred! Ultimately, we lost 10 years of time because a true comparison of coronary angioplasty to intravenous thrombolytic therapy did not occur at that time. Like the TIMI Investigators, the scientific community, including our group, became less interested in coronary angioplasty and more interested in intravenous thrombolytic therapy.

While the TIMI trial was being organized, Eric Topol from our group coordinated

Table 1 Angioplasty Versus Intracoronary Streptokinase

	PTCA	SK	*p*-Value
No. of patients	29	27	
Reperfusion	83%	85%	NS
Final stenosis	44 ± 10%	80 ± 7%	<0.001
Change in EF	+7 ± 0.1%	+0.5 ± 0.5%	<0.01
Thallium ischemia	12%	45%	<0.05

EF = Ejection fraction (contrast ventriculography).
Source: Ref. 10.

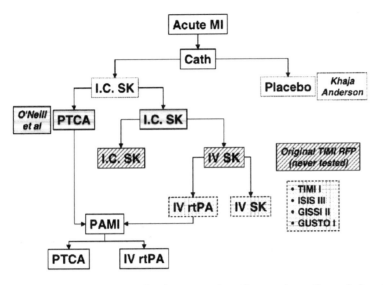

Figure 1   Logic diagram for the progression of comparison of reperfusion strategies.

a multicenter placebo-controlled trial of intravenous tPA (13). This study demonstrated that intravenous tPA was a highly effective thrombolytic agent. Since a catheterization-based reperfusion strategy was so labor intensive and logistically difficult, scientific interest turned to an intravenous approach. The mainstream scientific community wanted to further validate intravenous thrombolytic therapy. Thus, the focus of TIMI turned from a comparison of intracoronary versus intravenous streptokinase to a comparison of intravenous streptokinase to re-PA. Similarly, the GISSI and ISIS investigators launched comparisons of tPA versus streptokinase. Thus, the thrombolytic wars were launched. What was forgotten by many was that coronary angioplasty had not been systematically compared to intravenous lytics.

In 1986, our group diverged from the scientific mainstream. Although we were excited about the increased applicability of intravenous therapy, we remained concerned about those patients that failed to reperfuse and were concerned about the underlying stenosis that persisted after thrombolytic therapy. We were convinced of the superiority of PTCA but recognized that intravenous therapy would be more widely available.

At this point, Eric Topol, Robert Califf, Richard Stack, Dean Keriakes, Barry George, and I formed a working group. This group was entitled the Thrombolysis Angioplasty Myocardial Infarction (TAMI) trial. We wished to determine whether angioplasty had incremental value after thrombolytic therapy. We proposed a strategy that might marry the best of both approaches. Local administration of intravenous thrombolytic therapy would allow a widespread, early initiation of reperfusion therapy. Patients could then be transferred to regional centers and have catheterization performed. Since we were convinced of the value of an open artery, all patients with failed lytic therapy were treated with salvage PTCA. A major question existed about whether angioplasty was required for patients with patent vessels. For this reason, those patients with reflow established were randomized to immediate versus delayed angioplasty. Based on our previous randomized trial of angioplasty versus intracoronary streptokinase, we postulated that immediate

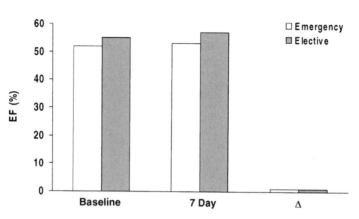

Figure 2 Contrast ventriculography was performed at initial catheterization and repeated 1 week later in patients randomized to emergency angioplasty versus delayed angioplasty. No difference in preservation of ventricular function was detected.

PTCA would provide more effective preservation of ventricular function. Contrast ventriculograms were performed at immediate catheterization and prior to hospital discharge. We were greatly surprised that no improvement in global or regional ventricular function existed for the group treated with immediate PTCA (Fig. 2). The TAMI-I trial is now labeled as a negative trial. Unfortunately, what is forgotten is that 50% of patients initially treated were not randomized (Fig. 3). In total, 25% of patients failed to reperfuse and underwent salvage PTCA and 25% of patients had extensive multivessel or left main

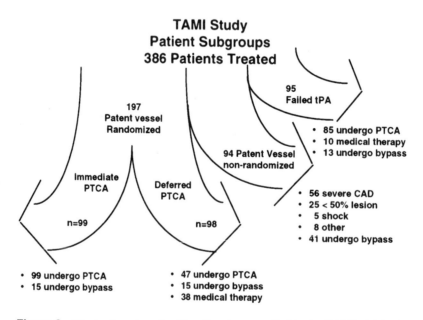

Figure 3 The treatment received by all patients enrolled in the TAMI trial is depicted. Note the large proportion of patients not randomized and the large proportion of patients undergoing surgery prior to discharge.

disease and underwent urgent bypass surgery. These patients probably benefited the most from this strategy, but because no randomization occurred, the incremental value of early catheterization could not be proven.

At the same time that the TAMI trial was conducted, the TIMI-IIA (14) and European Cooperative Studies (15) also tested early versus delayed intervention (Fig. 4). Not only was immediate catheterization ineffective, a disturbing trend toward higher mortality occurred for the immediate invasive approach. In retrospect, a variety of explanations for these results can be provided. First, these studies demonstrated that balloon angioplasty did not augment myocardial salvage after successful thrombolysis. This was the major scientific accomplishment of the TAMI-I trial. Second, combining the risk of hemorrhage of thrombolytic therapy and the risk of invasive procedures actually worsened clinical outcome. While we initially postulated that thrombolytic therapy could facilitate PTCA, in fact the converse was true; frequently what appeared to be an excellent angioplasty result led to abrupt rethrombosis. The mechanical result of angioplasty actually appeared to be harmed by thrombolysis. By 1989, after publication of the TIMI-IIB (16) trial, the cardiology community was largely convinced of the futility of mechanical reperfusion therapy.

A few committed investigators, including Geoffrey Hartzler, James O'Keefe, Donald Rothbaum, Bruce Brodie, Paul Overlie, Greg Stone, Robert Califf, Cindy Grines, and I, were still not convinced that primary angioplasty had undergone adequate systematic clinical evaluation. We were troubled by two questions. First, why were the early promising results of primary angioplasty therapy not translated to the studies of combined therapy? Second, primary angioplasty was criticized because by 1990 primary angioplasty literature included only a few single-institution nonrandomized studies and our initial small randomized trial. Insufficient data existed as to whether primary angioplasty could be adequately performed outside of Kansas City and Royal Oak.

We recognized that there was very little quality control data on direct PTCA. This was in 1990–1991. There certainly was a lot of anecdotal information. Hartzler's group had published an extraordinary amount from the Mid American Heart Institute (17). These

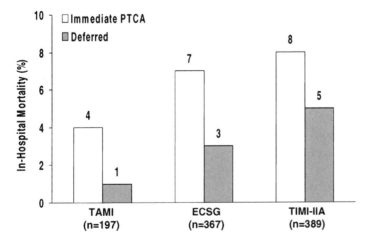

Figure 4   TAMI = Thrombolysis in Myocardial Infarction Trial; ECSG = European Cooperative Study Group; TIMI-IIA = Thrombolysis in Myocardial Infarction Study. Note the higher mortality for the patients treated with immediate angioplasty.

data were criticized because they were not core-lab controlled. Also, there was a real concern that self-reporting of positive results had occurred.

For this reason, the Primary Angioplasty Registry (PAR) was conducted (18). This was a prospective registry of five centers throughout the United States that pooled their data in 270 consecutive patients. Core-lab analysis of the angiograms and ventricular function was conducted at Duke University. We found that 97% of the patients had achieved TIMI-3 flow, and at 6 months 87% of the patients had a patent coronary artery (19). One thing that is really not emphasized in the literature is the fact that usually thrombolytic therapy is successful in 75–80% of the patients in restoring flow to the coronary arteries, but only 30–60% of the time is TIMI-2 flow achieved. Angioplasty appeared dramatically more effective in establishing TIMI-3 flow. Additionally, at 6 months, if those patients are followed with an aggressive anticoagulation strategy such as subcutaneous heparin or coumadin, there is still about a 30% reocclusion rate. So, if 100 arteries are treated with lytic therapy, 75 are going to be open acutely and 25 are going to reocclude. At 6 months, the patency rate would be about 50% with a pure lytic approach compared to about 87% patency for direct PTCA.

The other thing that was a little bit of a surprise and again really quite fascinating is the fact that there was a very substantial improvement in ventricular function in the PAR study. Initial ejection fraction was 51% and went up to 57% after the 6-month angiogram. There really is no other literature showing an improvement in global ventricular function for a large group of patients treated with thrombolytic therapy. There is a delayed improvement in ventricular function after PTCA therapy. Also, the vast majority of these patients had patent coronary arteries allowing for continued healing and improvement of ventricular function.

The reason for our persistence in exploring mechanical reperfusion in the face of mounting scientific opinion of the futility of this approach was multifactorial. First, our clinical impression about the benefit of this approach was at odds with the literature. Second, the explosion of angioplasty centers and the increase in trained operators suggested that this could become a broad-based reperfusion strategy if its clinical value was demonstrated. Most importantly, it appeared that angioplasty was superior to thrombolytic therapy in achieving arterial patency.

As we surveyed the carnage of the TAMI, TIMI-IIA, and ECS studies, we were struck by the disparity of our early excellent results with lone angioplasty therapy and the subsequent poor results of the combined studies. For that reason, we did a randomized study of sequential streptokinase versus lone angioplasty therapy. We chose streptokinase rather than tPA because at that time some data existed (20) suggesting that clot-specific agents were more detrimental than nonspecific agents for combined lytic/PTCA therapy.

In the SAMI trial (21), patients that came into William Beaumont Hospital and Moses Cone Hospital in North Carolina were randomized to treatment with a placebo or with intravenous streptokinase therapy before PTCA therapy. We thought this was going to be a winner! We thought that inducing a lytic state and allowing fibrin degradation products to be generated would actually have a beneficial antiplatelet effect. This would be better approach in optimizing the advantage of angioplasty and decreasing the reocclusion rate. Nevertheless, when this study was finished, we found no advantage in treating patients with streptokinase therapy (Table 2). Patients treated with streptokinase had more need for emergency bypass, a higher rate of vascular complications, a greater need for blood transfusions, a more prolonged length of stay at greater cost, and no advantage in terms of either immediate patency rate or patency rates at 6 months. In addition, no advan-

Table 2 Overall Results of SAMI Trial

	SK	Placebo	p-value
No. of patients	59	63	
PTCA success	98%	92%	NS
ER CABG	10%	1.6%	.03
Vascular events	29%	5%	.004
Transfusions	39%	8%	.0001
Hospital stay	9.3 ± 5	7.4 ± 4	.046
Hospital charges	25.1 ± 15.3 K	19.6 ± 7.2 K	<.02
6-month patency	89%	86%	NS

SK = Intravenous streptokinase; ER CABG = emergency bypass; K = 1000 dollars.
Source: Ref. 21.

tage with respect to preservation of ventricular function existed. This study really led us to question the incremental value of lytic therapy in treating these patients. More importantly, it led us to understand that perhaps we did throw the baby out with the bath water in the late 1980s in terms of mechanical approaches. It occurred to us that the lytic therapy actually was the culprit in terms of the poor outcomes for aggressive therapy compared to a strict thrombolytic approach. Based on the SAMI trial, we concluded that the optimal aggressive strategy would be to perform angioplasty without antecedent thrombolytic therapy. Other studies have corroborated these observations.

One of these is the important and very well done TAUSA study completed by John Ambrose (22). In this study, patients presenting with unstable angina or postinfarction angina were randomized to either placebo or to intracoronary urokinase administration. The hypothesis that lytic therapy would enhance the efficacy of angioplasty in a thrombolytic milieu was tested. The results of this study, like the SAMI trial, were very negative. Treatment with urokinase doubled the rate of recurrent ischemia and doubled the need for an emergency bypass. A much higher 12.9% rate of major cardiac events occurred for urokinase therapy and only a 6.3% rate of major cardiac events with placebo.

Insights into the mechanism for the deleterious effect of adjunctive lytic therapy came from the pathology series Bruce Waller put together from Indianapolis (23). He did autopsies on a number of patients who had mechanical intervention and examined the coronary arteries of patients treated with angioplasty alone or pretreated with thrombolytic therapy. An example of a vessel after combined therapy is depicted in Figure 5. Very extensive hemorrhage in the wall of the blood vessel is present. On the cross sections, one can see a very large intramural hematoma present that becomes occlusive of the coronary lumen. Perhaps this is why there is more recurrent ischemia and more need for emergency bypass surgery in these patients. The increase in major cardiac events may in fact be a pure mechanical problem associated with a very large hemorrhage occurring in the vasa vasorum of the blood vessel after intracoronary or intravenous thrombolytic therapy. Without antecedent lytic therapy a bland dissection without hemorrhage was found in the pathologic cross sections.

In 1992, we therefore concluded that lytic therapy worsened the outcome of infarct angioplasty. Data from Bruce Waller suggested that intramural hemorrhage of the treated blood vessel occurs after adjunctive thrombolytic therapy. Without antecedent lytic therapy, the artery has a very bland appearance. In addition, it is known that thrombin is a very potent mediator of platelet activation (24). All lytic therapy, no matter how fibrin-

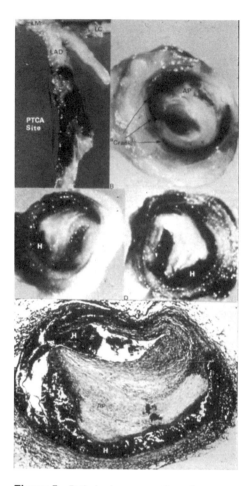

Figure 5 Pathologic cross section of a coronary artery from a patient who expired after combined thrombolytic therapy and angioplasty. Note the intramural hemorrhage visible microscopically (top left). Also note the plaque dissection (''crack'') present in the top right panel. Extensive hemorrhage that encroaches and obliterates the lumen is seen on the lower two panels. AP = Atherosclerotic plaque; H = hemorrhage.

specific, will liberate thrombin at the site of the occlusion. Finally, the combination of lytic therapy and catheterization increases the need for blood transfusions and increases vascular complications. The combined clinical and pathology findings strongly suggested that combination therapy was a very deleterious way of treating MI patients. The silver lining of the story was that one does not need to administer thrombolytic therapy to perform an optimal infarct angioplasty. A patient that has a high risk of intracranial bleeding or systemic bleeding can be very adequately and optimally treated without thrombolytic therapy. This is actually one major advantage of primary angioplasty.

The findings of the SAMI and TAUSA trials were the underpinnings for the PAMI trial (25). Our hypothesis was that optimal mechanical reperfusion had not been adequately tested against a pure intravenous lytic approach. In the PAMI trial, patients with symptom onset of less than 12 hours received heparin and aspirin and were randomized either to

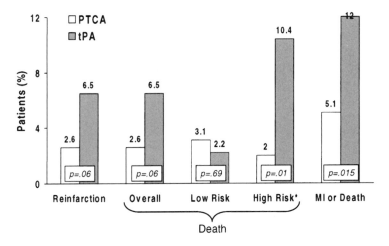

Figure 6 Overall outcome and subgroup outcome for the PAMI trial.

direct angioplasty or to intravenous tPA. One criticism of this study was the high rate of intracranial bleeding in the group of patients treated with tPA. This occurred not because we were unlucky or that we did not know how to use lytic agents but because we chose a very aggressive anticoagulation strategy and had no upper age limit for participation. The patients were treated with 10,000 units of heparin in the emergency room and given oral aspirin. We then tried to follow their ACTs very carefully to make sure that they were therapeutic. The main reason aggressive heparinization was used is that we felt angioplasty would be associated with a lower risk of recurring ischemia, and we would be criticized in retrospect by people arguing that lytic-treated patients were not optimally anticoagulated. Importantly, the overall mortality for tPA-treated patients was identical to that of the GUSTO trial.

At the time of the PAMI study, many questions were raised about the use of intra-

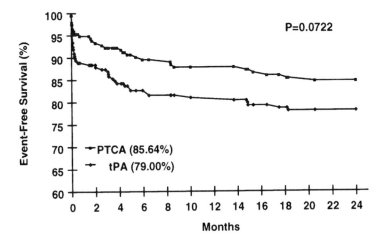

Figure 7 Long-term event-free survival for PTCA- and tPA-treated patients.

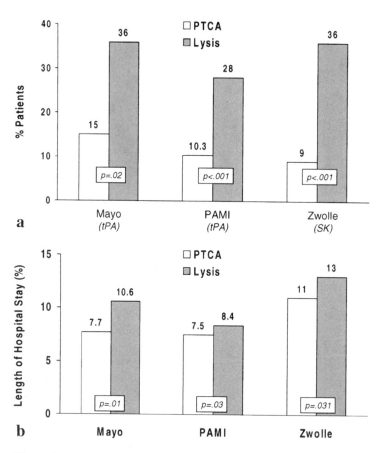

Figure 8 (a) Incidence of recurrent ischemia for PTCA- or lytic-treated patients. Note that recurrent ischemia in lytic-treated patients is comparable to contemporary thrombolytic trials such as GUSTO-I. (b) Length of stay tended to be lower for angioplasty-treated patients. For nonmedical reasons, the length of stay for MI is much longer in European countries.

venous heparin with tPA. The HART study (26) suggested that it was absolutely essential that tPA-treated patients also be treated with intravenous heparin. So, we did our best to try to use a very aggressive anticoagulation regimen to make sure the PAMI study could not be faulted by the fact that inadequate anticoagulation was what led to a suboptimal outcome for thrombolytics. The outcome of the PAMI study is depicted in Figure 6. The overall cumulative endpoint of death or reinfarction was significantly lower for patients treated with angioplasty compared to thrombolytic therapy. In this study, patients at high risk realized the greatest benefit. High risk was defined by the TIMI criteria as anterior MI, older age group, and admission heart rate greater than 100. In this high-risk group, 10% of the patients died if they were treated with lytic therapy and only 2% died if they were treated with angioplasty. The cumulative endpoint again, death or reinfarction, was 5% for the angioplasty group and 12% for the tPA-treated group. These patients were followed for a long period. We looked at reinfarction-free survival for the patients treated with angioplasty compared to those treated with thrombolytic therapy. We were concerned that perhaps restenosis might rear its ugly head at this point, and the initial benefit accrued to angioplasty might decline over time as the patients develop restenosis. Yet, the initial benefit remained over a prolonged period, and initial freedom from death or reinfarction was 80% for the tPA-treated group and 90% for the PTCA group (Fig. 7). So, there was a substantially better initial and long-term prognosis for the patients treated with angioplasty.

The Zwolle and Mayo Clinic trials of primary PTCA were reported concurrently with the PAMI trial. In aggregate, these studies demonstrated that angioplasty resulted in lower mortality, less recurrent ischemia and a lower length of stay compared to angioplasty therapy (Fig. 8). Ironically, the GUSTO trial and the GUSTO angiographic substudy have provided the greatest corroborative value to angioplasty therapy. These studies convincingly validated the open artery hypothesis and unequivocally demonstrated the crucial role of reestablishment of TIMI-3 flow in improving survival probability. Since primary angioplasty results in such superior rates of TIMI-3 flow compared to thrombolytic therapy, a superior outcome for angioplasty therapy is understandable.

Weaver et al. (27) have recently summarized the studies comparing thrombolysis to primary PTCA. A lower mortality rate, lower rate of death or nonfatal reinfarction, and a dramatically lower risk of stroke have been demonstrated. The challenge to the cardiovascular community will be to find ways to make this therapy available to a wider range of patients worldwide.

REFERENCES

1. Muller JE, Stone PH, Markis JE, Braunwald E. Let's not let the genie escape from the bottle—again. N Engl J Med 1981; 304:1294–1296.
2. Rentrop KP, Blanke H, Karsch KR, Wiegand V, Kostering H, Oster H, Leitz K. Acute myocardial infarction: intracoronary application of nitroglycerin and streptokinase. Clin Cardiol 1979; 2:354–363.
3. Rentrop KP, Feit F, Blanke H, Stecy P, Schneider R, Rey M, Horowitz S, Goldman M, Karsch K, Meilman H, Cohen M, Siegel S, Sanger J, Slater J, Gorlin R, Fox A, Fagerstrom R, Calhoun WF. Effects of intracoronary streptokinase and intracoronary nitroglycerin infusion on coronary angiographic patterns and mortality in patients with acute myocardial infarction. N Engl J Med 1984; 311:1457–1463.
4. Kennedy JW, Ritchie JL, Davis KB, Fritz JK. Western Washington randomized trial of intracoronary streptokinase in acute myocardial infarction. N Engl J Med 1983; 390:1477–1482.
5. Kennedy JW, Ritchie JL, Davis KB, Stadius ML, Maynard C, Fritz JK. The Western Washington randomized trial of intracoronary streptokinase in acute myocardial infarction: a 12-month follow-up report. N Engl J Med 1985; 312:1073–1078.
6. Anderson JL, Marshall HW, Bray BE, Lutz JR, Frederick PR, Yanowitz FG, Datz FL, Klausner SC, Hagan AD. A randomized trial of intracoronary streptokinase in the treatment of acute myocardial infarction. N Engl J Med 1983; 308:1312–1318.
7. Khaja F, Walton JA Jr., Brymer JF, Lo E, Osterberger L, O'Neill WW, Colfer HT, Weiss R, Lee T, Kurian T, Goldberg AD, Pitt B, Goldstein S. Intracoronary fibrinolytic therapy in acute myocardial infarction: report of a prospective randomized trial. N Engl J Med 1983; 308: 1305–1311.
8. O'Neill WW, Topol EJ, George BS, Kereiakes DJ, Abbotsmith CW, Boswick CJ, Califf RM. Improvement in left ventricular function after thrombolytic therapy and angioplasty: results of the TAMI study (abstr). Circulation 1987; 76:IV-259.
9. Hartzler GO, Rutherford BD, McConahay DR, Johnson WL, McCallister BD, Gura GM, Conn

RC, Crockett JE. Percutaneous transluminal coronary angioplasty with and without thrombolytic therapy for treatment of acute myocardial infarction. Am Heart J 1983; 106:965–973.

10. O'Neill W, Timmis GC, Bourdillon PD, Lai P, Gangadharan V, Walton J Jr., Ramos R, Laufer N, Gordon S, Schork A, Pitt B. A prospective randomized clinical trial of intracoronary streptokinase versus coronary angioplasty for acute myocardial infarction. N Engl J Med 1986; 314: 812–818.

11. Gruppo Italiano per lo Studio Della Streptochinasi Nell'Infarto Miocardico (GISSI). Effectiveness of intravenous thrombolytic treatment in acute myocardial infarction. Lancet 1986; 1: 397–402.

12. Verstraete M, Brower R, Collen D, Dunning A, Lubsen J, Michel P, Schofer J, Vanhaecke J, VanDeWerf F, Bleifeld W, Charbonnier C, DeBono D, Lennane R, Mathey D, Raynaud P, Vahanian A, VanDeKley G, VonEssen R. Double-blind randomized trial of intravenous tissue-type plasminogen activator versus placebo in acute myocardial infarction. Lancet 1985; 2: 965–969.

13. Collen D, Topol EJ, Tiefenbrunn AJ, Gold HK, Weisfeldt ML, Sobel BE, Leinbach RC, Brinker JA, Ludbrook PA, Yasuda I, Bulkley BH, Robison AK, Hutter A Jr., Bell WR, Spadaro JJ Jr., Khaw BA, Grossbard EB. Coronary thrombolysis with recombinant human tissue-type plasminogen activator: a prospective, randomized, placebo-controlled trial. Circulation 1984; 70:1012–1017.

14. Rogers WJ, Baim DS, Gore JM, Brown BG, Roberts R, Williams DO, Chesebro JH, Babb JD, Sheehan FH, Wackers FJTh, Zaret BL, Robertson TL, Passamani ER, Ross R, Knatterud GL, Braunwald E for the TIMI II-A Investigators. Comparison of immediate invasive, delayed invasive, and conservative strategies after tissue-type plasminogen activator: results of the Thrombolysis in Myocardial Infarction (TIMI) phase II-A trial. Circulation 1990; 81:1457–1476.

15. Simoons MV, Betriu A, Col J, vonEssen R, Lubsen J, Michel PL, Rutsch W, Schmidt W, Thery C, Vahanian A, Willems GM, Arnold AER, DeBono DP, Dougherty FC, Lambertz H, Meier B, Raynaud P, Sanz GA, Serruys PW, Uebis R, VanDeWerf F, Wood D, Verstraete M. Thrombolysis with tissue plasminogen activator in acute myocardial infarction: no additional benefit from immediate percutaneous coronary angioplasty. Lancet 1988; January:197–203.

16. Guerci A, Ross R. TIMI II and the role of angioplasty in acute myocardial infarction. N Engl J Med 1989;320:663–665.

17. O'Keefe JH, Rutherford BD, McConahay DR, Ligon RW, Johnson WL Jr, Giorgi LV, Crokett JE, McCallister BD, Conn RD, Gura GM, Good TH, Steinhaus DM, Bateman TM, Shimshak TM, Hartzler GO. Early and late results of coronary angioplasty without antecedent thrombolytic therapy for acute myocardial infarction. Am J Cardiol 1989; 64:1221–1230.

18. O'Neill WW, Brodie BR, Ivanhoe R, Knopf W, Taylor G, O'Keefe J, Grines CL, Weintraub R, Sickinger BG, Berdan LG, Tcheng JE, Woodlief LH, Strzelecki M, Hartzler G, Califf RM. Primary coronary angioplasty for acute myocardial infarction (the Primary Angioplasty Registry). Am J Cardiol 1994; 73:627–634.

19. Brodie BR, Grines CL, Ivanhoe R, Knopf W, Taylor G, O'Keefe J, Weintraub RA, Berdan LG, Tcheng JE, Woodlief LH, Califf RM, O'Neill WW. Six-month clinical and angiographic follow-up after direct angioplasty for acute myocardial infarction. Circulation 1994; 90:156–162.

20. Kowalski E, Lopec M, Wergrzynowicz A. Influence of fibrinogen degradation products (FDP) on platelet aggregation, adhesiveness and viscous metamorphous. Thromb Diath Haemorrh 1963; 10:406–423.

21. O'Neill WW, Weintraub R, Grines CL, Meany TB, Brodie BR, Friedman HZ, Ramos RG, Gangadharan V, Levin RN, Choksi N, Westveer DC, Strzelecki M, Timmis GC. A prospective, placebo-controlled, randomized trial of intravenous streptokinase and angioplasty versus lone angioplasty therapy of acute myocardial infarction. Circulation 1992; 86:1710–1717.

22. Ambrose JA, Orlandino DA, Sharma SK, Torre SR, Marmur JD, Israel DH, Ratner DE, Weiss MB, Hjemdahl-Monsen CE, Myler RK, Moses J, Unterecker WJ, Grunwald AM, Garrett JS, Cowley MJ, Anwar A, Sobolski J, for the TAUSA Investigators. Adjunctive thrombolytic therapy during angioplasty for ischemic rest angina: results of the TAUSA trial. Circulation 1984; 90:69–77.

23. Waller BF, Rothbaum DA, Pinkerton CA, Cowley MJ, Linnemeier TJ, Orr C, Irons M, Helmuth RA, Wills ER, Aust C. Status of the myocardium and infarct-related coronary artery in 19 necropsy patients with acute recanalization using pharmacologic (streptokinase, r-tissue plasminogen activator), mechanical (percutaneous transluminal coronary angioplasty) or combined types of reperfusion therapy. J Am Coll Cardiol 1987; 9:785–801.

24. Coller BS. Platelets and thrombolytic therapy. N Engl J Med 1990; 322:33–42.

25. Grines CL, Browne KF, Marco J, Rothbaum D, Stone GW, O'Keefe J, Overlie P, Donohue B, Chelliah N, Timmis GC, Vlietstra RE, Strzelecki M, Puchrowicz-Ochocki S, O'Neill WW, for the Primary Angioplasty in Myocardial Infarction Study Group (PAMI). A comparison of immediate angioplasty with thrombolytic therapy for acute myocardial infarction. N Engl J Med 1993; 328:673–679.

26. Hsia J, Hamilton WP, Kleiman N, Roberts R, Chaitman BR, Ross AM, for the Heparin-Aspirin Reperfusion Trial (HART) Investigators. A comparison between heparin and low-dose aspirin as adjunctive therapy with tissue plasminogen activator for acute myocardial infarction. N Engl J Med 1990; 323:1433–1437.

27. Weaver WD, Simes RJ, Betriu A, Grines CL, Zijlstra F, Garcia E, Grinfeld L, Gibbons RJ, Ribeiro EE, DeWood MA, Ribichini F. JAMA 1997; 278:2093–2098.

Index

About the Editors

IRA S. NASH is Associate Director of the Zena and Michael A. Wiener Cardiovascular Institute, Mount Sinai Medical Center, New York, and an Assistant Professor, Mount Sinai School of Medicine, New York. In addition to directing the quality assessment and improvement activities of the Cardiovascular Institute, he is the Director of the clinical elective in cardiology, Mount Sinai School of Medicine. The author, coauthor, editor, or coeditor of numerous research articles, editorials, abstracts, book chapters, and books, he is a Fellow of the American College of Cardiology. Dr. Nash received the A.B. degree (1980) summa cum laude from Harvard University, Cambridge, Massachusetts, and the M.D. degree (1984) cum laude from Harvard Medical School, Boston, Massachusetts, where he attended the Harvard-M.I.T. Program in Health Sciences and Technology.

VALENTIN FUSTER is Richard Gorlin Heart Research Foundation Professor of Cardiology, Mount Sinai School of Medicine, New York. Additionally, he is Dean for Academic Affairs and Director of the Zena and Michael A. Wiener Cardiovascular Institute, Mount Sinai Medical Center, New York. The author or coauthor of over 400 articles on the subjects of coronary artery disease, atherosclerosis, and thrombosis, he is the President of the American Heart Association, a member of the Advisory Council of the National Heart, Lung and Blood Institute, the Chairman of the Fellowship Training Directors Program of the American College of Cardiology, and Consulting Editor of the journals *Circulation* and *Circulation Research*. Dr. Fuster received the B.S. degree (1961) from Colegio Jesuitas, Barcelona, Spain, and the M.D. (1967) and Ph.D. (1971) degrees from Barcelona University, Spain, having done his research fellowship and postdoctoral thesis at the University of Edinburgh (1968–1971). He has received numerous international awards and he is Honoris Causa of five universities.